Care without Pathology

CARE WITHOUT PATHOLOGY

How Trans- Health Activists Are Changing Medicine

Christoph Hanssmann

MINNESOTA

University of Minnesota Press
Minneapolis
London

Chapter 3 was originally published as "Epidemiological Rage: Population, Biography, and State Responsibility in Trans- Health Activism," *Social Science & Medicine* 247 (February 2020): 112808, https://doi.org/10.1016/j.socscimed.2020.112808; copyright Elsevier 2020.

Published by the University of Minnesota Press
111 Third Avenue South, Suite 290
Minneapolis, MN 55401-2520
http://www.upress.umn.edu

ISBN 978-1-5179-1340-3 (hc)
ISBN 978-1-5179-1341-0 (pb)

A Cataloging-in-Publication record for this book is available from the Library of Congress.

Printed in the United States of America on acid-free paper

UMP BmB 2023

Contents

Introduction 1

1 Care without Pathology: Coordinating Depathologization 45

2 Unruly Terms: Negotiating Trans- Diagnoses 77

3 Epidemiological Rage: Population, Biography, and State Responsibility in Trans- Health Activism 111

4 Saving Lives, Saving Money: Investing in Trans- Lives 145

5 Crashing the Gate: Consent-Driven Care and Self-Determination 187

6 Extending Depathologization: The Coalitional Approach 229

Conclusion 255

Acknowledgments 273

Notes 281

Bibliography 327

Index 367

Introduction

In the week that I was writing what I thought were the final lines of this book, I received a flurry of texts. “What did you think about the manifesto?” It was the fall of 2022, and a new version of the care standards for the international provision of transgender health had just come out. The organization that has published these guidelines for the past four decades was hosting its annual conference for health-care providers in Montreal. During the opening session, one white transgender woman, a surgeon named Marci Bowers, introduced another—pediatrician Rachel Levine, assistant secretary for health for the U.S. Department of Health and Human Services. Before Levine could deliver her address, a group of transfeminine activists took the stage and the mic. They held a black banner with pink text spelling out the name of their collective—“Traps”[1]—and read a prepared manifesto to the audience that had gathered to listen to Levine reflect on the state of trans- health.[2] In it, they criticized the organization’s “infantilizing and stigmatizing tradition” of “organizing exclusive conferences around trans health for doctors, psychiatrists and other specialists far removed from our material realities” (Traps, n.d.). As they introduced their demands, they emphasized the prohibitive expense of accessing care:

> The moralistic and patriarchal stubbornness of doctors, scientists and the State to regulate our bodies causes unacceptable, sometimes fatal violence. The financial burden of transition, the absence of transfeminist leadership in community and hospital settings, the underfunding of scarce resources for transfeminine people, and extreme discrimination in employment place us in a precarious situation.

The group received a standing ovation from the audience. However, organizational staff hurried to stifle the message, turning off the event's livestream almost immediately and calling security.[3]

Nearly a decade before, in August 2013, I stood on the sidewalk in downtown Buenos Aires in front of the Hotel Bauen. I had come to Argentina to study how political organizing, health politics, and medical systems have shaped the emerging field of transgender health. The prior year, the nation had passed the Gender Identity Law, which its proponents called the world's first depathologized law related to trans- people.[4] In other words, the law defines people seeking gender-affirming care not as ill but as legitimately entitled to pursue such care of their own accord. Its provisions include access to trans- therapeutic care based solely on what people say they need. As I will discuss shortly, *trans- therapeutics* is the term I use to describe gender-affirming care that is specifically sought by trans- people. In addition to changing paradigms of access, the law also addressed financing across the full health-care system. At least on paper, access to coverage for trans- therapeutics includes people who use the publicly funded safety-net system for their health care in addition to those with public or private health insurance plans. The passage of the law marked a significant change from earlier models of care, which required lengthy psychiatric evaluation and a diagnosis of what at the time was called "Gender Identity Disorder."

The law has also replaced the convoluted bureaucratic process that was previously required for people to change the gender marker on their legal identity documents. Before, people's bodies had to match what state officials determined was the supposedly proper way for a body to look to be defined as "male" or "female." This usually meant that people had to prove that they had undergone surgery to change the appearance of their genitals and to remove reproductive organs. Before the passage of the law, these surgeries were extremely expensive and very hard to access. Furthermore, many people did not want them, or only wanted some and not others. As a result, many people did not qualify for a legal gender reclassification. Even in the rare cases that they did qualify, people generally had to go through a lengthy process in court to get approval for their legal identity documents to be changed to a gender that reflected how they lived. This meant a lot of time and steep legal fees, which were impossible for most people. However, people wanted legal documents that matched how they presented themselves—especially since they needed these documents to apply to jobs, to travel, to find places to live, or to access services and benefits.[5] With the Gender Identity Law, these document changes became much less burdensome, at least formally speaking. Surgery requirements and lawsuits were no longer necessary. Instead, a streamlined bureaucratic process was introduced into the national registration agency. After the law's passage, strict state-based requirements were no longer enforced, and people could change the gender on their identity documents based solely on what was called "self-perceived need."[6]

In my home country of the United States, gender-affirming care was changing, too. Large hospital systems, whose leadership had previously dismissed trans- therapeutics as illegitimate or experimental medicine, were beginning to open trans-focused clinics. For example, in New York City in 2016 alone, two large hospital systems—Mount Sinai and Northwell Health—opened integrated transgender health programs, offering everything from endocrine care and hair removal to surgeries and voice coaching. These integrated programs were often partly modeled on those innovated by public-health and community-based clinics in the late 1990s and early 2000s, emerging from structures put into place by HIV/AIDS activism and feminist health-care movements.[7] Fortune 500 companies were beginning to boast coverage for gender-affirming care as part of their employment-based insurance plans, especially as advocacy organizations began publicly tracking this information.[8] Yet for people with public forms of coverage—people whose care is covered by the government through programs like Medicaid, Medicare, prison- or jail-based health care, and many others—trans- therapeutics were actually becoming less accessible than they were before. Local, city, and state officials introduced policy campaigns and lawsuits to undermine public coverage for trans- therapeutic care, often pushing for these practices to be explicitly excluded from federal or state programs. Nine U.S. states now prohibit the use of Medicaid funds for all such forms of care, with six of these bans having been introduced in or after 2015.[9]

I became especially interested in New York State's pitched battle to win statewide Medicaid coverage for gender-affirming care for trans- people after its enduring legal exclusion stretching back to 1998. Trans- health activists and advocates, particularly those based in New York City, had worked to challenge this exclusion since the early 2000s. They finally won its repeal in 2015.

Over the next few years, I returned to Buenos Aires and New York City to spend time and speak with activists, advocates, and health-care providers. I was interested in how trans- health was emerging as a field in general, but I was especially focused on how the field was taking shape vis-à-vis public systems of care. Trans- health is an institutionalizing field, but its meanings are still contested; it means many things to many people. In my research, I set out to understand what people thought it meant specifically as a public good. To date, no book-length studies of which I am aware have centered these questions, despite the distinct ways that public forms of trans- health are taking shape. As nearly 19 percent of people in the United States are covered by Medicaid and 36 percent of people in Argentina are covered by the safety-net public hospital system as of 2022, this is a topic in pressing need of investigation. This book examines laws and regulations on different scales: specifically, a state regulation in New York and a national law in Argentina. In both places, though, I was most interested in the grassroots activism and provider practices that shaped the landscape of care and led to these changes.

Back to the sidewalk in front of the Buenos Aires hotel: I had just wrapped up a day at a sexuality studies conference that was taking place there. Outside, I met another scholar who was also attending. I told him I was studying the transnational emergence of trans- health, and he made it clear that he considered himself as an ally to transgender communities. I continued, mentioning that my focus was on public coverage for gender-affirming and other forms of trans- health care. He paused a moment before responding, "But isn't it very expensive, though?" Referring to gender-affirming care, he said, "I mean, *should* states really be paying for something like that?"

It was not the first time I had encountered such questions. In fact, I had spent the prior months wading through news articles and policy papers that contested public coverage for trans- health care, alluding to its cost or legitimacy. But I was surprised to hear such things from this queer scholar, who was attending a conference critically focused on sexuality and neoliberalism. I responded as I often do, asking why cost was the first concern to arise when it came to these particular care practices. Rarely is this the first question to emerge, for example, in discussions about the notoriously expensive care related to cancer treatment or organ transplantation. In these cases, the preservation of life and need for intervention are generally and implicitly recognized as priorities.[10] Concerns about the cost of care—and, particularly, how collective publics are implicated as taxpayers—surface mainly when moralizing (and often marginalizing) questions come to the fore. Further, questions of restraint seem to apply selectively to other recipients of public spending, as in the case of the U.S. military, which routinely receives at least half of the nation's full discretionary budget. He did not argue with any of these points, but neither did he relinquish his position that cost ought to be a central and primary consideration.

I detected no deliberate antagonism in his query. He represented himself as a queer activist and trans- ally. He was not taking a religious fundamentalist or masculinist authoritarian position that trans- therapeutics jeopardize the family form or a natural, hierarchical, biological order. Nor was he rehashing the antitrans- position that some people take from what they see as a more progressive position: that gender-affirming care is somehow antifeminist because it supposedly reasserts gender roles or puts too much stake in technology. Instead, his qualms were about the limits of sharing the costs of care. In the finitude of economic and care distribution, he was asking, is the cost of trans- therapeutics too much to ask? In other words, who counts as "the public," and who can claim care?

Some variation on his question, "Should states really be paying for something like that?," echoes across right-wing radio airwaves, syndicated television journalism, and social media debates. As my fellow conference-goer demonstrated, the question also circulates well beyond right-wing punditry. Across political spectra, journalists, lawmakers, policy wonks, and even trans- advocates may issue similar questions—perhaps to play devil's advocate or to express the difficult necessity of fiscal restraint. Whether from the political Left or Right, and whether delivered in a whisper or a shout, the question seems to serve as a badge of pragmatic rationality. Its askers seem eager to convey a judicious prudence and a refusal to be shaken by the whims of political correctness or the demands of the so-called woke masses. The implication, of course, is that certain forms of health care might be okay if people pay for them on their own. But for those without the means to do so? The askers suggest that material resources have limits, and public support for trans- therapeutics is perhaps too unfair a material strain on public coffers.

This book focuses on those who have pushed back against such claims and developed a notion of trans- health as a social need and a public good. The manifesto that Traps delivered was only the most recent of these bold activist claims. This group and others have asserted a claim to care in part by revising the questions that get asked about trans- people and our lives and in part by reframing the stakes of health-care access—especially for poor trans- people, trans- people who are Black, Indigenous, and people of color, *travestis,* and other people marginalized within infrastructures of care.[11] The activists, advocates, and health-care providers with whom I spoke undertook this while simultaneously centering the imperative to organize care around questions of need rather than pathology. They asked questions like, "What do trans- people require, medically and otherwise, to survive and to thrive?," instead of "What is trans- people's illness and how should it be addressed?" Finally, in contrast with the many important reflections in trans- studies that examine how biomedicine has shaped transness, this book looks to the ways that trans- activism has shaped biomedicine and care distribution—often in ways that go well beyond the bounds of what might be called "trans- health." Examining the different and contested ways that people in New York City and Buenos Aires defined and practiced trans- health, I demonstrate how these interventions have been a critical part of proposing new modes of orienting biomedical treatment. I refer to these practices as "care without pathology."

The Big Picture

When it comes to trans- politics, the last decade has been a strange one indeed. In the United States, trans- celebrities began gracing magazine covers and, at least in small measure, populating Hollywood casting lists. Simultaneously, *transgender* became a scapegoat for culture wars during the Trump administration. Executive efforts to define *transgender* out of existence, as the *New York Times* put it, summarily failed (Green, Benner, and Pear 2018). However, even after Trump's memorable exit from the White House, Christian fundamentalist legal advocacy groups like the Alliance Defending Freedom have been supplying antitrans- templates to state lawmakers, driving what has become a wholesale legislative bombardment against trans- people. Even as President Biden appointed Levine to the White House cabinet, in 2021 alone, more than one hundred antitrans- bills were proposed by over thirty state legislatures (Branigin and Kirkpatrick 2022). Health care and medicine have been the primary legislative targets, and proposed bills have gone so far as to propose criminal action against providers who provide trans- therapeutics to patients. To date, only a few of these have stuck. Nevertheless, these developments will likely provide cover for administrators in schools, insurance companies, prisons, courts, hospitals, immigration enforcement, and other institutions to double down on antitrans- and other exclusionary policies—even in states that are not directly affected by these proposed or approved laws.

Argentina's contemporary culture wars have not centered on transness as a defining wedge in the same way that they have in the United States. Nevertheless, activists were anxious that the 2015 election of right-wing pro-business candidate Mauricio Macri might mean a reversal of recent legislative wins, especially 2012's Gender Identity Law. As I mentioned before, the law's provisions included a guarantee to access for gender-affirming care across the health-care system, including in the safety-net systems provided by public hospitals.[12] Despite activists' fears, the law remained untouched. However, the series of austerity measures that Macri's administration rapidly installed gutted health care and other public programs, instead directing funds to international financial markets. As such, the forms of publicly subsidized gender-affirming care that were enshrined by the law were effectively nullified, along with many other forms of health-care access for poor Argentines. By 2019, many of the nation's residents were fed up with skyrocketing poverty and inflation, inadequate health coverage, the elimination of tens of thousands of public-sector jobs, and more. Protesters took to the streets to reject these policies and demand reinvestment in the nation's broader health and prosperity. Even after Macri's ouster later that year, current president Alberto Fernández's administration is navigating public-health crises following defunded infrastructures that were further strained by a global pandemic.

In the meantime, trans- health-care provision in Argentina, the United States, and elsewhere has been in a sustained (if profoundly incomplete) sea change. In the early 2000s, T. Benjamin Singer (2006) characterized this as a shift from pathology-driven models of transsexual medicine to community-health-driven models of care. This book discusses "transsexual medicine" as a specific field of medicine emerging in the mid-twentieth century, focusing on strictly binary gender transition for a small number of people and requiring lengthy and intensive surveillance and authorization by medical and psychiatric providers.[13] In Singer's (2006) account, gender nonnormativity and particularly transness were largely defined through frameworks of psychiatric or criminal pathology through most of the twentieth century. In a crescendo of activism that seemed to crest around the turn of the twenty-first century, trans- people forcefully resisted pathologization. In place of illness, abnormality, or disturbance, they instead proposed frameworks of difference, variation, or spectra. They also insisted on coverage for biomedical care, which many people considered to facilitate wellness. This has provided a new blueprint not only for trans- health but for biomedical practice more generally. Activism is thus changing conversations about biomedicine, even if pathologization still remains at the core of many of its practices.

Activists' visions are beginning to diffuse into the mainstream—even as they have been met by a forceful backlash. The uptake of these visions is sharply uneven, but in certain sectors, depathologization has increasingly come to characterize emergent forms of trans- health. In recent years, this approach to care has guided changes in laws, regulations, policies, care protocols, and diagnostic classifications. Depathologization has shaped care practices through Argentina's Gender Identity Law, the World Health Organization's *International Classification of Diseases and Related Health Problems,* and (to some extent) the American Psychiatric Association's *Diagnostic and Statistical Manual,* just to name a few. If pathologization defined the field of transsexual medicine in the twentieth century, depathologization is the North Star toward which activists are pressing for transformation in contemporary frameworks of trans- health.

If the degree to which trans- activism has shifted the terrain of debate has been surprising, so has the intensity of the backlash—and perhaps also its sources. Right-wing fundamentalist lobbies are predictable detractors. They are following the blueprint of reactionary antiabortion politics when it comes to trans- health, specifically by passing laws enabling providers to object to delivering trans- therapeutic care and criminalizing those who offer such care (especially when it comes to providers who work with trans- youth). In South America, right-wing political movements are similarly pushing back on what they call "gender ideology." The 2018 election of Brazilian president Jair Bolsonaro provided a national stage for an aggressive antisocialist nationalism that defined "gender ideology" as among its primary targets. At a 2019 speech to the United Nations, Bolsonaro singled out education systems for disputing the supposedly biological fact of sex difference. Joining these oppositional ranks has been a small but clamorous group calling themselves "gender-critical" feminists. This group sees themselves as saving people from trans- politics, which they consider brainwashing. They (erroneously) view transmasculine people as being fooled by patriarchy into becoming men to avoid being targets of sexism and transfeminine people as entitled men who are trying to own womanhood by feminizing themselves (Bassi and LaFleur 2022).[14] Their stridently antitrans- politics alongside their insistence on their feminist commitments have led many to refer to them as "trans-exclusionary radical feminists" or TERFs. While perhaps somewhat less vocal in the Global South, TERFs in the United States and Europe have argued that "gender" is troublingly replacing "biological sex" and therefore obscuring what they contend is the biological fact of girlhood and womanhood. Curiously enough, these positions contravene the sustained critiques of biological essentialism that many feminist analyses have advanced over the last seventy years.[15] Yet their claims to antitrans- feminism have occasioned a sustained association with Christian fundamentalist moralism, giving rise to a starkly peculiar coalition.

Right-wing proponents of supposed family values and self-identified feminists who oppose the changes for which trans- activists are pushing share very little, save for an unshakable infatuation with the biological myths of sex binarism. However, many of the nurses, doctors, social workers, and therapists who work directly with trans- patients seem to be less certain about the supposed self-evident truth of biological sex. Professional associations that develop guidelines and diagnoses are also slowly and inconsistently revising some of their positions about transness being a pathological condition in need of strict authoritative management. As new models of care have begun to gain limited traction, there have been some changes to the way things used to work. As I described before, the previous way was to have nontrans- experts decide who really counts as trans-.[16] What activists call "depathologized care" moves away from authorities being the ones to drive these decisions. Instead, at least for some providers, care responds to who trans- people say we are and what we say we need.

In addition to some people still doing things the former way, some are looking for new ways to assert expertise or authority. Some providers who hang on to the former way truly believe that there is something deeply wrong with their patients, but others are simply hesitant to lose a clear-cut theory of transness.[17] This has driven some to seek other theories of transness, including through research on potential biological indicators in, for example, brain structure and function.[18] As such, research about the biological basis for transness seems to give providers a new way of doing things the former (expert-driven) way.

According to many activists, though, depathologized care offers another way forward. Certain care providers are (gradually, and sometimes begrudgingly or conditionally) accepting the opacity and radical heterogeneity of transness.[19] By this, I mean not only that trans- people are very different from each other but that we may not—or cannot—know how or why people are trans-. Yet activists assert that people know a lot about what they need, and health-care providers' roles can be in listening carefully and responding to these needs. As such, some forms of trans- health have begun to center people's knowledge of themselves as a primary basis for care.

Even as trans- depathologization has begun to take root, there remain analysts who are unsure if the institutionalization of trans- health practice might be counterproductive. They wonder if perhaps a better approach to depathologization would involve the abolition of trans- health as a discernible field. These voices rightly assert that many people access gender-affirming care and that, quantitatively speaking, most of them are nontrans-. These forms of gender-affirming care—whether freely chosen or forced on patients—are often covered by insurance for nontrans- people, even though this is resolutely not the case for trans- people.[20] This being the case, why should we work so hard to build a field that doubles down on the exceptional status of trans- people rather than simply work to ensure our inclusion as rightful subjects of gender-affirming care, just like anyone else who might (consensually) seek it? This is a provocation that remains unresolved in this book, given its concern with how activists have confronted institutional medicine in large part through negotiation and institutionalization. Yet, it remains a question that animates some of the ambivalence that activists bring to the normative question of what trans- interactions with medicine ought to look like.

It is impossible to tell a single story about trans- health, and depathologized care remains the exception rather than the rule. Still, I suggest that the interventions of trans- health activists—alongside other health activists—have occasioned a reevaluation of health-care practice and biomedical knowledge more generally. Specifically, activists have conceptualized care without pathology, which is a key topic of this book. In addition, they have placed struggles over the distribution of care at the center, particularly when it comes to questions of public financing. The contentiousness that surrounds trans- health—from across political constellations—has thrust to the fore debates about public support for care. Like many forms of biomedical care, not all members of the public may need access to gender-affirming care—and among those who do, very few may be trans-. As a contested form of care, though, trans- therapeutics have raised new questions about what it means to support health collectively, even when individuals within those collectives have distinct needs.

This book works to interrogate the emergence of trans- health. In particular, it focuses on trans- health in its public form and through its transnational institutionalization within the thicket of global trans- politics. In so doing, it asks a series of questions related to the ways that trans- health activists and advocates (and some providers) have challenged hierarchical frameworks and logics of biomedical care distribution. For example, if medicine pathologizes to treat, how might we understand depathologization in practice? How does depathologization affect care coverage, particularly for low-income people who seek it? How does trans- health vary by location, health-care infrastructure, and social movement histories? In what ways have activists and providers clashed or collaborated? How do trans- health activist movements reframe the ways that providers and the public view trans- health? Finally, in what ways do trans- activists and trans- health providers view their work in the broader landscape of health-care provision and justice-based struggles? In what follows, I seek to answer these questions by analyzing ethnographic interviews and observations, legal and regulatory documents, activist materials and art, and documents and classificatory schema used in care provision. While trans- health is far from monolithic, *Care without Pathology* aims to chart some of the paths it is taking in its partial divergence from twentieth-century transsexual medicine.

No Safety in Terminology

In advocacy and education circles, the umbrella has become the preferred metaphor through which to discuss transness. In this sense, *transgender* (and sometimes the foreshortened form *trans*) figures as a catchall under which the many and proliferating forms of gender nonnormativity—including so-called local variations—can be grouped. Despite its popularity, some activists and scholars reject these universalizing aspirations. Drawing on subaltern, decolonial, and anticolonial theorizing, they call for *transgender*'s provincialization.[21] Yet, there remain loose networks, both situated and transnational, that organize under the banner of transness, even when this diverges from people's understanding of themselves. Travestis are among the many groups who have been thrust under the transgender umbrella, despite their clear claims to the contrary (and I will say more about this group shortly). Yet they still agitate, work, and protest alongside people who call themselves "transgender." Amid these complexities, what might we name these collectives?

In addition to geographies of transness, temporalities also make it difficult to settle on terminology, as its pace of change remains dizzying. In the quarter-century that I have called myself "transgender," I have watched its related terms multiply and shift at breakneck speed. Language is an engine of change, and these transformations reflect the political dynamism of trans- politics. At the same time, terminologies reflect the uneven fields of power through which they travel. As an author, I must navigate this contested linguistic landscape in the present. My aim is to use terms that will be both accessible to readers and acknowledge geographic, conceptual, linguistic, and other limitations. However, their meanings are sure to keep shifting. As Stuart Hall (1997, 299) warns, "I am trying to persuade you that the word is the medium in which power works. There is no safety in terminology. . . . Don't clutch onto the word, but do clutch on to certain ideas about it."[22]

With these provisos in place, I will now introduce the terminological choices I have made in this book and briefly discuss my reasons for doing so. When I use the term *trans-*, I refer to collectives that exceed, break, or cross binary or normative sex/gender systems. In general, I use *trans-* in its hyphenated form rather than *transgender.* Susan Stryker, Paisley Currah, and Lisa Jean Moore (2008, 11) propose this as a term that "resists premature foreclosure by attachment to any single suffix."[23] I must confess that I am ambivalent about the term—as one colleague mentioned, it looks like a typo. Another found it unsightly. However, in its somewhat fragmentary quality, it is perhaps apt in undertaking the challenging work of describing this heterogeneous collective and reducing the universalizing collapse of *transgender.* I lean into the ugliness and awkwardness of the hyphen in part to remind readers of the irksome persistence of universalizing terms for those who do not find shelter under *transgender*'s presumptive umbrella.[24] In addition to *trans-,* I also mobilize terms that study respondents use to define themselves, such as *travesti.* Occasionally, I generalize by using terms such as *gender/sexual nonnormativity*—despite its clumsiness and unwelcome stabilization of the referential norm against which it is defined. The inadequacy of these efforts is among the many reasons I consider terms such as *trans-*—alongside the book's other terminological choices—to be under erasure.[25] None of the terms I mobilize are in hierarchical relation with the others, nor is one strictly separate from or reducible to the others.

When I use the term *travesti,* I refer to its politically reclaimed use by largely working-class sex/gender nonnormative femme or transfeminine people in Argentina. Travestis are typically racialized as nonwhite Mestiza, Afro-descendant, or Indigenous and are often rural-to-urban migrants from the provinces. Travestis in Argentina have been systematically criminalized through the regulation of public space and conduct, especially through their association with sex work. Throughout the 1990s, they worked to illuminate perilous conditions of life linked to marginalization and criminalization, largely through political resistance to the policing of public space (Berkins and Fernández 2005; Fernández 2004; Cutuli 2012, 2013, 2015; Farji Neer 2017; Simonetto and Butierrez 2022). While travestis generally disidentify with *transgender* (and generally also *transsexual*), they often collaborate with people who describe themselves as such. Travesti theorists emphasize their disidentification from *transgender* at multiple levels, including the latter's insistence on separating gender from sexuality—a division that travesti subjectivity actively blurs.[26] *Travesti* is a term that escapes English translation, though some authors reductively and erroneously translate it as *transvestite.*

Activists and advocates also take other approaches to naming these collectives. For example, in the recent past, activists in the Global South appended an asterisk as a cheeky addendum to the ostensible umbrella of *trans* in part to enable access to global funding for transgender organizing, despite their disidentification with the term (International Gay and Lesbian Human Rights Commission 2005). The asterisk was a momentary addendum of choice in the United States as well, though this term carries a different and somewhat freighted legacy in the Global North–based blogosphere.[27] In Argentina, some groups have turned to the tactic of "multiplying the *T*'s"—insisting on the tripled *transgénero, transexual,* and *travesti.*[28] Historian Howard Chiang (2021) terms the nonreductive continuities of sex/gender variance "transtopia," and I have endeavored to take a similar conceptual approach.[29]

Some might argue that simply hyphenating *trans* does little to displace *transgender*'s stubborn ethnocentric conceit, and they are likely correct. It remains impossible to use the term *trans-*—hyphenations, asterisks, or other modifications notwithstanding—and *not* be caught in webs of neocolonial meaning-making. Yet, in its movement, the translations and proliferations of *trans-* have taken on new meaning and forged concrete political solidarities. This has also occurred in the realm of transnational queer/*cuir* politics, which complicate notions of linguistic imperialism that presume the direct portability of terms and concepts.[30] In addition, these refusals of ethnocentric subordination confront the hubris of universalizing terms like *trans* or *queer,* forcing a reckoning with their geographical and political specificity. *Care without Pathology* strives to highlight how activists and advocates resist neocolonial impulses not only through creative linguistic reworkings and refusals of *transgender* but also through shifts to systems-focused rather than identity-focused coalition-based work.

Settling on a term to describe the varying technologies through which people might enact or embody transness is just as challenging. These include but are not limited to varying surgeries, the use of exogenous hormones, hair removal, body contouring, and voice coaching. People might pursue these within or outside the realm of biomedicine (sometimes through means that are criminalized) and in varying combinations. In aggregate, these technologies have been called "gender-confirming care," "gender-affirming care," and "trans- therapeutics," among other things. Each comes with its own histories and baggage.[31] Here, I tend to use the term *trans- therapeutics* for several reasons.[32] First, it decenters gender as its primary or singular object of intervention. Second, in avoiding *confirmation* or *affirmation,* it reduces the implication of a linear or completable process. Third, *therapeutics* refers to a varying array of treatments, therapies, drugs, or procedures that function within broader logics of health and wellness. Finally, it refers specifically to a broader series of technologies as they are specifically accessed by trans- people and travestis.

In this book, I also frequently refer to *trans- health* as a means of describing trans- therapeutics. This relates in large part with the way trans- therapeutics have come to define the practices related to trans- health. However, *trans- health* in fact names a much broader set of phenomena. For example, trans- health also includes the basic and specialty care that trans- people and travestis access on a regular basis, even beyond trans- therapeutics. In this sense, trans- health is simply any form of health care that is accessed by trans- people (trans- therapeutic or not). *Trans- health* also refers to the generalized political claims that people make to assert the need for sufficient conditions of existence. There is permeability between each of these levels of meaning. Nonetheless, trans- therapeutics has become the primary domain of struggle through which more generalized discussions of care provision and care politics have taken shape. This book empirically follows these currents to focus on trans- therapeutics. Unfortunately, doing so also risks reproducing this reductive gesture. I remain hopeful that the book's conclusions still offer reflections on trans- health that engage its broader connotations.

Methods and Methodology

This book's analyses are based on multisited ethnographic data and various other data sources. Between 2012 and 2018, I conducted ethnographic interviews and observations and collected document-based data in the form of regulations, laws, diagnostic manuals, clinical care protocols and guidelines, professional standards, websites, and activist art and publications. My ethnographic research spanned multiple sites and spaces of interest—clinics, organizations, protest sites, news and online media, and conferences. Nearly all of these were concentrated in two metropolitan cities: New York City and Buenos Aires.[33] Although there were other potentially generative locales in which to ground the work, I selected these cities for several reasons: in each site, self-identified trans- health experts—both providers and activists—worked in both local and transnational collaboration; each city/region was in the midst of an important set of regulatory and legal transformations regarding public provision of trans- health; and these sites spanned the Global North and South, which enabled transhemispheric discursive inquiry.

Theory-Methods Packages

The decision to structure the study transhemispherically was influenced by what Susan Leigh Star (1989) calls "theory-methods packages." This refers to the ways that methodological choices and theoretical orientations are in mutual relation.[34] Transnational and decolonial feminist inquiry and science and technology studies (STS) form a large part of my theoretical approach to this work—and thus also to its methodological conceptualization.[35] Transnational and decolonial feminisms emphasize the uneven currents of power and resistance that shape life and politics. These theoretical approaches emphasize the diffuse and historically rooted forces that shape these currents over and above the structuring work of the nation-state as such. Decolonial feminisms focus particular attention on how histories of colonization have shaped epistemologies. These seek to intervene in the mythology of the Global North (or West) as a center of knowledge and modernity. For its part, STS interrogates how knowledge and expertise materialize, change, and endure—and within this, how things become facts, particularly in and through technoscience and biomedicine.[36] One of STS's emblematic approaches has been to study up to account for the practices of experts and producers of privileged knowledge. Feminist STS recognizes and integrates less traditionalist or linear forms of expert knowledge production, which has led to methodologies characterized by "studying across" (as well as "standing with") (TallBear 2014). Feminist STS also attunes to the "background" work of infrastructures and organizing systems (Star 1999). Each of these theoretical perspectives was critical to how I structured this study methodologically.

The study's dual-sited, transhemispheric structure involves comparative elements, but I do not regard this as a comparative case study. Rather, I aim to trace discursive processes of knowledge production, attuning to the relations and interactions within and between sites, geographic regions, and distinct infrastructures. In her cross-hemispheric historical work on race in the Americas, Juliet Hooker (2017) discusses the limitations of comparison. Her study mobilizes "South-to-South" or "hemispheric juxtaposition," which differs from the "studying across" approach I take here (4). Nevertheless, I share her concerns about comparative approaches. In addition to treating sites as discrete or separate, she asserts, comparative methodologies construct and hierarchize the differences they purport to analyze (13). In "studying across," I strive to resist the trappings of comparative analysis.

While I use the terms *Global North* and *Global South* to raise into relief the power differentials that shape transhemispheric knowledge production, it remains crucial to note that these terms perform their own collapses. Economies of knowledge are of course uneven within as well as across these sites—with racialized class, academic credentials, and fluency in English, among other things, influencing who can produce supposedly legitimate knowledge. In addition, flows of migration—chosen or not—complicate the seeming stability of geographic location. These terms are crucial to transhemispheric inquiry but, like so many other terms utilized in this book, also remain under erasure.

I was trained as a sociologist, and this has shaped the way I approach research. Describing methodology often involves making visible the sometimes-tacit assumptions about knowledge that dwell in disciplines and trajectories of training. In the vein of interpretivist qualitative sociological analysis, I study mostly nonnumerical data and draw conclusions that focus on how meanings come to be shared or contested. This led me to adopt an approach called "situational analysis" in this study (Clarke 2005). This is an extension of grounded theory, which is one of the central paradigms of qualitative research. Grounded theory does not start with a specific hypothesis but instead invites iterative theorizing across a range of sites. These methodologies center action and interaction rather than subjects, resulting in a broad and often messy field of inquiry. Barney G. Glaser and Anselm L. Strauss (1967) developed grounded theory to address a generalized question: What is going on here? Situational analysis extends this approach by assuming that there is not one specific truth that can be captured in answering this question, but much can be gained by accounting for the many elements involved in meaning-making. The situation of trans- health is both unruly and uncontainable, and situational analysis accounts for such messiness.

Trans- health's multiplicity also pertains to geopolitics. In an early conversation in my fieldwork, an activist in Buenos Aires commented that Global North–based scholars often study the Global South as a source of data rather than theory. Yet there are rich theoretical analyses emanating from the Southern Cone that are relevant to expansive notions of trans- health politics but that are not yet central to Global North–based debates—though they ought to be. As such, I aimed to read, engage, and mobilize these theoretical works in my analyses. In addition, spending time with activists has influenced how I frame questions related to trans- health. Argentine scholar and activist Cecilia Palmeiro (2020, 4) calls this "collective intelligence," which she asserts emerges through manifestos, direct actions, interviews, and popular assemblies to "produce theory out of practice." This book engages analyses that are in large part enabled by such work.

One of the methodological limits of this book is its central focus on metropolitan cities. As a growing number of scholars note, studies of trans- and queer life, politics, and subjectivity focus largely on urban existence or migration—a phenomenon that Scott Herring (2010) terms "metronormativity."[37] Given this book's focus on mass action, metropolitan sites offered a high concentration of people and robust, easily identifiable forms of political mobilization. However, this de-emphasizes the rural and suburban instantiations of trans- health, which is likely to differ significantly from the accounts that I present in this book.

Study Methods

Between 2013 and 2016, I interviewed thirty-four health-care providers and activists/advocates, evenly split across both study site and role. Both prior to and after this period of fieldwork (between 2012 and 2018), I also collected document-based data. Over the ethnographic course of the study, I spent three noncontinuous months conducting fieldwork in each city, becoming acquainted with trans- health landscapes in each site.[38] In so doing, I became acquainted with sites that were frequented by trans- health activists. I followed them to political actions, summits, films, and artistic performances. I also collected advocacy materials, activist editorials, blog posts, ad campaigns, visual images, and videos. In addition, I became familiar with sites related to trans- health-care provision. I visited hospitals, community clinics, and therapists' offices. I also attended clinical trainings, went to provider conferences, and tracked changes to diagnostic classifications, care guidelines and protocols, and regulatory policies concerning trans- health.

Over the course of fieldwork, I took detailed field notes during and after observations and interactions with respondents. I also wrote reflective and analytic memos across the full trajectory of data collection and analysis. Using ATLAS.ti qualitative analysis software, I thematically organized and coded transcripts, field notes, and other key data sources. Mobilizing Adele Clarke's (2005) cartographic approaches to data analysis, I developed multiple visual maps to chart and track the shifting situations of trans- health's emergence. I struggled to maintain an up-to-date archive of these materials, as the field was changing (and continues to change) with lightning speed. As such, I (mostly) stopped collecting data in 2018, despite ongoing shifts.

Ethnographic Study Sources

For this study, I interviewed two primary groups: (1) those who engage in activism or advocacy related to trans- health and (2) those who provide health care to trans- people. Recruitment in each ethnographic site used stratified purposeful sampling to identify potential respondents, followed by theoretical sampling (Creswell 2006, 125–27). I used flyers to advertise the study in activist meeting sites and clinics, and key respondents helped distribute these. The clinics I focused on generally ran specific trans- health programs, so providers were more likely to be familiar with (and, in many instances, particularly supportive of) trans- patients and trans- health.[39] Activist recruitment focused on social movement work in trans- health in particular.

While I group these together, I maintain some differentiation between "activists" and "advocates." Self-identified trans- activists worked in various ways to bring about changes in trans- health, whether in temporary formal roles of institutional consultation or in street-based protests. Professional advocates also advocated for changes to trans- health and politics, but they primarily worked in institutionalized (and often paid) roles as attorneys or leaders of nonprofits. Labor scholar Jane F. McAlevey (2016) contrasts advocacy methods of social change with broad-based, cross-class grassroots organizing. For McAlevey, advocacy structures maintain power relations by working on behalf of people, while grassroots organizing is led by those directly affected by the conditions they address. The distinction I draw here is somewhat less rigid, as there is permeability between each of these roles in trans- health. Many advocates also call themselves activists, and indeed some became advocates through involvement in grassroots activism. However, I note the distinction in role when it is important or evident. Otherwise, I tend to use the language of "activism," since this is how most people I interviewed and observed describe themselves.

The health-care providers I interviewed worked in a variety of roles. They included nurses, nurse practitioners, social workers, physicians, psychologists, and psychiatrists. All were involved in the direct provision of care for trans- patients, and some were also involved in professional associations related to trans- health. Some providers also understood themselves to be activists—I mention this when discussing respondents who understood themselves in this way. However, I generally default to their role as providers in analyzing ethnographic data.

Increasing collaboration between these groups has, in some regard, made the boundaries demarcating them somewhat more permeable. For example, in the past decade, an increasing number of trans- activists seem to be pursuing professionalized roles as providers or advocates. In addition, some health-care providers have become politicized in their interactions with trans- patients. This permeability presents a challenge in terms of clearly naming people's roles. However, the roles in which people were acting markedly affected the positions they took. For example, some of the respondents with whom I spoke shared that their professional role—for example, as an attorney—necessitated taking positions on trans- health that may have been in partial or total conflict with their beliefs as an activist.[40]

I rarely include demographic data to describe the individuals I interviewed and observed. I am somewhat ambivalent about this decision, because I think it matters. People's subject positions with respect to race, gender identity, sexuality, disability, and immigrant status (among other things) were relevant to their views in both implicit and explicit ways. However, identifiability in this study is already a major concern. Trans- health is a small and controversial field, and even using pseudonyms does not guarantee anonymity. Especially given the growing scrutiny on its practices by opponents of trans- access to health care, I aim to protect respondents' confidentiality—including by limiting the details I share about them. That said, it remains important to note some of the demographic variation among the groups I interview.[41] In aggregate, the group of people I interviewed ranged in age from their twenties to midsixties. Of those who shared their self-identified race, a little over half identified as Black, Indigenous, or people of color. Self-identified activists were nearly all trans-, while advocates also included self-identified nontrans- allies. Most advocates, if they did not identify as trans-, identified as queer, cuir, *lesbiana,* lesbian, gay, *puto,* bisexual, or otherwise sexually nonnormative. Among care providers, only three were trans- or travesti. However, a majority also identified along lines of sexual nonnormativity in the United States. In Buenos Aires, just fewer than half of providers identified in this manner.

Study Sites

Buenos Aires, the capital of Argentina, is home to about three million of the nation's nearly forty-six million inhabitants. While not part of the city proper, its outlying urban areas contain an additional ten million inhabitants. The nation has a three-tier health system, which comprises a robust safety-net system made up of public hospitals. Depending on changing economic conditions, this serves between a third and half of the nation's residents (who generally lack formal coverage). The nation's member-based systems include a large employment-based insurance system (Obras Sociales), which is run by labor unions and financed largely by employee and employer taxes, and a smaller and more expensive private insurance sector that covers those with more wealth.

Buenos Aires has a reputation as a particularly European city in a partially Europeanized nation—which scholars argue is in large part due to the lingering discursive effect of the nation's whitening regimes and concerted authoritarian efforts to erase Indigeneity and Blackness (E. D. Edwards 2020; Hein 2020). These histories influence the way race has been administratively defined to emphasize whiteness, which has led to a claim that the nation is 97 percent white or European (including Mestizos). Xenophobia and class-based subordination often carry implications of Indigeneity or Blackness, which stem from early nationalist discourse. There is pointed conflict around the question of public social support systems, which often takes place through debates about Peronism, dating back to Juan and later Eva Perón's populist national policies (Elena 2011).

The recent history of social movements in Buenos Aires is significantly shaped by the nation's brutal military dictatorship that lasted from 1976 to 1983. During this time, an estimated thirty-thousand people—mostly leftists and young activists, or those who were suspected to be involved in revolutionary activity—were kidnapped or murdered by state or paramilitary forces. In the intervening time, international frameworks of human rights have become an important site for confronting state power and violence. In the past decades, some of these confrontations have emphasized the specificity of queer and trans- subjectivities, though not without controversy (Rizki 2020). As previously mentioned, collective resistance among travestis grew in the 1990s, especially in response to criminalization through police edicts, which forbade wearing clothes of the supposedly opposite sex or soliciting sex work. As travesti activists made clear, informal economies were often the only means of survival, but this work exposed them to other dangers through police violence or imprisonment. When Buenos Aires became an autonomous district, a new code was adopted in 1998 that instead criminalized "disorder" and "public scandal"—enabling arbitrary arrests and fines. The city explicitly prohibited sex work shortly thereafter, and travestis were targeted by all these regulations.[42] Travesti activism and trans- activism grew in Buenos Aires, confronting sustained criminalization and demanding redress.

Inequities nevertheless persisted, and in the first decade of the 2000s, trans- and travesti activists turned their attention to challenges associated with health access, legal gender reclassification, and legal name change. They also began collectively agitating for access to formal employment sectors and reparations for targeted state violence during the dictatorship. Prior to 2012, gender reclassification required court orders and extended judicial processes, since national laws prohibited the practice of trans- therapeutic medicine and name changes that supposedly "give rise to misunderstandings with respect to a person's sex."[43] Before the passage of the Gender Identity Law, gender reclassification also required irreversible sterilizing surgeries, to which Argentine scholar Martín De Mauro Rucovsky (2019, 227) wryly referred as the "political promise of a . . . shared future where monsters would not multiply." The law's passage was celebrated by activists, but it also brought about some odd political posturing. For example, the relatively supportive (if perhaps pandering) stance of former president Cristina Fernández de Kirchner led to a press conference during which trans- people and travestis were publicly granted new IDs. One of these honored recipients was summarily and curiously patted on the head by President Fernández de Kirchner.

As for the other study site, New York City contains 8.5 million of New York State's 19 million inhabitants (and the United States' 333 million). Unlike New York State more generally, white people make up the minority of residents in New York City. Historically, New York City's experiments with robust social safety nets have been vilified for producing economic crises, though scholars suggest these had more to do with systematic divestment on the part of wealthy New Yorkers (Phillips-Fein 2017).

The United States has an even more fragmented health-care system than Argentina, and Medicaid is only one of several public programs that subsidizes health care for low-income people. About a third of people in New York State have Medicaid. In the United States, public forms of health care are nearly as fragmented as private forms. The largest portion of publicly subsidized care is provided by Medicaid and Medicare—two federal programs that are each administered by the same federal agency (the Centers for Medicaid and Medicare Services) but that differ markedly in their structure and organization.[44] In 1981, Medicare issued a moratorium on funding trans- therapeutics, which was not lifted until 2014.[45] Federal Medicare rules tend to inform state Medicaid policies, but there is not a universal enforceable policy related to trans- therapeutics because the latter are determined state by state. Different states' Medicaid programs have divergent policies on trans- therapeutic coverage, ranging from explicit inclusion to categorical exclusion. During the course of my fieldwork, New York changed its rule excluding trans- therapeutic care and added an explicit provision for coverage in 2015.

The passage of the Affordable Care Act (ACA) in the United States also had a marked effect on trans- therapeutic provision in the United States more generally. This law enacted provisions prohibiting medical discrimination based on sex.[46] There was some confusion as to whether this rule included gender identity as part of sex discrimination, and the Obama administration, reluctant to take a stand on the matter, kept mum for some time. Six years later, after persistent pressure from activists and advocates, the U.S. Department of Health and Human Services finally issued a memo confirming that gender identity discrimination was indeed prohibited under the ACA.[47] This stipulation came under scrutiny during the Trump administration when a memo surfaced that they planned to reinterpret this rule and to narrow the definition of *sex discrimination* to apply only to "biological sex." This was among the Trump administration's efforts to "define transgender out of existence" (Green, Benner, and Pear 2018). The Biden administration has maintained gender identity's inclusion as being protected from discrimination, but it will likely be targeted once again.

Meanwhile, the changes brought about by the ACA, as well as Medicare and Medicaid coverage, introduced new revenue opportunities for large health-care systems. This was especially true for systems that could provide surgical care, unlike the community clinics that had long provided subsidized care for hormone-based and primary care for trans- people alongside surgical referrals to a small number of private surgeons. For example, in 2016, shortly after the ACA clarified legal corroboration for gender-affirming care and after Medicare and Medicaid reimbursements became available for trans- therapeutics, the Mount Sinai Hospital system in New York City opened a Center for Transgender Medicine and Surgery.

When it comes to social movements, New York City boasts the storied legacy of the Stonewall Rebellion. Despite taking place after several other similar rebellions, Stonewall became synonymous with queer liberation struggles. New York City also has a long history of health-care activism, particularly related to HIV/AIDS in the 1990s. This, combined with feminist health movements, in part shaped the landscape of community health clinics in the city—including those providing care for LGBTQ+ patients. Politically, the city has also been the site of significant tension after former mayor Rudy Giuliani's efforts (alongside police chief William Bratton) to formally implement quality of life policing in the early 1990s—a framework of policing that drastically expanded police harassment, criminalization, and violence against poor people, people of color, and people with disabilities. Queer and trans- youth of color were singled out for harassment, and some organizing projects in the city responded directly to these racialized and classed forms of antiqueer and antitrans- marginalization. As a majority people of color city, New York also has a robust history of queer and working-class social movements. The fact that multiple trans- organizations have emerged within this milieu has enabled relatively more expansive openings for trans- advocacy to coalesce with health, housing, and economic justice and anticriminalization movements.[48]

These descriptions, of course, only scratch the surface, but they nevertheless provide some ethnographic grounding on which the remainder of the book will build. In what follows, I discuss some of the primary scholarly conversations to which *Care without Pathology* contributes.

Sick of It All: Pathologization and Depathologization

If there is one concept upon which trans- activists, trans- studies scholars, and trans- supportive providers can generally agree, it is depathologization. In my research, respondents used the term *depathologized* to refer to the laws, diagnoses, or clinical relationships to which they thought trans- health should aspire. However, as a position of resistance, depathologization is not always explicit about the *pathologizing* forces it aims to counter. *Care without Pathology* works to identify these ranging forces and interrogate what proponents of depathologization understand themselves to be working against. As such, this book resists the dominant trend in trans- studies, which positions depathologization as a rejoinder to the unique ways that psychiatric pathologization has affected trans- people. Instead, it asks what happens when transness is only one among many targets for far-reaching and entrenched processes of pathologization and how depathologization practices resist these forces in a broader sense.

As such, chapter 1 argues that trans- health's growing institutionalization as a field has staged new debates about medical power. Within this, trans- therapeutics are moving toward becoming a wellness-based rather than a curative project. In the chapter, I show how activist interventions disrupted techniques of diagnostic individualization not only in their formal classificatory definitions but also in the *enactment* of clinical and medical care. I discuss how depathologization movements are not necessarily equivalent to demedicalization, even though popular narratives treat gay and lesbian demedicalization projects in the United States in the 1970s as a blueprint for trans- depathologization efforts. By synthesizing trans- health with other care-based depathologization efforts—centrally feminist health and disability activism—I show how trans- depathologization works in practice through care without pathology. This phrase originates with a group of activist providers (Informed Consent for Access to Trans Health Care), and I extend it to describe the ultimate objectives of trans- health activists related to depathologization. Building on these insights, I argue that certain social movements—for example, reproductive justice, the Latin American feminist Green Tide (Marea Verde) movement, and disability justice—contest pathologization beyond the singular realm of health care by highlighting connections between biomedical care, criminalization, immiseration, and state violence.[49]

Depathologization activism and scholarship have focused largely on health and medicine. The very notion of gender nonnormativity as relevant to and appropriately managed by medical providers originates largely in early to mid-twentieth-century European and U.S. sexology (Meyerowitz 2002).[50] Indeed, pathologizing forces in medicine have a great deal to do with defining conditions as illnesses. However, pathologization is something different from medicalization—a sociological term that describes how conditions are defined as being within the jurisdiction of medicine. Pathologization, in contrast, also involves the implication of abnormality, and frequently also subordination, marginalization, or criminality (Haritaworn 2015; Salessi 1995; Gill-Peterson 2018; Gupta 2019). As such, a meaningful engagement of depathologization politics means paying attention to pathologizing processes that were set into motion far prior to the period of study. I cannot fully do justice to these histories. However, my research builds on work in anticolonial and decolonial trans- studies—largely archivally based—that deftly takes up this endeavor.[51] There are three interwoven strands of pathologization that are especially worth noting: racialized eugenics, psychiatric praxis, and legal and regulatory control.

It is difficult to overstate the significance of late nineteenth- and twentieth-century eugenics in shaping the pathologizing classifications through which care practices have been constructed. Despite their different expressions in the United States and Argentina, Lamarckian paradigms of heritability and nation-building were prominent forces shaping medical and scientific classification, sexological praxis, and public-health infrastructure.[52] These accounts proposed binary sex and heterosexuality as pinnacles of the achievement of civilization. Lamarckian frameworks and their successors thus regarded the supposed failure to achieve these as reflecting "unfitness," which generally tracked along lines of race, class, and disability. Such commitments were expressed in different beliefs, policies, and practices, but they generally formed the conditions within which sex (and eventually gender) became foundational for racialized regimes of eugenics, statecraft, and the biopolitical technologies of health (Amin 2018; Foucault 1990; Haritaworn 2015; Schuller 2018).

In the United States, the notion of biological race and white supremacist nationalism took center stage in eugenic theory. The Argentine eugenic movement was no less racializing, but it more prominently emphasized Catholic familial moralism and authoritarian nationalism (Miranda 2018; Stepan 1991).[53] In each site, proponents of eugenics disparaged sexual and gender variance as threats to the nation in their ostensible reflection of biological inferiority or evolutionary failure. The imbrications of race, economic class, disability, and sex/gender far precede eugenics, but this era marked a point during which notions of health became central to these relations. These distinct sedimented legacies have in part formed the present conditions of trans- and travesti life in New York City, Buenos Aires, and well beyond.

For its part, psychiatric praxis has taken divergent paths in the United States and Argentina. Psychoanalysis in the United States is often associated with elitism, which is not necessarily the case in Argentina.[54] The field is far from a monolith in either site, but in the last four decades, the United States has largely adopted a biomedical psychiatric model that focuses on diagnosing specific mental illnesses. Some scholars (Kirk and Kutchins 1992; Lakoff 2006) attribute this to administrative structures governing health financing and the intensified importance of specific diagnoses to justify specific treatments (and coverage schema). Argentina, in contrast, maintains a Lacanian psychodynamic focus that has generally steered clear of the emphasis on diagnostic classification that dominates U.S. psychiatric practice. As Andrew Lakoff (2006) points out, Argentine mental-health professionals generally bristled at the diagnostic turn. They objected first to the implication that psychiatric and psychological care could be diagnostically standardized and, second, to the privatization of care with which they associated the *Diagnostic and Statistical Manual* (*DSM*).[55]

Despite these differences, psychiatric regimes in both the United States and Argentina took pathologizing approaches to variation in sexuality and gender through the late nineteenth and twentieth centuries (Drescher 2020; Farji Neer 2018; Gill-Peterson 2018). Despite their less diagnostically oriented approach, Lacanian psychodynamics have generally regarded sexual/gendered nonnormativity as perverse. Indeed, in Argentina, psychiatrists colluded with law enforcement in the nation to produce criminalizing frameworks restricting public space from travestis (Fernández 2004, 34).[56] In the United States and Europe, psychiatric notions of sex, gender, and sexuality emerged in large part from European sexological views. Richard von Krafft-Ebing's 1886 *Psychopathia Sexualis* and notions of "sexual inversion" were particularly influential in shaping modern psychiatric nosologies (Drescher 2020). More recently, psychiatric classifications—specifically the notion of gender nonnormativity as a mental illness—have been mobilized as justifications for such things as the termination of parental visitation rights (Minter 2018).

As such, legal domains also play a central role in regimes of pathologization. In both study sites, ideas about gender and sexuality—which have of course been defined through racialized subordination, paradigms of disablement, and notions of nationalist virtue—are expressed within administrative, civil, criminal, and family law (among many others). In Argentina, these range from the criminalizing edicts that enabled arbitrary expulsion of travestis from public space to the nation's pre-2012 administrative requirements for sterilizing surgeries as a precondition for legal gender reclassification. In the United States, they include sex-work-focused crimes such as solicitation charges or possession of condoms, which has led to what activists have termed "walking while trans" statutes (Kelly 2021).[57] Until the 2010s, surgical requirements also imposed barriers to gender reclassification for federal identification (such as passports). Several states and U.S.

territories still require surgeries for reclassification, though these provisions have relaxed somewhat over time in some places due to advocacy by trans- activists.

Concerns about pathologization focus on biomedicine. However, panning out from this view reveals the interwoven paradigms of normalization, particularly as they take shape over the nineteenth and twentieth centuries. These include expressions of white supremacy, anti-Blackness, colonial knowledge, eugenics, criminalization of public space, dictatorial rule, and other modes of domination and authority that are relevant to defining pathologies and norms.[58] Pathologization is therefore as present in criminal, civil, and administrative law as it is in diagnostic manuals, classificatory systems, and care standards—a point that I take up in more detail in chapter 2.[59] Psychiatric pathologization of transness has been particularly foundational to twentieth-century transsexual medicine (shuster 2021; Thompson and King 2015; Meyerowitz 2002). Accordingly, this is the main target of trans- depathologization activisms (Burke 2011, 20). Yet these narrowly focused depathologization campaigns run the risk of intensifying pathologization's effects for some people while alleviating them for others.[60]

Depathologization activists have played a formative role in shaping ideas and practices related to trans- health in New York City, Buenos Aires, and transnationally. Currently, their critiques have become impossible to ignore, even for the most recalcitrant providers (Pearce 2018; shuster 2021; Suess, Espineira, and Walters 2014). Trans- activists and advocates, as well as providers who stand with them, now readily contribute to determining trans- health practice—even through pointed paradigmatic conflicts.[61] While many of these debates focus on health care, resistance to pathologization often takes place within a much more expansive field. For example, the activist coalition involved in drafting the Gender Identity Law took a fourfold approach to "depathologize, decriminalize, destigmatize, and deauthorize judicial authority" from transness (Rosendo et al. 2016).[62] In this book, I argue that depathologization activists have targeted interwoven forms of pathologization in both narrow and expansive registers—including through coalitional depathologization activism.

In this sense, "care without pathology" is not necessarily an exaltation of trans- wellness or a means of asserting sanity and health against debility and illness—at least it is not *only* this to all who engage it. Cameron Awkward-Rich (2022), Hil Malatino (2022), and Andrea Long Chu (2018) argue that bad, dissociative, negative, and depressed feelings and conditions are not only consistent with but also constitutive of transness. Awkward-Rich names this "trans maladjustment," in part as a means of generatively resisting trans- disavowals of sickness. Certainly for some, care without pathology was about affirmation, a claim to health, and the outright rejection of transness as illness. For others, though, care without pathology had more to do with material demands for conditions that enable life for those who have, in different ways, been rendered ill through varying paradigms of the social or made to disappear from public spaces. This latter form of care without pathology does not require distance from maladjustment or bad feelings, but instead it entails confrontation with the forces that do violence to pathologized forms of life.

Considering Boring Things: Classification and Infrastructure

Regardless of how people identify themselves, transness is distributed via bureaucratic, classificatory, and infrastructural means—and diagnoses play key roles in this. *Care without Pathology* thus plumbs the depths of diagnostic classification manuals, care protocols, and medical coding systems to trace how trans- health has revised meanings and practices related to transness. These texts are resources that some might describe as boring things. Feminist STS scholar Susan Leigh Star (2002, 108) playfully characterizes her scholarly interest in classification, standardization, and infrastructure by claiming her membership in the "Society of People Interested in Boring Things." *Care without Pathology* likewise shines a light on these boring things (and their ersatz claims to political neutrality), demonstrating that these are in fact sites through which power often circulates most intensely—and sometimes most brutally.[63]

I am not particularly concerned with who is or is not in fact trans- as a truth claim, but I realize that being identified as trans- affects people's life chances and affects access to (or freedom from) biomedical care. Spending time with diagnostic classifications means constantly coming up against the question of who counts as trans-. Historically, practitioners of transsexual medicine pursued this question anxiously and doggedly, and for many, this heated curiosity has not abated. For some, though, classifications have taken on importance that extends beyond or even displaces what they say about those to whom they were applied. As I spoke with activists, advocates, and providers who fought for public access to trans- health, it was clear that classifications were instead most important in the way they facilitated actions—particularly, reimbursement for the costs of care (at least in the United States). In this sense, classification mattered to people involved in trans- health, even if it mattered in different ways than it had before. Yet, as I argue in chapter 2, analyses of trans- health must develop a more nuanced and robust engagement with the work of classification to account for the distinctions between formal classifications, how classifications work in practice, and how classifications become tangled up with other seemingly unrelated classificatory schema.

In chapter 2, I thus examine how providers and activists revised pathologizing psychiatric diagnoses and (at least partially) reconceptualized transness as a benign variation. Many of the central debates in trans- health hinge on the trans- diagnosis, its validity, its ability to capture gender nonnormativity, and its ability to bring about specific outcomes for both providers and patients. The trans- diagnosis does not exist in the singular but is rather a gloss on the many distinct and shifting diagnoses that appear in varying psychiatric and medical classificatory systems throughout the world. The pathologizing impulse of these classificatory genealogies becomes a central tension in some of the conflicts defining trans- health as an emergent field. The depathologized diagnoses that resulted from negotiated revisions also aimed to facilitate access to care that would still be defined as medically necessary. Tracing these diagnoses across different iterations of the *Diagnostic and Statistical Manual* and the *International Classification of Diseases,* I show how these terms, definitions, and classifications became sites of contestation and negotiation between providers and activists. Drawing on revision processes for each resource, I analyze diagnoses through infrastructures of medical practice, health-care financing bureaucracies, and scientific research, tracing how revisions transferred focus from individual pathology to social concepts of distress or gender incongruence. In so doing, I describe how diagnoses still stuck to people differently depending on race, geographic location, access to wealth, citizenship, age, and much more. All of these also affected claims to recognition and legitimacy.[64]

In the realm of biomedicine, gender nonnormativity has taken many forms and names. These include Transsexualism, Gender Identity Disorder, Gender Dysphoria, and Gender Incongruence, in addition to variations that invoke the specificity of age, sexual orientation, and other forms of difference. Most are still defined as psychiatric conditions, but activists and providers have worked to establish nonpsychiatric classifications (which I discuss at length in the opening chapters of the book). Changing definitions range in scale from localized clinical policies to international classification systems and treatment protocols—and each of these seems to be under near-constant revision. Such definitional changes not only shift ideas about transness but also bring about reprinted manuals, revised coding schemas, new human rights imperatives, and changes to gender reclassification laws. Finding a relatively stable and universal diagnostic classification—or at least one that can work well enough—seems to be a primary objective of the restless redefining.

Diagnostic struggles are complicated by the fact that health-care financing systems are organized around medical classifications. In other words, care can generally be covered only when there is a diagnostic code to which it can be attached. People who advocate for depathologization come up against this when they want to eliminate diagnostic classifications while maintaining links to care and coverage. I describe this tension as the "illness–care conundrum," which I discuss in the first chapter. Rather than dispose of classifications, depathologization activists and advocates worked to change diagnostic content to preserve the codes that provided a link to covered care (or at least potentially covered care).

As they relate to trans- health, financing systems receive a fair amount of attention from policy analysts but are not as frequently engaged on a theoretical level. *Care without Pathology* emphasizes economic concerns not only to show their behind-the-scenes centrality in shaping depathologization struggles but also to highlight political economy in trans- health more generally. For example, health-care bureaucracies, financing schema, guidelines, and protocols all had considerable implications for care coverage. Considering these within a broader landscape of health politics meant tangling with the austerity regimes characterizing trans- health as excessively costly and nonessential, especially for stakeholders that focused on the public provision of care.

This also meant contending with the stratified systems of care within which trans- health operates. As trans- studies scholar Aren Z. Aizura (2018) points out, it is crucial to consider the economic and medico-legal infrastructures that produce trans- people as "consumers" versus "patients." These dynamics set the scene, he asserts, for medical tourism, selective commodification, racialized stratification, and exclusion within transnational markets of care provision. For example, the shift to comprehensive centers for trans- health within large health-care systems in the United States reflects not only social shifts but also the fact that trans- therapeutics have "become intelligible to US health markets as monetizable" (171). These mostly privatized care systems stand to benefit financially from the inclusion of trans- subjectivities into legitimated domains of biomedicine. As Aizura claims, these explicitly trans- affirmative programs are situated within systems that approach movements for universal and free health access with suspicion, if not outward resistance. In this sense, trans- health practices differ radically across economic as well as diagnostic infrastructures of biomedicine and health-care financing.

Casting Claims to Care: Trans- Health and Social Movements

Returning to the moment in Buenos Aires in 2013 when I politely clashed with another scholar about who might be entitled to public forms of care, I noted the strangeness of having this debate in front of the Hotel Bauen—the site of the conference and the place where he was staying. The hotel had closed during Argentina's 2001 economic crisis, and in the following years, its former employees had recuperated the business. Reopened as a worker-owned cooperative, the hotel became a popular site for activist meetings. The Bauen was one of many reclaimed and recuperated hotels. About thirty city blocks due west, in the Villa Crespo neighborhood, a hotel called Gondolín was reclaimed around the same time—not by workers but by the travestis who were staying there.[65] To this day, it continues as a site for communal living for travestis in the city. The Bauen and the Gondolín were among the many models for collectively run cooperatives in the nation. In addition to providing shelter, the recuperated workplace model also became important for travestis who had been systematically excluded from formal labor markets for decades.[66] The Hotel Bauen and many other worker-owned cooperatives became targets for right-wing politicians and champions of vertically integrated and wage-stratified business models.

The conference itself was cosponsored by the University of Buenos Aires, a tuition-free university that is open to all. Its universal-access approach to education and its reputation as a haven for leftist thought has also placed it in the crosshairs of right-wing and neoliberal governments for the better part of the twentieth and twenty-first centuries.

In other words, we stood at a point on the map of the city that represented a brick-and-mortar rejoinder to both austerity and authoritarianism. Yet there we were, debating the very questions that animate austerity politics: What are the limits of collectivized care, and who should be excluded from its reach? In fact, the very trans- health movements I was studying in Buenos Aires and New York City were in the process of refusing and inverting such questions. Rather than interrogating the fiscal limits of care, they asserted that austerity regimes were simply extensions of the violence of pathologization in the first instance. These activists pushed back on economic claims through critiques of distributive inequity and by defining robust forms of trans- health as a social good.[67] Instead of asking who should be excluded from care, they inquired into the ways that massive upward transfers of wealth—and not social spending—had produced scarcity for many.[68]

Collectives therefore engaged what Vek Lewis and Dan Irving (2017) call "trans political economy."[69] Their critiques of these dynamics were at their most pointed when it came to public forms of care provision. *Care without Pathology* traces how trans- health activism not only reckoned with the pathologization of trans- people but also engaged varied struggles related to resource distribution, health inequity, and feminist, racial, and disability justice. Social movement studies, particularly those centered in the United States, have tended to parse movements linked to class solidarity from those related to identity formations—the latter of which are generally called "new social movements" (Laraña, Johnston, and Gusfield 1994). Social movement theorizing in and from the Global South, in contrast, has largely engaged the ways economic and cultural struggles coemerge (Garretón 2002; Álvarez et al. 2017). Likewise, during my fieldwork, the activists who advocated for depathologized trans- health, especially in its public form, organized across constellations of meaning that saw social structure, economic distribution, and relative subject position as interconnected rather than discrete. This was especially evident in how coalitional depathologization activists took up issues of debt. *Care without Pathology* thus discusses how activists understood issues as diverse as sovereign debt repayment, reparations for state violence, and taxation as central concerns for trans- health and politics.

In this sense, trans- health movements—at least those that focused squarely on racialized and economic stratification—were grappling with pathologization as it has been shaped by racial capitalism or, more precisely, what David Theo Goldberg (2009) calls "racial neoliberalism."[70] In chapters 3 and 4, I discuss how activists focused on questions of economic distribution, inclusive of its racialized and racializing dynamics, to resist radical disinvestment from collective forms of care. Some activists were explicit about the ways racial injustice shaped access to public forms of trans- health, while for others these were more implicit. The latter was especially relevant in Buenos Aires, where paradigms of racialization followed different trajectories than those in the United

States.[71] Activist critiques of racial capitalism and neoliberalism were key to the community-based research and advocacy campaigns in Buenos Aires and New York City that I trace in chapters 3 and 4. In these chapters, I argue that activists in each site sought to adopt techniques of data analysis to redefine health and contest the structural violence, pathologization, racism, and immiseration that unevenly shaped conditions of life for trans- people and travestis.

In chapter 3, I analyze travesti and trans- activist-led community-based studies conducted in Argentina in the early 2000s, which blended quantitative and narrative biographical data. I call these "epidemiological biographies," and I analyze how they defined criminalization, state violence, and immiseration as primary conditions endangering trans- and travesti health and life expectancy. I argue that these studies made state violence against trans- people legible through logics of population health, even as the concept of "population" also emerged from techniques of state control. These community-based studies had a considerable effect on national trans- health politics and provided an evidentiary basis for the passage of Argentina's Gender Identity Law in 2012.

These community-based studies emerged in part through collective political action that reformulated dominant modes of statistical aggregation. This statistical turn—which I call "statistical collectivization"—produced contradictory effects. At one level, it obscured differential conditions of criminalization and violence. At another, it directed attention to the racialized, classed, sexualized, and gendered ways that travestis were marginalized and prioritized materially distributive regulation over and above civil protections. Through these contradictory actions, social movements reformulated dominant notions of health by challenging state securitization and contesting state power.

In chapter 4, I argue that activists and advocates in New York also engaged in statistical collectivization, but in a way that promoted the advantages of cost savings associated with state coverage for trans- therapeutics. As was the case in Buenos Aires, they used statistical data to foreground how structural violence and inequity affect trans- health. However, they also pointed to speculative cost savings associated with expanding public coverage for trans- therapeutics, given the likelihood of preventing mental-health crises and suicide attempts. As such, I refer to these as "economized epidemiological biographies."

Working with and against logics of austerity, activists and advocates contested long-standing claims by state administrators and popular media that trans- therapeutics were too specialized, politicized, or expensive for public financing. They also made ethical claims that defined trans- therapeutics as the "regular healthcare that non-trans people receive every day when they need it" (GLAAD and Sylvia Rivera Law Project 2013a) and worked to define the Medicaid exclusion as an expression of state racism. The combined actions of public media and direct-action campaigns and legal challenges led to the elimination of the Medicaid exclusion for trans- therapeutic coverage. I draw on Michelle Murphy's (2017) concerns with the utility of population and what they see as its inevitable "economization of life" to analyze the contradictions between New York activists' strategic claims for cost efficiency and justice-based ethical imperatives.

The Medicaid fight that I examined in New York was relatively unusual within U.S.-based trans- advocacy, since it focused on material redistribution rather than antidiscrimination.[72] In contrast, Argentine activists' work to shift material access to health care was part of a series of demands among trans- and travesti activists around employment and educational access, as well as reparations for state-sanctioned violence during the military dictatorship of 1976–83.[73]

Finally, neoliberalism's uptake across the Americas had very different effects by nation and region, and this influenced how trans- and travesti activists engaged their transnationally facing work.[74] These confrontations with neoliberalism influenced how vulture funds, psychiatric imperialism, geopolitics, and philanthropy—in addition to depathologization—became central tensions in transnational activism and advocacy. For example, depathologization activists took up notions of self-determination and autonomy in the antigatekeeping activism I discuss in chapters 1 and 5, but for transnationally engaged activists, these terms took on broader connotations linked to anti-imperialism. In chapter 5, I focus on informed consent protocols to show how these multivalent meanings became important for trans- people and travestis seeking more decision-making autonomy in clinical care. Coordinating work both within clinics and between different national infrastructures of health, activists worked to develop consent-driven care frameworks to confront subordination, whether explicitly or symbolically. These negotiations were enabled by what Susan Leigh Star (1993) calls "cooperation without consensus."

However, the clinical protocols that activists helped to develop fell short of the revolution that they might have desired. In fact, while cooperation in these realms may reflect certain changes in authority, practice, and power dynamics within biomedicine, it also reflects how gender nonnormativity has become a flexible site for economic, affective, and political investment. Before the consolidation of many of these transformations, Marxist trans- studies scholar Dan Irving (2009, 395) critiqued the figure of the "self-made man" at the heart of self-determination in trans- health and politics:

> It is critical to grasp the significant governing role that economic discourse plays in mediating the construction of hegemonic transsexual masculinity in order to begin to disentangle the various power relations existing within the current conceptualization of sex/gender self-determination. As critical scholars and activists, do we know what we are demanding when we articulate the need for sex/gender self-determination within neoliberal capitalist society?

This book takes up Irving's provocation to understand what activists, providers, and scholars were demanding in foregrounding self-determination. Certainly, some respondents were more concerned with the singularity of depathologizing transness than they were with confronting the pathologization of racialized poverty. However, many of the people with whom I spoke saw themselves as demanding something much deeper than just gaining entry into biomedical entrepreneurialism.[75] Even amid the nascent growth of trans- therapeutics as an economic industry, depathologization activists saw trans- health as one site from which to confront inequities and exclusions in care and distributive politics.

State of Flux: Biopolitics and Legal Intervention

Many trans- health activists with whom I spoke worked on trans- health by intervening in clinical care, but others focused on changing state, national, and municipal laws and regulations. Trans- health remains a contested field, and the legitimacy of trans- therapeutic practices have often been in question. As such, legal decisions about its status affect decisions about care provision and coverage. Public and private hospitals, clinics, and third-party payors have long defined trans- therapeutics as "cosmetic" or "experimental" and have used this to justify coverage exclusions (Baker and Cray 2013). In *Care without Pathology,* I focus primarily on analyzing two examples of legal or regulatory change that address public coverage for trans- therapeutics: Argentina's federal Gender Identity Law and New York State's Medicaid rules for service coverage.

As I mentioned at the outset, the Gender Identity Law passed in Argentina in 2012. The content was drafted by a coalition of trans- and travesti activists and allies that called themselves the Frente Nacional por la Ley de Identidad de Género (the National Front for the Gender Identity Law), or the Frente (Hollar 2018; De Mauro Rucovsky 2019; Sabsay 2016). It was hailed as groundbreaking by the international media (though curiously underreported in the United States), and even Argentine activists were somewhat surprised by its unanimous passage in the Senate.[76] The law combined provisions governing legal gender reclassification with provisions on health access and coverage. It eliminated surgical and diagnostic requirements, and care providers and judges were no longer in charge of deciding who would receive trans- therapeutic care (which activists refer to as "gatekeeping"). Instead, it formally guaranteed coverage for desired care and introduced a framework of informed consent, which I discuss in chapter 5.[77]

The law also applied to minors who had parental support, and other minors could pursue a court order to access care even without parental consent. The Gender Identity Law became an international model not only in its depathologizing structure but also in its bundling of health care and administrative legal identification change. Various nations, particularly in Europe and South

America, followed its lead.[78] However, in the years following its passage, activists struggled to translate the law's symbolic import into concrete changes for trans- people and travestis in Argentina, especially when it came to the law's provisions with respect to health care.[79] In this book, I focus on this legal struggle not only because it was the first of its kind but also because it was led by trans- and travesti activists as a part of a broader set of materially redistributive fights.

In the United States, Medicaid policies that regulate care coverage for low-income people have been a target for trans- activists and advocates striving to expand access to trans- therapeutic care. In 2015, New York's Department of Health formally lifted its sixteen-year exclusion clause for what they called "gender-confirming care" for trans- people. The rule was changed amid a class-action lawsuit, and it initially introduced coverage for a limited number of procedures. However, it set limits on procedures that were considered cosmetic and limited eligibility to adults. Advocates kept pressing and in 2016 won an expanded set of covered procedures and coverage for minors.[80] In chapter 4, I focus on New York's Medicaid fight. I do so in large part because it was preceded by a lengthy multipronged struggle led by both grassroots activists and legal advocates to expand access to trans- therapeutics for low-income people.

In *Care without Pathology,* I trace these legal and regulatory projects, dissimilar as they are in scale and objective, to gain insights into how activists and advocates made claims about the social and material imperatives for collective trans- flourishing. While the Argentine law passed legislatively, changes to U.S. Medicare and state Medicaid programs stemmed from legal challenges and closed-door regulatory decisions. Nevertheless, each of these changes reflected sustained organizing efforts to contest how austerity regimes shaped the administration and stratification of trans- health. I am concerned less with these laws as objects and more with the political organizing that preceded their uptake.[81] As I reflect on these struggles, I ask what compromises people made, how they engaged the limits of law, and how they marshaled their political commitments into legal tactics.

This book dwells in the domain of laws, state health bureaucracies, and public budgets as its empirical focus, but its broader concerns and desires extend beyond these. In my ethnographic study, state and municipal governments defined what counted as public forms of care through their monopolies on taxation, budgeting, and apportionment. This was why state systems became the targets for activist campaigns to expand care distribution. States are not, of course, the only imaginable mode of care collectivization. In the past decade, we have witnessed climate disasters and a global pandemic baldly expose the limits of many state infrastructures in effectively providing care, relief, and repair. A longer view reveals these as enduring dynamics of violence. Mutual aid networks emerge from a long and varied history and, in many sites, have sought to address and respond to these failures. Currently, forms of mutual aid are once again providing sites of refuge for those who suffer systematic abandonment or targeting (or both).[82]

In chapter 6, I argue that coalitional depathologization activism was a means of engaging these more expansive political desires. Here, I foreground the subset of activists with whom I spoke who were explicit about confronting the dynamics of state violence, racial capitalism and neoliberalism, and imperialism. Defining their work as "extending depathologization," I show how their efforts and objectives transcended the bounds of trans- health and strove to enact radical transformations in care relations, state responsibility, and the broader conditions of life. Coalitional depathologization activists raised into relief the histories of harm that led to pathologization, and they insisted on doing so with pointed attention to macroeconomics, colonization, and racialization (among other things). Not only did they demand nonhierarchical notions of clinical care, but they also applied these demands for horizontalism to geopolitics.

In their attunement to how trans- health advances more expansive demands for access, distribution, and coalition, these activists evoked what scholars describe as transnational feminisms (Grewal and Caplan 1994; Swarr and Nagar 2010). They also drew on notions of transfeminism as a "politics of resistance and alliance [that considers] domination to be a multilayered system that produces cross-oppressions, including transphobia" (OUTrans, n.d.).[83] As such, I suggest that transnational depathologization activism, in some forms, might be best described as transnational transfeminism. Such approaches may chart a path not only for depathologization but also for the eventual enactment of broader health-care infrastructures that are accessible to and that care well for everyone—and perhaps that even change the terms of medicine to fit the vision of care without pathology.

This book necessarily navigates tensions between mass movements grappling for political power vis-à-vis present-day infrastructures and those prefigurative-facing movements that seek to create microcosms of the worlds they seek to manifest. These are not mutually exclusive, but they often collide in their representation of what makes up a political objective and what defines success for movements. Federal, state, provincial, and municipal governments are currently at the center of distributive debates, so depathologization activists trained their attention on these—even if they had more expansive political desires. As an ethnographer, I did the same.

Despite these limits, focusing on states, laws, and public infrastructure care provides an empirical basis through which to confront the strange textures of contemporary biopolitical regimes.[84] The distribution of health care is among the key sites through which the division between those marked for life and those marked for death is adjudicated. However, this does not mean that health remains confined within the walls of clinics and hospitals. Contemporary health politics mark something much more diffuse.[85] *Care without Pathology* examines the conditions, claims, and effects of these transformations—from the clinic rooms to boardrooms to streets. It frames questions of health not only around the questions of bodies and their care but also through macroeconomics, neoliberal politics, redistribution, redress for state violence, and social movement demands for new and different worlds.

1 Care without Pathology

Coordinating Depathologization

In 2012, a group of transgender celebrities—including British transgender rabbinical student Maxwell Zachs and Canadian transgender beauty queen Jenna Talackova—started a petition to request that the World Health Organization (WHO) remove "transsexualism" from its chapter on mental illness in the *International Classification of Diseases* (*ICD*). Circulating via Change.org with the title "We are Trans* Not Sick," the petition gained 91,019 signatories internationally (Zachs et al. 2012). Its sponsors were from North America and Europe, and different versions circulated in Spanish, French, English, and German. In Zachs and colleagues' (2012) version (the one that circulated in the United States), the petition's brief introduction asserted that "gender is not an illness, it is just a part of who I am." He described the 1990 removal of the classification of "homosexuality" from the *ICD* as a parallel precedent. However, he emphasized the need to maintain some form of diagnostic classification as a bridge to care. As Zachs and the other petitioners asserted, "This doesn't mean that we should be excluded from the health system: pregnant women are not sick, but they have medical protocols and assistance. The same should happen with trans people." The demand, therefore, was that the *ICD* do away with "transsexualism" as a mental-health condition and simultaneously develop a "classification that allows trans people to get the medical help they need."

In 2011, a year before the petition circulated, the transnational trans advocacy organization Global Action for Trans Equality (GATE) met to address this very tension between depathologization and the need for care coverage. This group was aware that the WHO was already convening a working group to explore how to develop a new, nonpsychiatric diagnostic classification for transness as part of *ICD-11,* the revision to 1990's *ICD-10.* In anticipation, GATE convened a group of mostly trans multidisciplinary experts in The Hague to issue recommendations to the WHO. Participants came from South and North America, East and Southeast Asia, Europe, and several other regions. Their priorities were to simultaneously depathologize transness, maintain access to coverage for trans- therapeutics across disparate health-care systems and strata, and ensure applicability across transnational expressions of gender nonnormativity.

Emphasizing covered access to care, GATE's advisory proposed a diagnostic model that could be tailored to localized needs, communities, and—perhaps most critically—varied health coverage infrastructures. This decentralized, flexible model was termed the "Starfish Model," for its capacity to exist in separable parts. While it was not ultimately adopted, the WHO's formal *ICD-11* revision team cited the report's recommendations, emphasizing diagnostic flexibility to maximize possibilities for care coverage. I detail this process more fully in the next chapter.

As the Change.org petition and the GATE recommendations exemplify, activists, advocates, and a growing number of health-care providers asserted that being trans- could not be equated with sickness. Correspondingly, they asserted trans- health was a wellness-based rather than a curative project. Yet access to care coverage remained a persistent challenge that depended on health-care infrastructures that were shaped by a range of forces and interests. Many proponents of depathologization ran up against the illness–care conundrum, or the need for a diagnostic classification to justify coverage eligibility. As I discuss in the Introduction, Argentina's 2012 Gender Identity Law addressed this conundrum through its national coverage guarantee, at least in theory. In the United States, however, state, federal, and private insurance regulations varied wildly—and publicly subsidized trans- therapeutics were the subject of pointed public debate and controversy. Yet for activists, it was not enough for biomedicine to relinquish the idea of trans- people as being mentally ill. It was crucial, they argued, for trans- people to have access to affordable, quality health care—including trans- therapeutics. In other words, they wanted care without pathology.

"Care without pathology" is in fact a phrase that is featured on the website of Informed Consent for Access to Trans Health Care, or ICATH (n.d.). This loose network, which no longer appears to be active, included mostly trans- therapists and providers who circulated tools, letter templates, and messaging to reduce gatekeeping in trans- health care. The website draws on this phrase only briefly to describe the position that the group took on trans- health-care provision as a set of practices that should not require pathologization. In this chapter and throughout the book, I extend this claim theoretically and consider its broader interventions in care relations and politics.

As a concept, care without pathology raises pressing questions about biomedical practice in a general sense: If medicine must pathologize in order to treat, what would be involved in a depathologized health-care practice? Given that the work of health-care providers is to diagnose and treat, what happens when their patients assert knowledge and directives about what enhances their own wellness? Finally, how flexible are paradigms of care given the reimbursement and coverage schemas that organize diagnostic and treatment protocols? This chapter will set out the stakes for addressing how these questions have been taken up both within and beyond trans- health and will thus serve to map out the terrain that I will cover in the rest of the book. The subsequent chapters will reflect on the concepts it covers and the questions it raises in more depth and detail.

In this chapter, I assert that "care without pathology" distinguishes trans- health from lesbian and gay depathologization movements' approach to biomedicine, which sought to disentangle themselves from biomedical regimes. Instead, depathologizing projects in trans- health seek funded, nonhierarchical trans- therapeutic care and seek to organize this as a wellness project rather than a curative treatment for illness. For activists, this also involves the elimination of psychiatric and pathologizing diagnoses (which I discuss in detail in chapter 2) and gatekeeping practices, which they aim to address through consent-driven care (which I build on in chapter 5). Taken together, these analyses aim to define and describe what trans- activists mean by *depathologization* and to explore the concrete means by which they have worked with providers to enact it though clinical practice.

Next, I discuss the illness–care conundrum as one of the more intransigent barriers for depathologization activists (at least for those whose health-care systems require diagnoses for reimbursement). Within this, I assert that medical gatekeeping, in addition to its specific relevance to trans- therapeutics, is also as a cost-control method for health-care provision.

Finally, I discuss trans- health activists' embrace of care without pathology as putting it in close kin relation with reproductive justice, Green Tide (Marea Verde) feminists, and disability justice, among other movements. Unlike lesbian and gay depathologization activists, these movements do not necessarily desire a full separation from biomedicine, though they certainly seek transformed relations of care within it. I ask what comes into view by taking this approach to remapping the legacies, trajectories, and objectives of trans- depathologization. In this section, I also discuss the conceptual coalitional relations that take shape between these movements. I conclude by describing how some depathologization activists—who I call "coalitional depathologization" activists—make these coalitional connections concrete within their movement work by extending depathologization. I discuss this group in greater depth in the final chapter of the book.

A Theory of Care without Pathology

Positions on depathologization that I describe in this chapter are generally aligned with the paradigm of "care without pathology." In general terms, this notion describes care practices that work to transform relations of biomedical power while retaining access to covered or subsidized biomedical or perimedical therapeutics. Among the groups that I observed, people who favored depathologization enacted care without pathology by revising biomedical knowledge in the form of diagnoses or care protocols. Others worked to modify bureaucracies of health reimbursement or financing regulations. A few choreographed clinical work-arounds to ensure access while avoiding pathologizing diagnoses or sidestepping coverage exclusions (I address some of these approaches in the following chapter). Among all of those I observed, proponents of trans- depathologization sought to transform the relations of biomedical care rather than seeking wholesale extraction or separation from medicine—and ongoing depathologization projects follow a similar trajectory. In this manner, trans- depathologization converges more closely with feminist health and disability activism than with the demedicalizing objectives of late twentieth-century gay and lesbian depsychopathologization movements. This chapter explores those resonances, concluding that they converge not only through the phenomenon of care without pathology but also through broader shared desires for health justice.

Trans- health activist and public-health scholar Amets Suess (2015, 219) calls trans- depathologization "a paradigm shift from a conceptualization of gender transition as a mental disorder towards its recognition as a human right." In the past decade, trans- depathologization has begun to shape mainstream biomedicine at a transnational scale—though not without contestation. For the past thirty years or more, travesti and trans- scholars and activists have confronted pathologizing medicolegal knowledge about gender nonnormativity. Sandy Stone's (1992, 167) "The 'Empire' Strikes Back: A Posttranssexual Manifesto" characterizes encounters between health-care providers and trans- people as taking place "across a diagnostic battlefield" through which clinicians act as "gatekeepers for cultural norms." Activists and scholars Lohana Berkins and Josefina Fernández (2005, 55) emphasize the simultaneous imputation of illness and criminality related to pathologization: "To have a travesti identity . . . is synonymous with criminality." Over time, such confrontations have condensed into specific depathologization demands from trans- health activists in local and transnational formations, such as GATE, Stop Trans Pathologization (STP), and ICATH, among others.

As a result of these persistent efforts to address pathologization, activists are increasingly—though unevenly—enrolled as lay experts and community advisers. Flagrant antagonism between medical gatekeepers and trans- communities is inconsistently giving way to Susan Leigh Star's (1993) notion of "cooperation without consensus," which enables groups with conflicting positions to work together. This increasing collaboration has partially shifted the dominant gaze when it comes to care and opens up the space for trans- health to contend more openly with the notion that racialized transphobia shapes both biomedical practice and the world. In this sense, certain activists have illuminated (and worked to force the field to contend with) the implicit and explicit connections between clinical encounters and the broader conditions of the body politic that Alondra Nelson (2011) calls "social health."

In a general sense, depathologization projects address power relations in biomedical care by contesting subordinating and entrenched knowledge about illness, pathology, and normativity. Activists thus work to counter what psychiatrist and ethicist Erik Schneider (2018, 170) calls "definitional sovereignty." However, demedicalization—the removal of practices, conditions, or modes of being from the jurisdiction of medicine—is not equivalent to most forms of depathologization within trans- health. Many trans- and gender nonnormative people consider biomedical technologies to be an important element of sexed/gendered embodiment and enactment and work to "preserve medicalization" even as they contest its pathologizing terms (Burke 2011, 189). Because access remains a central concern, proponents of trans- depathologization define trans- therapeutics as a social good and medical necessity rather than a private market commodity. However, they generally assert that the provision of such therapeutics should be based on self-determination rather than pathologization or illness.

This is the vision advanced by depathologization activists, who claim transphobia as the "illness" most profoundly affecting the lives of trans- people (Stop Trans Pathologization 2012).[1] Relative to ICATH's vision to develop infrastructures of informed-consent-driven rather than diagnostically driven care (discussed in more detail in chapter 5), the group's website promotes "care without pathology" (ICATH, n.d.). The website content expands on this only briefly as "a departure from the system that uses [diagnoses] as a means for accessing gender-confirming health care" and emphasizes the consistency of this approach with gender-affirming care for nontrans- people. In the remainder of this chapter, I extend ICATH's concept of care without pathology as a broader political claim and intervention in hierarchical politics of care.[2]

"Diagnosis Means There's Something Wrong with You": The Illness–Care Conundrum

Talia, a nurse practitioner in New York City, became involved in trans- health in the early 2000s. Not only did she think that patients knew best what they needed, she also saw her role as being one that supported their wellness rather than directing their treatment. She was especially frustrated about the expectation that she should apply psychiatric diagnoses to trans- patients to facilitate therapeutic coverage. "I still don't think that, as a nurse practitioner, I should really be diagnosing people with things out of the *DSM*" (interview, August 3, 2013). The clinic in which she worked had adopted a protocol that required only informed consent on the part of patients rather than verification letters from mental-health providers. I discuss these informed consent processes in depth in chapter 5. Despite Talia's clinic not requiring letters from psychiatrists or psychologists, she and most of her colleagues strove to use some version of a diagnostic classification for trans- patients to facilitate coverage for care.

Our conversation took place while New York State's Medicaid program still prohibited coverage for trans- therapeutics—an exclusion I discuss in detail in chapter 4. This exclusion was introduced in 1998 and formally prohibited state Medicaid funds from being used for any care related to trans- therapeutics. At the time, a number of public and private insurance programs did offer such coverage, although this was nearly always contingent on receiving a *DSM*-based diagnosis of Gender Identity Disorder (or, after 2013, Gender Dysphoria). Yet due to New York's regulatory exclusion, even a formal psychiatric diagnosis would not enable many poor patients to access subsidized care for hormone treatments, surgeries, or related forms of care.

Since Talia's patients were almost entirely covered by Medicaid, she rarely used the psychiatric diagnosis since it would not help with payment for care. Instead, she regularly risked her license by using a work-around that was common among health-care providers treating trans- patients on Medicaid. "For billing purposes, I just use Endocrine Disorder-NOS [Not Otherwise Specified] 259.9" (interview, August 3, 2013).[3] As I will discuss further in the following chapter, this *ICD*-based code diagnoses disorders in which people produce too little or too much of an endocrine hormone. Some New York–based providers mentioned that certain clinics or systems of care had adopted Endocrine Disorder-NOS as part of a standard protocol for diagnosing trans- patients. Talia and other providers justified the legitimacy of its use by explaining that trans- patients could indeed be understood to have a hormone imbalance, though most realized that insurance payors might see this as a fraudulent claim. However, Talia did not find either coding approach—the *ICD*-based Endocrine Disorder or the *DSM*-based Gender Identity Disorder/Gender Dysphoria—to be ideal, since both indicated a pathological state. "We actually view people as being generally healthy. Diagnosis means there's something wrong with you. [Why do] we still have to assign a code to health? Why can't we just use V70.0—the code you use for a well visit—for all of our trans- health and have that cover everything?" (interview, August 3, 2013). In other words, Talia wondered why she was required to diagnose wellness.

I interviewed Marcus at a restaurant in the Bronx in the summer of 2013. A social worker who was working in a New York trans- health clinic, he echoed Talia's dissatisfaction with this predicament. "You're coming in for care, [so] you always have to have a diagnosis. . . . I don't like it. I don't know how to have alternatives within the system that we have" (interview, July 23, 2013). As providers caring for poor patients who would not likely be able to access costly therapeutics without coverage, Talia and Marcus emphasized that diagnostic revision or declassification (the process of removing diagnostic classifications) was only part of the story of trans- depathologization. Health-care access and coverage were also central concerns—and the danger of their patients or clients losing access to current or future coverage for therapeutics kept them from wanting to do away with diagnoses entirely (even in the form of work-arounds, such as Endocrine Disorder). While they both wished for a system in which patients could obtain the therapeutics they needed without a diagnosis, they also recognized that access to covered or subsidized treatment in most health-care coverage systems required a code or diagnosis.

I refer to the constraints that Talia and Marcus identify as an "illness–care conundrum" to describe the difficulty of providing or accessing care in the absence of a specific and diagnosable illness. The tight links between pathology, diagnosis, and the legitimacy of treatment shaped Talia's inability to use a V70.0 well visit code to care for her trans- patients and Marcus's need to diagnose in the absence of an alternative bridge to care. Most medical institutions—certainly those in the United States—require some form of diagnosis to provide access to covered or subsidized care. While preventive care, including in Medicaid programs, is generally covered, prescribing medications generally requires the identification of a problem or chief complaint on the part of a patient. Usually this occurs through a diagnostic code, not simply a visit code. When it comes to trans- therapeutics, reimbursement or subsidies for costly care are the main reasons that many activists, advocates, and supportive providers oppose declassification, or getting rid of a diagnosis altogether. In this sense, trans- therapeutics for people with wealth have long been depathologized, as diagnostic requirements need not be met for elective out-of-pocket care. But for most middle- and low-income people in the United States and Argentina who seek health care through insurance or government-financed health programs, out-of-pocket care can be prohibitively expensive.

Even with a diagnosis, only recently have United States–based public and private payors even begun to reliably reimburse for trans- therapeutics. Throughout the early 2000s, private insurance companies slowly but steadily increased coverage for such care, citing medical and scientific evidence about medical necessity. State Medicaid programs, however, were slow to eliminate exclusions, and advocates assert that public financing in fact diminished during this period (Spade et al. 2009). The federal Medicare program in the United States removed a blanket exclusion on trans- therapeutics in 2014, thirty-three years after instituting it. Some shifts in public financing accompanied the passage of the Affordable Care Act in the United States, which enacted provisions prohibiting discrimination in Section 1557 of the law. After some confusion, the U.S. Department of Health and Human Services explicitly articulated that discrimination on the basis of sex also included gender identity.[4] For depathologization activists and advocates, such expansion of the possibility for reimbursement or subsidized trans- therapeutics in the United States (though still contested) only increases the stakes of having a reliable form of diagnostic classification linked to care. Thus, the illness–care conundrum is as pronounced as ever. These contingencies set the stage for activists, advocates, and supportive providers to press for changes to diagnostic classifications that are at once depathologizing and an effective bridge to care. I explore these classificatory revisions in more detail in the next chapter.

Given its intransigence in the United States, it is important to understand that the infrastructural relation between diagnosis, code, care, and coverage is not so tightly linked in all sites of care provision. In Argentina, for example, the passage of the Gender Identity Law eliminated all diagnostic requirements for gender-confirming care. The sole requirement to qualify for covered care was not a diagnosis or code but simply "self-perceived need" by those seeking trans- therapeutic care (Theumer 2020).[5] In Argentina's case, links between diagnosis and treatment remain important in health-care practice more generally. However, the health system's somewhat higher degree of centralization relative to the United States renders the link a bit more flexible, since the national Ministry of Health sets standards for regulation. While the system remains highly fragmented and managed at a provincial rather than national level, the Ministry of Health can effectively set the terms for covered health benefits—including those that do not require diagnosis. As such, coverage for trans- therapeutics is legally guaranteed across the three-tier system, including in the nation's safety-net system of public hospitals. In practice, this guarantee was unfortunately limited first by a three-year delay on the part of the Ministry of Health to issue concrete regulations to guide practices and financing and next by a near-evisceration of the public-health system under the austerity measures enacted by the Macri administration from 2015 to 2019. Nevertheless, the diagnostic (or, rather, antidiagnostic) provisions of the Gender Identity Law set a standard to which transnational activists looked for guidance in the realm of depathologizing trans- health, although not all health infrastructures could accommodate this approach.

As I will discuss in chapter 2, both the clinical roles and classificatory criteria involved in establishing diagnosis as a bridge to trans- therapeutics are somewhat unusual within the broader field of biomedical practice. In accordance with professional standards of care, trans- experiences are usually narrated by trans- people to psychotherapists—often called "gatekeepers" by trans- activists. These standards are explicitly set out in documents like the World Professional Association for Transgender Health's (WPATH) *Standards of Care*. In turn, psychotherapists are charged with ascertaining whether these feelings qualify as a medical need rather than simply a desire. The threshold of medical necessity here is the line that divides the types of care that are at least potentially or partially eligible for coverage, subsidy, or reimbursement from those that patients are expected to cover on their own.

When it comes to trans- therapeutics, the notion of medical necessity has been one of the most controversial and debated points structuring care. While there is a thriving plastic surgery industry that operates largely on out-of-pocket payments from patients, insurance or state subsidies still cover some forms of plastic surgery, such as reconstruction after tissue damage. To qualify for coverage, there is an important difference in whether people seek "reconstructive" or "aesthetic" surgeries (Heyes and Latham 2018). As Eric Plemons (2010, 320) explains, this distinction is a particularly crucial and contentious one for trans- therapeutics, because it also maps onto whether or not a procedure is considered "medically necessary." Depending on ranging regulations and policies, medical necessity might (though does not always) bring about care coverage or subsidized costs for hormone prescriptions, genital, body, or facial surgeries, hair removal, voice coaching, or other trans- therapeutic practices.[6] These provisions of course also range by health-care system. Argentina's Gender Identity Law requires funding for most trans- therapeutic surgeries, so when it comes to this study, the distinction between "reconstructive" and "aesthetic" is currently most relevant in the United States. However, what counts as "medically necessary" became a heated point of debate in the long process of regulating and implementing the Gender Identity Law's health-care provisions—a process that was not finalized until 2015 (Farji Neer 2018).[7]

The stringent psychotherapeutic gatekeeping requirements and pathologizing impulses of twentieth-century transsexual medicine—and its transitory passage into the twenty-first century—reverberate in contemporary debates about the role of psychotherapists in trans- health. These often center on struggles over what transness is, who can decide, and how biomedicine should be involved. The rate of change is slow, in part because the psychopathologizing logics of transsexual medicine form the basis for the medical and administrative infrastructures (including diagnoses, standards of care, insurance reimbursement procedures, policies, and regulations) upon which trans- health practices are built. Yet many of the trans- health providers with whom I spoke—most of whom understood themselves to be particularly supportive of trans- people and politics—soundly refused both pathologizing and gatekeeping approaches. They did not see their work to consist in diagnosing illness to bring about a future state of wellness. Rather, they claimed they were diagnosing (or perhaps simply assessing) *wellness.* In providing trans- therapeutics, care providers saw themselves as facilitating the flourishing of wellness in a world that is itself pathologically cruel toward trans- people.[8]

Remapping Trans- Depathologization's Kin Relations

In this section, I redraw the social movement family tree that represents trans- depathologization's emergence chiefly through histories of gay depsychopathologization. Looking instead to feminist health and disability activisms, I suggest that tracing these other branches of depathologization's kin relations sheds new light on each of their commitments—specifically their shared investments in care without pathology. Analysts frequently offer up the depsychopathologization of homosexuality as a blueprint for trans- depathologization, whether as parallel or historical precedent (Drescher 2010, 2020).[9]

Resonances between each of these depathologization movements are indeed strong and stem both from their intertwined histories of pathologization and from their techniques of resistance. Psychiatry's pathologization of queerness emerged in large part from U.S. and European sexological research on "sexual inversion" in the nineteenth and twentieth centuries. As Jules Gill-Peterson (2018, 79) asserts, this genealogy of knowledge produced racialized pathologization of gender/sex/sexuality and, at least for white subjects, the possibility of "normative cure." *Homosexuality* was gradually defined as its own unique subset of so-called inversion in the early twentieth century. The psychiatric promise of "cure" led to its diagnostic entry into the *DSM* in the early 1950s.

In the 1960s and early 1970s, gay liberation movements became increasingly organized and politically active, and the American Psychiatric Association (APA) became one of their targets. This had to do not only with its pathologization of nonnormative sexualities but also with the APA's endorsement of conversion therapies—which often included electroconvulsive and other invasive and traumatizing supposed treatments. In the early 1970s, activists began infiltrating the APA's annual conference as both presenters and as protesters. At the 1972 convention, a panel of gay and lesbian activists and a costumed and masked gay psychiatrist using the pseudonym "Dr. H. Anonymous" held a panel entitled "Lifestyles of Nonpatient Homosexuals." In their presentation, they urged the APA to depsychopathologize queerness and remove homosexuality as a diagnosis in the *DSM*—a demand that was met the following year.[10]

Analysts, such as psychiatrist Jack Drescher (2010, 2020), who explore the links between these movements take care to differentiate the stakes of lesbian and gay versus trans- depathologization projects—especially the extent to which the illness–care conundrum uniquely structures trans- health. Indeed, trans- depathologization has involved not only redefining what transness is or is not but also shifting how its care guidelines, financing schemas, treatment protocols, and clinical practices should be organized to count as depathologized forms of care. Sociologist Mary Burke (2011) points out that the claims of trans- health activists only become legible in the process of distinguishing medicalization (which activists may desire) from pathologization (which social movement activists resoundingly reject). Likewise, in my study, proponents of depathologization did not demand a release from medicine's jurisdiction—at least in terms of access to care. In fact, for some activists, expanding medicalization and maintaining biomedical legitimacy were among their key demands. As Anya (interview, January 12, 2016), a New York–based advocate, commented, "It's really important . . . that we advocate for all health care that's necessary. I think trans- health care is totally necessary and should be covered."

However, study respondents made it clear that retaining access to care did not mean accepting the conditions on which trans- health had to date been premised. Anya (interview, January 12, 2016) asserted that trans- people should have access to the following:

> Anything that makes you feel affirmed in your gender identity and expression. So definitely for a lot of people it's hormones and different kinds of surgeries. . . . [But] just like access to reproductive health care in an affirming way is important, not having . . . any forced surgeries but having autonomy in the way that you choose the health care that you want or don't want.

In this regard, proponents of trans- depathologization sought a thorough revision of the practices and power relations that constitute trans- health's practice guidelines, clinical dynamics, modes of access to care, and means of financing care. Specifically, they worked to level the relationship between provider and patient—or at least argue for the necessity of this leveling—by foregrounding self-determination.

Such work draws directly from activists and scholars who have criticized other forms of pathologization in science and medicine. *Depathologization* is not always the specific term under or around which groups organize, but it refers to a mode of health activism that contests the terms on which certain bodies, social practices, subjectivities, or conditions are viewed as pathological or nonnormative. Feminist activists, for example, seek to redefine women (and sometimes other feminized people) as healthy and nonpathological, countering scientific and medical notions about the inherent inferiority or illness of feminized bodies (Ehrenreich and English 1973; Martin 1987; Murphy 2012; Tarzibachi 2017). Relatedly, reproductive justice activists contest how racialized sexism and ableism is enacted in relations of clinical care and how eugenic pathologization underwrites practices such as forced sterilization (Luna 2009; Ross 2006; Silliman et al. 2004). Disability activists frequently and explicitly use the term *pathologization,* centrally critiquing notions of the "norm" in health care and medicine. They frame the norm as the falsely naturalized state against which people with disabilities are viewed to be ill, pathological, or deficient (Clare 2017; Schweik 2009). None of these advance a position that health care is inherently destructive, though each regards biomedical practices and techniques as being shaped by and through pathologizing and hierarchical relations of power.

Through their frequently subjugating encounters with medicine, feminist health and disability activists have developed the mode of theory in practice that Argentine-born and U.S.-based philosopher María Lugones (2003, 210) calls "streetwalker theorizing." "It is in this line of vision, street-level, among embodied subjects," Lugones explains, that this form of knowledge-making takes place and leads to "a rather large sense of the terrain and its social intricacies" (209). I suggest that some trans- activists have extended activist theorizing about care without pathology to draw coalitional and epistemological connections between movements and people who are defined as inferior, ill, or criminal. Among these different groups of activists, synthetic theorizing about depathologization required an equally expansive account of pathologization and its legacies, exceptions, and bureaucratic expressions (Kafer 2013).

In the petition to the WHO that is quoted at the beginning of this chapter, Maxwell Zachs and fellow authors (2012) name pregnancy as an exemplar of care without pathology on which trans- health might be modeled. As Zachs et al. assert, "Pregnant women are not sick, but they have medical protocols and assistance." Indeed, "normal pregnancy" is one of the few medical encounters for which there is fairly reliable coverage for a potentially nondiagnostic *ICD* code: Z34.00 codes an "encounter for supervision of a normal first pregnancy, unspecified trimester" (*ICD-10*). GATE's aforementioned Starfish Model worked to develop a similar visit code for clinical encounters for trans- therapeutics. Z-codes make up an *ICD* chapter on "factors influencing health status and contact with health services" (*ICD-10*). Few of these Z-codes are covered without an accompanying diagnosis, though "normal pregnancy" is a common exception. While people involved in the *ICD* diagnostic revision discussed Z-codes as a promising means of care without pathology, in the end they decided that various public and private insurance systems were less reliable or consistent in reimbursing visit codes than they were diagnostic codes.

Sociologist K. K. Barker's (1998) account of medicalized pregnancy, however, might call prenatal care and birth into question as a paragon of care without pathology. She points out that pregnancy's relatively recent entry into biomedicine was accompanied by its transition into a "disease model" (1069). Even beyond diagnosis, Barker describes the central problematic of the clinical relation: "The pregnant woman's ability to know her own body through experience . . . to ensure her health had become essentially superfluous in contrast to her new, primary patient status" (1074). While many activists share these related concerns about excessive medical control, overuse of surgical techniques, and overreliance on hospital settings for births, few advocate a full break from medicine's involvement in pregnancy. Instead, most activists or scholars propose a renegotiation of the conditions and practices of care provision, focusing on autonomy and sustained contestation of medical paternalism (N. Edwards 2005; Kukla et al. 2009).

Others caution that the notions of autonomy and choice are all but impossible to exercise in coercive legal and biomedical regimes, particularly those within which a cascade of differentially applied laws and policies govern pregnancy far prior to the clinical encounter. As Shellee Colen (1995) asserts, pregnancy is differentially pathologized at the level of population—a phenomenon she calls "stratified reproduction." For childbearing or potentially childbearing Black, Indigenous, Latinx, and other people of color, the convergence of racialization, criminalization, and medicalization has culminated in selectively antinatalist policies and practices, including forced or coerced sterilization. Eugenic and posteugenic regimes have identified these groups, as well as poor white people and people with disabilities, as enacting degenerating influences on national and transnational populations. In this regard, racist and ableist pathologization of "kinds" of people also has a bearing on the conditions and relations of clinical care. In her ethnography of a public and a private obstetric ward in New York City, anthropologist Khiara M. Bridges (2011) analyzes differential medical management of pregnancies among poor, Black expectant parents. In addition to pathologizing pregnancy, she also observes the accompanying medicalization of racialized poverty: "The poor [are] treated as biological dangers within the body politic" (16). As Bridges's work illustrates, histories of colonial and racial science and medicine both reinforce and reproduce the unevenness of pathologization in daily clinical practice.

Reproductive justice (RJ) movements in the United States have responded directly to these multilayered phenomena of pathologization by linking claims for biomedical self-determination to necessary shifts in broader social and political conditions that foster or compromise health. As a movement conceived and advanced by Black feminists in the United States, RJ has departed from individual choice-based reproductive rights paradigms by addressing the differential collective harms of gendered/sexualized racism. SisterSong (n.d.), a formative United States–based RJ organization, has in the past defined *reproductive justice* as the freedom "to maintain bodily autonomy, have children, not have children, and parent the children we have in safe and sustainable communities" (quoted in Loder et al. 2020). They distinguish this from choice-based approaches to reproductive health, arguing that these conceal the eugenic and racist practices that systematically work to prevent Black people (as well as a host of other targeted groups) from having children. SisterSong's Loretta Ross (2006) describes how this framework was inspired in large part by Global South–based activists that U.S. women of color activists encountered during international convenings. Through these dialogues, activists identified and elaborated a "framework that aligned reproductive rights with social justice in an intersectional way" and that "bridg[ed] the multiple domestic and global movements" within which they were active (16).

In this sense, RJ approaches emphasize the need for more breadth in reproductive politics. For example, they assert that access to safe, high-quality health care is central to these politics, but so is freedom from state violence, sufficient food, and access to clean air and water. Its synthetic approach articulates collective self-determination in a manner that also echoes the socialist and anti-imperialist claims of Black Power movements—specifically, collective control on the part of exploited groups over life conditions and apart from the repressive or subjugating forces of state control.

In Argentina, the language of reproductive justice has less traction, but certain activists' multilayered approaches to politicized resistance bear much similarity. For example, RJ's broad approach is mirrored in the Latin American feminist movement often described as the Green Tide (Marea Verde), so named for the green neckerchiefs protesters often wear during demonstrations. The movement, which has a robust presence in Argentina and the Southern Cone, has largely centered on demands for free, safe, and legal abortion for all (Sutton 2020; McReynolds-Pérez 2017).[11] The movement also confronts state and interpersonal violence against women and trans- people through its claims to "Ni Una Menos," or "Not One Less" (also discussed in chapter 3) (Palmeiro 2018). Members of the Green Tide do not see these as separate but rather as intertwined issues relevant to bodily autonomy, freedom from debt, and freedom from state violence. As Sara Motta (2019), Verónica Gago and colleagues (2018), and Cecilia Palmeiro (2020) assert, Green Tide feminists organized International Women's Strikes to call attention to the economic violence of austerity, state violence against Black and Indigenous activists, gendered violence more generally, and access to quality reproductive health care. Like the politics organizing RJ movements, Latin American feminists in the Green Tide understand feminist autonomy and self-determination—rather than one specific issue, such as abortion access—as being at the heart of their endeavors.[12]

Notably, some Argentine analysts have outlined several of the tensions between Green Tide activists and trans- /travesti activists (neither of which are mutually exclusive groups). Geographer Francisco Fernández Romero (2021) in fact draws directly on RJ frameworks to describe how some people involved in the campaign for free, safe, and legal abortion were less than eager for trans- people to take active roles in leadership and vision. He describes the heated response to a 2014 presentation by Argentine philosopher Blas Radi, in which he argued that trans- men should be included in exchanges about reproductive rights as potentially childbearing subjects. In the subsequent discussion, some campaign members expressed strong concerns that such a shift might decenter women and displace the campaign's primary focus. Such tensions reveal the ways that even synthetic and coalition-focused social movements are not free from producing marginalizing exclusions. Nevertheless, trans- and travesti activists maintained a strong presence in the campaign, likely prompting the adoption of gender-neutral language in the legislation of abortion access (Fernández Romero 2021). I will return to these coalitional collaborations and tensions in the final chapter of this book.

Despite such fissures, the claims of Green Tide activists move across scale and range from individual bodily autonomy to anti-imperialist national and Indigenous sovereignty. For both feminist RJ and Green Tide activists, the actualization of self-determination lies on a political horizon rather than in the here and now. Still, such politics form an imperative and a vision for transformation in care relations that would necessarily be accompanied by radical transformations of economic, political, and social relations writ large.

Some disability activists and scholars in the United States and Argentina draw similar parallels between ranging dynamics of subjugation. Similar to RJ and Green Tide activists (and often among their ranks), disability activists link forces of economic and racialized exploitation, eugenic and coercive elements of medical power, and "ideologies of cure" (Clare 2017, 15). Concomitantly, they take care to develop critiques and political visions that account for the mutual and simultaneous operation of these intertwined forces and the possibilities for structural shifts. For example, even as some critique the "medical industrial complex," activists generally express a yearning for transformations to relations of care (Mingus 2015). Yet they see these transformations as necessitating expansive and sweeping political changes to economic distribution, racialized pathologization, and criminalization (Erevelles 2015; Mitchell and Snyder 2003; REDI n.d.; Orgullo Disca n.d.; Schrader and Penillas 2012; Sins Invalid n.d.).

Pathologization forms a central target of these critiques, and the necessity for care forms a crucial vision—yet these are frequently difficult to untangle. For example, Eli Clare (2017, 41) describes his ambivalence about diagnosis and its relation to both healing and violence: "Diagnosis wields immense power. It can provide us access to vital medical technology or shame us, reveal a path towards less pain or get us locked up. It opens doors and slams them shut." For Clare, diagnosis projects disorder onto variation or difference and produces problems in need of a medical fix. This curative approach, he asserts, has authorized sustained forms of violence under the cover of "care" and "treatment." At the same time, Clare asserts, diagnosis also sometimes becomes a bridge to needed forms of care.

For Argentine sociologist and disability activist Eduardo Joly (2010), one of the effects of pathologization is the exclusion of people with disabilities from both the economy and working-class movements—despite what he sees as their intuitive solidarities with the latter. Joly, who was active in anti-imperialist and youth movements as a student, founded Fundación Rumbos in Buenos Aires in part to highlight these exclusions and build class-conscious self-advocacy models for disability activism. Buenos Aires–based Orgullo Disca (Disability Pride) (n.d.) is similarly concerned with anticapitalism, but unlike Fundación Rumbos, the group situates itself explicitly within feminist and transfeminist struggles. Such a political lens is particularly evident in their vociferous critiques of paternalism—including guardianship—as an impediment to independent living, political mobilization, and depathologization.[13] In 2020, member Eire Pandemonium posted an essay on the group's blog entitled "Disability and Rebellion: We Have Tired of Guardianship" ("Discapacidad y Rebeldía: Nos hemos cansado de tutelaje"). Pandemonium (2020) claims a political autonomy that seeks to transcend reformist advocacy in disability politics: "You can't be a guardian to rebellion, and disabled people and queers are not going to stop until we see society burn to its foundations in order to rebuild it without stairs, or psychiatric hospitals, or ICDs, or prisons, or barriers."[14]

United States–based activist Mia Mingus (2015) combines a resistance to biomedical "cure" with an embrace of community-based care and intersectional mobilization in her mobilization of disability justice. Central to these efforts, she asserts, is the imperative to link antihierarchical notions of wellness, health, disability, and care to all liberation struggles.[15] Mingus (2015) expresses a desire "for more healers that don't continue to perpetuate ableist notions of how bodies should be (or strive to be) and for disabled folks who don't have to only know 'healing' as a violent word because of our histories of forced healing, cures and fixing." Mingus emphasizes that disability justice and other movements must ask what "true wellness and care look like for our communities," while at once resisting the eugenic, coercive, and pathologizing forces enacted by the medical-industrial complex.

Care without pathology, in these accounts, draws from disability justice and other social movement frameworks that call for the "leadership of those most impacted" by the dynamics of marginalization (Berne et al. 2018). Extending "nothing about us without us"—the disability activist maxim (Charlton 2000)—disability justice paradigms advocate political transformation led by "those who know the most about these systems [of oppression] and how they work" (Berne et al. 2018, 227). Mingus (2015) and Clare (2017) likewise strive to marshal expansive notions of healing and the embodied knowledge of people with disabilities against the "defectiveness" logic that they say underwrites biomedicine in its current forms. Neither one dismisses the prospects of medicine's healing capacities; as Clare writes, "At its best, diagnosis affirms our distress, orients us to what's happening in our body-minds, helps make meaning out of chaotic visceral experiences" (41). If Clare expresses an ambivalent and tempered credence in the potential of medical practices, Mingus (2015) voices a sanguine view of the objectives of certain (if few) care providers: "I get excited about practitioners who have accessible spaces and practices that can hold all kinds of bodies and minds."

"Nothing about us without us" thus becomes a guide for reimagining social life vis-à-vis care. For Joly, this might mean reimagining class struggle from the vantage point of those systematically deemed "unproductive." For Pandemonium, it might mean a radical reconfiguration of collective life with people with disabilities, trans- people, and queer people at the center. For Clare and Mingus, it might involve developing formations of care and support that actively reject dynamics of racialized violence and eugenics at all levels. Taken together, these are some of the constellations forming the key concept of this book: care without pathology.

At its broadest, care without pathology is an aspirational configuration of care that disavows multiple materializations of violence, from eugenics to white supremacy to austerity regimes under late capitalism. It seeks relations of horizontal collaboration within healing or care practices and views present manifestations of biomedicine as generally incompatible with these objectives, shaped as they are by varying forms of subjugation. Self-determination or bodily autonomy are key concepts for proponents of depathologization. I will discuss these complex and contested terms in more detail in chapter 5. As Amanda (interview, January 23, 2016), an attorney and advocate based in New York, described, autonomy in trans- health means that it is "up to [the person pursuing care] to make that decision with guidance. . . . So there [is] no gatekeeper anymore." Self-determination, in this regard, is an antidote to the most blatantly coercive forms of care that gatekeeping describes. As reproductive justice and disability justice paradigms assert, however, decisions proceed in scenarios of coercion that dominate biomedical practices and the legal, economic, and political fields in which they operate. In a more expansive register, therefore, *self-determination* might point to a collective articulation of political transformation rather than a claim to "free choice" within the operations of for-profit systems of care and persistent conditions of abbreviated life (Stanley 2014).

The Fight against Medical Gatekeeping

For trans- health activists, gatekeeping has come to characterize an obsolete, condescending, and pathologizing way to structure access to trans- therapeutics. As Walter Bockting and colleagues (2004, 277) write, gatekeeping psychotherapists act as "arbiters of who has access to sex reassignment and when such candidates are ready."[16] Currently, many surgeons and prescribing physicians in the United States and elsewhere require letters of authorization from licensed mental-health providers before proceeding with trans- therapeutic care. This was also the case in Argentina prior to the passage of the Gender Identity Law. These guidelines are codified in WPATH's *Standards of Care* (2011), which advises providers that trans- people be required to obtain one letter of referral to initiate hormone use or mastectomy and two to access genital and other surgeries.

New York–based trans- advocate Claire (interview, January 14, 2016) pointed out that these requirements contrast with equivalent practices among nontrans- people seeking medical care. As she observed:

> [Trans- health] isn't special health care . . . it's the same health care that many people access every day. . . . The hormone therapy that I receive is the same that some cis women in menopause receive, or at other points in their lives for whatever reason, and same goes for testosterone. There are cis men that access that as well. So things like that and surgeries often can be similar to things that cis people receive as well. Trans health care has been sensationalized. . . . We wanted to just challenge that and question that mental-health evaluation should not be necessary for standard forms of hormone therapy. (Interview, January 14, 2016)

Human rights advocates Eszter Kismödi, Mauro Cabral, and Jack Byrne (2016, 385) call this a "double standard," asserting that it "reinforces gender hierarchies and medical authority while undermining transgender people's self-determination." Among the activists and advocates I observed and interviewed, eliminating this double standard was one of the primary justifications for consent-driven rather than gatekeeping-driven models of trans- health-care provision.

During our interview, Amanda (interview, January 23, 2016) observed that, despite the particular ire directed at gatekeeping practices in trans- health, "health is a gatekeeper industry." Amanda's point—that medical gatekeeping is a financial model within which trans- health gatekeeping takes place—is not consistently raised in broader discussions about trans- health. Nevertheless, it is important to consider the more general forms of gatekeeping to shed light on its particular materializations in trans- health. In a wide-ranging sense, medical gatekeeping positions primary-care providers or other first points of contact in medical systems to evaluate and authorize patients' need for specialty care before making referrals, in contrast with the free access arrangement of self-referral. Its logic is the provision of just and appropriate care provision against a backdrop of budget constraints and a presumption that patients tend toward medical overutilization (Willems 2001). Increasingly stringent forms of medical gatekeeping were one response to a precipitous national rise in health spending in the United States in the 1980s, which some health economists defined as a problem of "waste" in care provision. Health organizations use gatekeeping models to contain utilization rates as well as expenditures, though research is inconsistent in demonstrating its effectiveness in either regard (Velasco Garrido, Zentner, and Busse 2011). Health services researchers also assert that gatekeeping practices correspond with lower levels of trust in primary-care providers (Haas et al. 2003).

Although gatekeeping practices are not universal across health systems in the United States or Argentina, they have become commonsense cost-containment practices in some locales, especially within managed care organizations.[17] In the United States in the 1980s, rising health-care costs led to a set of debates about how to curb supposedly unnecessary care. At the time, its installation into the logic of managed care was highly contested. As medical ethicist and physician Edmund Pellegrino argued in 1986, gatekeeping raised "ethically perilous" questions about "medical rationing" (23). Yet Pellegrino also described some forms of what he called "morally licit rationing," such as "purely cosmetic surgery" (40). As discussed in the Introduction, this delegitimizing claim about surgical trans- therapeutics—that they are "cosmetic"—has been the basis upon which many health regulations and policies have excluded coverage, even when clinician gatekeepers diagnostically authorize eligibility for trans- therapeutics.

Such debates about cost containment and exclusions in health care seem on the surface to be centered on balance sheets. However, these in fact unfold against the backdrop of sustained global and domestic neoliberal reforms that have sought to pin sovereign debt to the ostensible excesses of the social spending of governments, particularly on those who policymakers scapegoat as biopolitical drains on economies and populations. Tracing the United States Tea Party's political ploy to block implementation of the Affordable Care Act (ACA) in 2013, Jenna Loyd (2017) shows how the racialized figure of the undeserving "free rider" played an outsized role in these debates, even if it was not always explicitly invoked. Recycling the 1980s-era story of the "welfare queen," Tea Party politicians sounded the alarm that the ACA would overspend on the "undeserving" and wreak havoc on the nation's economy and very identity. This, she argues, was a displacement of the debts of racism onto those who have been most subject to its effects (73). As she further emphasizes, the ACA was only the latest in a long line of national health reforms that have expanded health access for some while reproducing racialized, classed, and other inequities (71).

Gatekeeping in trans- health is embedded within these broader practices of medical gatekeeping, selective exclusion, and white supremacist narratives of "deservingness." From the perspective of trans- activists and advocates, though, gatekeeping practices specific to trans- medicine are particularly nefarious. Transsexual medicine, from the mid-twentieth century through the early 2000s, stringently limited therapeutics such as hormone use and surgeries to prevent what they regarded as disingenuous or fraudulent—not just "unnecessary"—utilization.[18] The transsexual patient was, by definition, suspect: in early versions of the HBIGDA (later, WPATH) *Standards of Care,* which were initially circulated in 1979, the act of directly requesting such therapeutics contraindicated their provision.[19] Furthermore, patients' legitimacy and "trustworthiness" were evaluated based on racialized and classed gender norms, often according to the individual discretion of physicians and psychiatrists (Skidmore 2011; Gill-Peterson 2018). Provider suspicions also extended into concerns about their potential patients' future actions. As Beans Velocci (2021) shows, requisite psychiatric screening was introduced in large part to protect physicians from their fears of malpractice suits and vindictive patients. These apprehensions also make plain the indivisibility of ableism and transphobia, as gender normativity was considered evidence of mental and somatic wellness. Assumed "deviance" from gendered standards therefore indicated a divergence from compulsory able-bodiedness and able-mindedness, lending to providers' belief that patients were not to be trusted. These were the views that led to a standardized emphasis on sustained psychiatric or psychological evaluation and diagnosis of pathological state in advance of referring people for trans- therapeutic care—and these dynamics continue to shape paradigms of trans- health.

Proponents of trans- depathologization, including respondents in this study, seek to eliminate various modes of gatekeeping set up by the WPATH *Standards of Care* (2011). Among other sites of intervention, activists and advocates argue against the need for obligatory therapy, psychiatric diagnoses, letters of authorization, and limitations on coverage for care that is regarded as medically unnecessary (such as facial feminization surgeries). Some activists, advocates, and providers worked to displace gatekeeping-driven models by developing protocols for informed-consent-driven care. Subsequent chapters take up in more detail some of the challenges to gatekeeping models, whether through classificatory reform, interventions in billing practices, or shifts in care models or guidelines. Through these varying interventions, proponents of trans- depathologization contest the standards that frame gender normativity as equivalent to bodily health and mental wellness and that define trans- therapeutics as illegitimate or elective health care. They do so by revising not only the roles of care provision in practice (i.e., who ultimately makes decisions about care) but also the infrastructures on which practices typically run. And as Susan Leigh Star and Karen Ruhleder (1996, 113) point out, this involves "wrestl[ing] with the inertia of the installed base" of transsexual medicine. For most respondents in my study, this wrestling involved making fundamental changes to care standards and guidelines, medical diagnoses, and financing schemas.

For a few respondents, though, tangling with trans- health infrastructures went beyond clinics, diagnostic manuals, and billing offices. They saw trans- health infrastructures as additionally running on other "installed bases," including criminal law and its historical imbrications with medical classification.[20] In our interview, Amanda (interview, January 23, 2016) emphasized that the "intersection of criminalization and trans- health care" has profoundly shaped care provision for poor people and people of color. As attorneys Pooja Gehi and Gabriel Arkles (2007) point out, criminalization is associated with trans- health care in the United States in wide-ranging and highly stratified ways. These authors explain the double bind of law and medicine for trans- people: gender reclassification and other laws require evidence of trans- therapeutic procedures or processes, but medical systems such as Medicaid regularly deny access to trans- therapeutics, claiming it is not sound medicine. Gehi and Arkles argue that this double bind has far-reaching effects on poor people with Medicaid.

Given Loyd's (2017) arguments about austerity and the reproduction of exclusions from health care, even gaining access to Medicaid is a struggle conditioned by notions of "deservingness." Such programs have often sought to exclude those defined as "criminals" or to criminalize poor people seeking access to medical care, generally speaking. This is compounded by the fact that given general and trans-specific exclusions from care, many poor and undocumented trans- people have pursued criminalized means of trans- therapeutics and worked to fund expensive unfunded care through informal and criminalized labor markets (as I discuss in chapter 5). Furthermore, disparities in trans- criminalization are exacerbated by racialized, gendered, and sexualized profiling on the part of police and false arrests based on mismatches between perceived gender and legal identification (Carpenter and Marshall 2017; Cutuli 2012; Gehi and Arkles 2007; Ritchie 2017). Racialized sex/gender nonnormativity in these circumstances is so potently associated with criminality as to be archetypical (Mogul, Ritchie, and Whitlock 2011).[21]

As I discuss in chapter 3, criminalization has also affected trans- health-care provision in Buenos Aires and Argentina more generally, albeit in distinct ways. As Argentine historian Jorge Salessi (1995) asserts, sexual/gender nonnormativity in Argentine history was simultaneously produced as both a crime and a clinical pathology in the broader landscape of national transformations in immigration, labor, racialization, and class struggle.[22] Anthropologist Josefina Fernández (2004) demonstrates that these legacies were extended by provincial police edicts, which were used to arrest and detain mostly poor travestis and trans- people beginning in the last military dictatorship (1976–1983). These did not criminalize sexual/gender nonnormativity per se but were broadly interpretable regulations that criminalized "scandal," often in the form of sexual solicitation. According to the late activist and author Néstor Perlongher (2004), "These so-called police edicts—which are not exactly laws but internal police regulations—enable anyone to be detained on suspicion of sex work, homosexuality, vagrancy, drunkenness, etc. and to be kept in jail without the intervention of a judge for up to 30 days in Buenos Aires and 90 days in Córdoba!"[23] After sustained protest on the part of travesti-led groups, regulations have changed, but criminalization persists (Cutuli 2011, 2012).

However, misdemeanor and contraventional codes in municipalities and provinces throughout Argentina remain in use to arbitrarily arrest and detain travestis for varied ostensible transgressions (a phenomenon that geographer Francisco Fernández Romero [2020] calls the "indirect criminalization" of "walking while travesti"). Argentine anthropologist María Soledad Cutuli (2017) describes the recent emergence of the figure of the "narcotravesti"—the ostensibly drug-trafficking migrant travesti—a fictional media image that leads to selective criminalization of travestis on charges supposedly unrelated to their racialized sex/gender presentation. Travesti activists point to these forms of sustained criminalization as central to the need for state-based reparations, which I will describe in chapter 3.

What, though, do these legacies of criminalization have to do with trans- health care, and specifically with gatekeeping? For study respondents, these trajectories shaped access to health-care provision at several levels. First and foremost, the medicolegal criminalization of sex/gender nonnormativity was fundamentally linked to the scrutiny and suspicion through deception, threat, and predation (Mogul, Ritchie, and Whitlock 2011, 68). For activist groups like STP, GATE, and ICATH, depathologization and antigatekeeping activism has been about contesting the structural distrust that produces the double standard of gatekeeping in trans- health care. For some advocates in the study, this critique also extended to gender-reclassification regulations and legal gender documentation. Amanda (interview, January 23, 2016) described being part of conversations related to the rollout of New York City's municipal identification card:

> We advocated strongly for self-determined gender. . . . [All the advocates] were on board with the idea, but still the policy makers were like, "Isn't that going to mean anybody can just go and get a card that says whatever? What if I want to use that for the purposes of committing fraud?"

For other study respondents, criminalization shaped the broader conditions of health and wellness. Some providers, like New York–based nurse practitioner Jacob (interview, January 26, 2016), described how sustained suspicion strained patient–provider relationships: "I think you need a lot more time with patients that need to develop trust. . . . And I now know we just don't have that time." For people like Mark (interview, January 15, 2016), an attorney and advocate in New York, "criminal law becomes a driver of different things, including incarceration. . . . But also criminalizing condoms [and] sex work obviously has a huge impact on health outcomes." He further explained that racialized criminalization of sex work landed many trans- women in jail or prison, where they were subject to even more intensely stringent and punitive gatekeeping regulations when it came to trans- therapeutics.

To understand this more fully, it is important to briefly discuss the nature of prison- and jail-based health care. These are systems unto themselves in both the United States and Argentina. In both sites, prisons may be run by states, provinces, or federally, and in the United States, the institutions might be public or private. As such, systems of imprisonment, as well as the health-care services that operate within them, are fragmented and have varying policies. In the United States, guidelines for prison- and jail-based health have existed since the 1970s.[24] Despite these standards, access to even the most basic forms of care can be an issue, especially if this involves care outside the prison or jail. In New York, for example, people frequently miss scheduled necessary medical visits because they are not provided escorts to take them to appointments. The quality of care inside prisons and jails is also a persistent issue of concern.[25] In 2014, New York State settled a lawsuit with a private company that was contracted to provide care to jails in thirteen counties for systematic understaffing and providing substandard care (Office of the Attorney General 2014). In Argentina, understaffing and inadequate care are also serious problems. For example, when people who were locked up were surveyed in 2019, 55 percent in Buenos Aires prisons and 31 percent in federally run prisons said they had not received medical care when they were sick (CELIV 2020, 27). Some advocates recommend removing health administration from prison authorities and placing it under the broader Ministry of Health (Prison Insider 2020). It is within this set of existing constraints that trans- people who are locked up attempt to access trans- therapeutics, and the policies that guide these outside of prisons and jails do not always apply within them.

During our interview, Amanda (interview, January 23, 2016) explained how trans- people who access and use hormones outside of medical supervision "stand the risk of being punished or criminalized for using hormones in a way that is not seen as legitimate." She added that "the person that [this is] going to affect first is the person who is in prison." Here, she was referring to the United States Federal Bureau of Prisons' blanket "freeze-frame" policy, in which incarcerated people are not eligible for trans- therapeutics while in prison beyond the formal prescribed care they were receiving upon imprisonment. Even for people who had long used hormones, this meant they would no longer have access to these without having received a medical prescription—even though care exclusions often meant that people resorted to procuring hormones through informal economies.[26] While the freeze-frame policy was formally overturned in 2011, Amanda and other advocates noted that they frequently received complaints and inquiries from trans- people who were imprisoned stating that they were repeatedly denied trans- therapeutic care based on the whims of those who controlled access to care.

As Joaquín (interview, August 3, 2015), a Buenos Aires–based advocate, mentioned, the activism that led up to the Gender Identity Law was coordinated in large part by travesti-led groups that had taken an active role in mobilizing resistance to police edicts in the

1990s. "There's a long, long history of struggle, so this fight was not something new for them." As he explained, these sustained fights against criminalization and their connection to claims for access to health and wellness shaped the campaign. It hinged on four interrelated principles: destigmatization, depathologization, decriminalization, and dejudicialization. The last three pertained directly to antigatekeeping measures in medicine, criminal law, and administrative law and advanced self-determination as a key intervention to gatekeeping writ large.

While much work in trans- studies has focused on gatekeeping as a phenomenon internal to medical practice, the views of my respondents posit that it has a much more expansive (and insidious) reach. Correspondingly, the work of depathologization aims to intervene in gatekeeping regimes not only through revision of care guidelines, classifications, and reimbursement practices (which I will discuss in chapter 2) but also through sweeping claims against criminalization and in favor of redistribution and collective self-determination (which I will expand on in chapters 3 through 6).

The concept of care without pathology was initially developed by activist providers to describe antigatekeeping models for trans- health care (and I will explore their work more directly in chapter 5).[27] This chapter extends care without pathology into a more capacious frame. In an expansive sense, it signals efforts to address and contest power relations in biomedical practice—not only in the realm of trans- health but also more generally. Through this frame, this chapter examines the genealogy of trans- health and depathologization in a different light. Specifically, it interrogates what we find when we look to relations between movements that center not only *depathologization* as an objective but also a strong vision for what good care relations and accessible care infrastructures would look like. These are the objectives that are at the root of expansive trans- health movements. The remainder of this book explores different ways that activists, advocates, and some providers have sought to enact these.

Care without pathology also enables a more sweeping analysis of depathologization. Depathologization has too frequently been historicized through a singular antecedent in the declassification of queer sexualities as psychiatric illnesses. As I show in this chapter, feminist health and disability activism and scholarship—particularly reproductive justice, Green Tide feminism, and disability justice paradigms—are in closer alignment with trans- health's depathologization claims.[28] Specifically, these have looked to biomedical care and the pathologizing practices that often compose it as things to systematically *transform* rather than evade or discard.

One of the ways that the trans- health activists and advocates (as well as some providers) in the study aimed to transform hierarchical and pathologizing relations of care was to address the patronizing dynamics of medical gatekeeping in trans- health. They strove to materialize these transformations through varying interventions in diagnostic practices, reimbursement and financing schemas, and standards of care. For activists, advocates, and certain supportive providers, these interventions fell under the banner of depathologization, which became a center of gravity for trans- health activism. This orientation, which I term "coalitional depathologization," was one of the ways that some trans- health activists mobilized depathologization and care without pathology in their most sweeping senses. I will explore coalitional depathologization in more depth in the final chapter. However, first it is necessary to delve into the ways that trans- health relates to themes of classification, collectivization, and care. I will turn to each of these in the chapters that follow. In chapter 2, I will discuss how various interventions in diagnostic classifications formed one angle of resistance against pathologization and brought about sustained collaboration—albeit tense and uneven—between providers, activists, and advocates. First, though, I draw on secondary and primary archival sources to discuss the prehistory of trans- pathologization. This will be necessary in forming a more expansive account of depathologization in what follows.

2 Unruly Terms

Negotiating Trans- Diagnoses

Clarissa, a newly practicing nurse practitioner in New York, described some of her various difficulties with medical charting as she cared for trans- patients. We sat in the kitchen of her first-floor apartment as she explained to me:

> There's no template for a trans- person. . . . There's not even a question, it's just male/female. And all the providers, they're like, just write it in the notes. Or in the *problem list,* is where it would go. (Interview, July 25, 2013)

Why did this matter to her? As a new provider, she hoped to support trans- patients as they sought various forms of trans- health: basic health care, specialty care unrelated to transness, and trans- therapeutic care. As a queer-identified person who shared community with trans- people, she knew that providers frequently made uninformed assumptions about their trans- patients that led to frustrating, humiliating, and at times hazardous experiences in care settings.[1] Indeed, many of us who have been trans- or intersex patients in waiting rooms have encountered the absurdity of negotiating a pink or blue intake form as a classificatory conundrum that, at best, provokes sidelong glances from other patients. Clarissa thought that providers being aware of a patient's trans-status might help prevent or ameliorate these outcomes. She also wanted to make sure that trans- patients were offered support as they decided whether and how to pursue and affordably access trans- therapeutics. Without a way to express their sex and gender accurately on their charts, she wondered, how would her trans-patients get care that was sufficient to their needs?

The impossibility of recording her patients' expressed gender on the electronic medical chart stood in stark contrast to the array of diagnostic codes on the chart that she could use to mark the supposed condition of a patient's gender nonnormativity. Providers like Clarissa thus faced a peculiar and remarkably mundane problem when it came to charting basic patient demographics: Should she check "male" or "female"? Why could she only designate patients' transness with a diagnosis for a psychiatric condition rather than a specific experience of sex/gender? And why was the problem list a suitable place to qualify the particulars of a patient's trans- history or present?[2]

The trans- diagnosis entered biomedical care in a formal sense relatively recently. Trans-sexualism as a diagnosis was introduced to the World Health Organization's *International Classification of Diseases* (*ICD*) in the late 1970s. The American Psychiatric Association's (APA) *Diagnostic and Statistical Manual* (*DSM*) was not far behind, adding Transsexualism and Gender Identity Disorder of Childhood to its pages in 1980. Throughout the course of its brief but contentious classificatory life, the trans- diagnosis has been a lightning rod for controversy and a target for modification. In the four decades since its formal classificatory birth, the nomenclature, description, criteria, differential diagnosis, and etiology of trans- diagnoses have been under continual revision.

Most recently and perhaps most notably, the World Health Organization decided in 2019 to jettison Gender Identity Disorder (which replaced Trans-sexualism in 1992) from the *ICD*'s chapter on mental health and illness. A substantially revised and reconceptualized description now accompanies a new classificatory diagnosis of Gender Incongruence, which is placed in a chapter on sexual health. In a media interview, Australia-based psychologist and advocate Sam Winter commented, "This is a historic move. An end to a classification that was a historical artifact, had little basis in science, and had massive consequences for the lives of trans people" (quoted in Fitzsimmons 2018). For transnational depathologization advocates like Winter, the change reflected the belated but decisive arrival of clinical language to accompany depathologizing shifts in trans- health practice.

Classificatory revision has therefore been one of the main sites of change marking the emergence of trans- health. During revision processes, activists and advocates organized to get the message of heterogeneity across to providers and professional organizations. They asserted that people had very different experiences of transness. They also argued that the administrative and biomedical infrastructures they had to navigate (even if they did not identify as transgender) were distinct and varied, and thus required flexibility and attention to financial as well as biomedical access. Some supportive providers had taken this heterogeneity seriously for some time, but the formalized process of diagnostic revision required broader consensus on the issue. Responding to entreaties of activists, providers and professional organizations yielded ground on the diagnostic imperative to supposedly accurately typify trans- diagnoses. Instead, they placed somewhat more emphasis on how trans- people understood their own experiences, stresses, and needs. Eventually, this resulted in the emergence of depathologized diagnoses that focused more on facilitating access to care than they did on establishing a standardized "truth" of transness. In this sense, the utility of diagnosis underwent a marked change.

The stakes of classification are high. As I discussed in chapter 1, trans- people are in a double bind when it comes to medicine. This dilemma involves the delegitimization and inaccessibility of trans- health paired with the requirements for medical authorization that were (until very recently) almost uniformly required for legal gender reclassification. Prior to the passage of the Gender Identity Law in Argentina, genital surgical requirements were stringently enacted. In the United States, there has been a trend toward relaxation in surgical requirements for gender reclassification at the federal and state levels, although requirements still range across states. In addition, the legitimacy of trans- health is under escalating attack, raising questions about the durability of these developments. Changing the diagnostic terms of health care is therefore of paramount importance for activists, advocates, and supportive providers. This has raised pointed questions about what diagnoses are good for. When it comes to trans- diagnoses, providers have historically mobilized these to sort "true transsexuals" from suspected charlatans.[3] For trans- people, they have been a painful means to an end, occasionally and inequitably enabling access to care. These stakes came to the fore in diagnostic depathologization, though questions remained about the extent to which it has shifted care in practice.

There is of course no *single* diagnosis that defines or describes transness. In fact, the multiple names, concepts, and codes that are incorporated by the gloss of the "trans- diagnosis" sometimes differ so drastically as to seem incommensurate. In combination, these make up a patchwork of efforts—both historical and present—that aim to name, define, describe, and contain transness into terms that are relevant to therapeusis. These diagnoses have been put to work in various ways, whether to pathologize, to exclude from care, to foster access to insurance coverage, or to assist patients in administrative efforts like gender reclassification.

Trans- studies scholars and depathologization activists have spent the last several decades scrutinizing landscapes of diagnostic classification. Some define it as a bureaucratic iron cage; others as a means of taming uncertainty and exerting expertise; and still others as a mode of biomedically enacted social control (Burke 2011; Eisfeld 2014; Suess Schwend 2020; shuster 2021). More recently, scholars are examining "trans-affirmative" domains of care to examine how diagnostic classification can be turned into a bridge to address the illness–care conundrum (Johnson 2018; Travers 2019). Each of these explanations rings true and provides an important explanatory account of the many facets of "classification and its consequences" (Bowker and Star 1999). However, the story of trans- health does not begin and end with trans- diagnoses. Other diagnoses and classifications also matter to trans- health practice and to trans- people's access to trans- therapeutic care. For example, the providers I observed and with whom I spoke also used diagnostic work-arounds (such as Endocrine Disorder) to enable care coverage. They also sometimes navigated trans- therapeutic care provision within broader classificatory infrastructures of care—struggling, for example, with how to accomplish the seemingly simple act of listing "sex" on a patient's medical record. So-called comorbid conditions mattered, too. Providers' assessments of mental health and other issues combined with trans- diagnoses in ways that affected trans- therapeutic care in stratified ways.

To bring a laser-focus to trans- diagnoses, then—as some trans- studies scholars and activists do—is to overlook how it works in practice. But even for those who take a broader view of diagnostic practice, the emphasis on classification still looms large. It is certainly worth the effort to understand the classificatory politics of trans- health, but most studies to date focus too squarely on the short life of the trans- diagnosis itself rather than the protracted historical dynamics from which it was birthed.[4] This view produces accounts of pathologization that are somewhat thin and that represent trans- pathologization along a single axis rather than as part of a web of pathologizing phenomena within which it is entangled. In addition to these historical omissions, much work on depathologization neglects what Kimberlé Crenshaw (1989) terms "intersectionality" in the legal domain.[5] Many accounts of depathologization—particularly those focused within the United States—also neglect the radically different mechanisms of diagnosis and care coverage within distinct care infrastructures. In both regards, trans- diagnoses are mobilized in distinct ways and stick to people differently. They are modulated by poverty, race, disability, nationality, exposure to criminalization, and participation in sex work—just to name a few. In both the historical and present sense, pathologization (as well as resistance to it) is therefore multiple, layered, and malleable.

This chapter focuses on how activists, advocates, and providers enact classificatory depathologization and adapt to changes in trans- diagnoses. Based on data from interviews, observations, and recent archives, it centers on how people coordinated with each other and with classificatory organizations to address trans- pathologization while maintaining a bridge to covered care across a multitude of health-care infrastructures. Earlier refutations of trans- pathologization were formed in an ambiance of mutual hostility and mistrust of Sandy Stone's (1992, 167) "diagnostic battlefield" between trans- people and providers, as mentioned in chapter 1. However, as depathologization movements gained momentum and credibility across the early 2000s, these dynamics became increasingly collaborative—albeit still sharply stratified.

I assert that trans- studies and activism would generally benefit from demoting classificatory concerns—especially in their single-axis form—from their current starring role. However, it remains worthwhile to follow the troubling history of medicalized efforts to contain the heterogeneity of transness, as well as the myriad ways that proponents of trans- depathologization have pushed back on ill-fated attempts to tame the radical variance of transness within diagnoses. Even as depathologization activists and advocates rejected the hubris of biomedical efforts to contain transness, though, their own confrontations with pathologization neglected some of the diffuse effects of these unruly forces. In bringing an unwavering focus on *stigma* to debates about care infrastructures, they often neglected a more synthetic analysis of trans- pathologization. This likely came as a precondition for collaborating with professional organizations, but it inaugurated stratified and stratifying implications for how depathologization could be taken up in practice.

In this chapter, I pursue each of these three threads—pathologizing histories, revised diagnoses, and the limitations of classificatory depathologization—and weave them together to illustrate some of the tensions in diagnostically focused trans- health activism. First, I draw on archival data from classificatory manuals and schema to trace the meandering recent history of the trans- diagnosis across the past four decades. I also supplement this with more protracted historical reflections from secondary sources. Second, I draw on ethnographic data to examine how activists, advocates, and supportive providers worked on and with diagnoses. Specifically, I show how each of these groups sought to maintain bridges to care coverage while abating the stigma of mental illness.

Focusing on diagnostic work both inside and outside of the clinic, I show how some providers worked to enact depathologization against the limitations of care infrastructures and reimbursement schema to try to care well for their patients. This coordinated work among activists, advocates, and providers reflects the partial shift to depathologized relations of care in trans- health practice. Finally, I step back to analyze classificatory revision in the broader milieu of social movements in the early twenty-first century and reflect on some of the constraints that activists, advocates, and providers encountered—and in some measure replicated—in their work to depathologize trans- diagnoses. In so doing, I turn to the figure of unruliness—first as a means of describing the radical variability and opacity of transness, then as a concept through which to represent diffuse forms of pathologization, and finally as a political orientation to social movements.

This discussion skews somewhat toward the United States, since the Gender Identity Law obviated the requirement for diagnostic classification for trans- therapeutics in Argentina in 2012. For reasons that will be clear, however, I show how these classifications have high stakes even for those who are no longer formally subject to them.

The primary data sources for this chapter include classificatory manuals and online materials, archival activist sources, and ethnographic data. Specifically, I examined five versions of the *Diagnostic and Statistical Manual* from 1980 to 2013 and three versions of the *International Classification of Diseases* from 1979 to 2019.[6] I also drew on web-based data published online by the American Psychiatric Association during the process leading up to the publication of the *DSM-5* (APA 2013) and by the World Health Organization leading up to the *ICD-11* in 2019. I read and qualitatively coded diagnostic classifications and online debates related to the trans- diagnoses in each classification system, additionally noting their shifting placements within each system. I was also a participant-observer in the beta phase of the *ICD* revision, in which users could read a public preview of proposed revisions on an internet platform and submit public comments. Finally, I examined archival activist materials related to diagnostic and broader classificatory activism and drew on ethnographic interviews and observations with activists, advocates, and care providers. For the first section of this chapter, I also drew on secondary sources to explore racialized histories of trans- health leading to the present.

Throughout the research process, I wrote analytic memos, generated positional and social worlds/arenas maps (Clarke 2005), and developed other graphical representations of classificatory shifts in and adjacent to biomedicine over the last several decades.

Caught Up in Classifications

The Prehistory of Diagnostic Depathologization

Currently, it is a given in trans- studies that scientific and medical practitioners have colluded with other powerful actors to develop classifications—generally pathologizing ones—as they have endeavored to identify and regulate the bounds of transness (shuster 2021; Thompson and King 2015; Meyerowitz 2002). However, scholars differ somewhat in how they historicize these pathologizing eventualities. Some locate the pathologization of sex/gender in colonial gender systems, others in United States and European sexological paradigms, and others in systems of forced captivity, enslavement, and state repression.[7] At stake across all of these is the nature of the racialized sex binary and its defense. Pathologizing or subordinating accounts of sex/gender nonnormativity have therefore sprung from a diverse set of supposedly expert fields across several centuries and continents (albeit in distinct ways). Sexology, criminology, anthropology, psychiatry, statecraft, and racial science—among others—have all had a hand in enunciating and materializing the hierarchies that haunt contemporary debates about pathologization.

My training is not in historical methods, and as a result I conducted limited work in historical archives for this project. It nevertheless remains important to situate some of these prehistories. While I can scarcely do justice to each of these trajectories, I draw below on secondary sources to develop an abridged prehistory of trans- diagnoses.[8]

Sexology is an interdisciplinary medical field that examines human sexuality and sexual behavior. Originating in Europe in the nineteenth century and eventually migrating to the United States, its articulation as a field marks a point at which sex and sexuality became primary objects within medicine. Previously, sexual behavior was a primarily juridical concern (Foucault 1990). Pathologization was sexology's bread and butter, as is apparent in the publication of two books that share the same title: *Psychopathia Sexualis* (the first by Heinrich Kaan in 1844 and the second by Richard von Krafft-Ebing in 1886). Nineteenth- and early twentieth-century sexologists in the United States and Europe exercised what can only be called a frantic classificatory exuberance as they developed the pathologizing diagnostic notions of sexual inversion, intersexuality, hermaphroditism, transvestism, and others. Underwriting this classificatory surfeit were roiling racialized anxieties about the sex binary's stability. Jules Gill-Peterson's (2018, 60) nuanced treatment of the twentieth-century archive of transness reveals a fretful panic about the relationship of sex differentiation to white supremacy. For nineteenth-century racial science, sex differentiation signaled the zenith of evolution—which eugenicist researchers equated with whiteness. Even as sexology tended not to mobilize explicitly racialized terms, its fidelities to racial science were more than evident—and indeed, the field's racial anxieties seemed only to intensify over the twentieth century (Somerville 2000; Gill-Peterson 2018; Schuller 2018).

It therefore comes as no surprise that medical practices became sites of racial formation and control. These sites included experiments on intersex children and the development of diagnostic and clinical protocols that racialized "plasticity"—in the form of embodied malleability—as the "eugenic alterability of sex as phenotype" (Gill-Peterson 2018, 67). As a "synonym for whiteness," this notion of plasticity racialized trans- life and had exclusionary effects on clinical access for trans- people (27). Around the mid-twentieth century in the United States, sexological theories became especially animated within psychology and psychiatry. The persistent elusiveness of sex classification eventually drove psychologist John Money to develop a concept of "gender" in the first instance and led psychiatrist Robert Stoller to extend this into "gender identity" (Meyerowitz 2002). These histories formed the landscape of twentieth-century transsexual medicine, and they remain sedimented within the contemporary classificatory schema of trans- health and politics more broadly.

Sexology was by far a less dominant discourse in Argentina.

Nevertheless, the early twentieth century saw an alliance form in the nation between government actors, psychiatrists, physicians, and criminologists (Ben and Acha 2001; Salessi 1995). In 1902, Argentine concerns with xenophobic public hygiene and the pathologization of working classes were taken up in an interdisciplinary periodical called the *Archives of Criminology, Forensic Medicine, and Psychiatry* (*Archivos de Criminología, Medicina Legal, and Psiquiatra*). At this point in history, state actors involved in Argentine nation-building were increasingly distressed about crime and sexual hygiene. This reached a fever pitch in their consternation about sex work and homoerotic expression. In the early twentieth century, these became targets of a repressive state apparatus that combined eugenicist fears of degeneration with racialized and classed xenophobia. The *Archives of Criminology, Forensic Medicine, and Psychiatry* thus concretized what became an enduring alliance between medical and juridical sectors—a coalition that has largely persisted to the present day.

Pathologization may seem to be the sole province of biomedicine, but other fields of knowledge (including but not limited to criminology) have also contributed to the accretions that produce transness as pathology. For example, throughout the twentieth century, Global North–based anthropologists approached the notion of the "third gender" with pointed curiosity.[9] Binary sex figured as the implicitly modern backdrop against which they represented sex/gender variance as antiquated, uncivilized, provincial, or exotic.[10] These accounts solidified notions of civilization and modernity as materialized through and against racialized gender. The colonizing impulse of twentieth-century anthropological accounts is resuscitated in trans- politics, as supposedly localized forms of gender expression—usually Indigenous or of the Global South—are subordinated to the presumptively universal figure of "transgender."

Structures of racialized subordination also form the broader pathologizing webs within which trans- pathologization also figures. For example, regimes of enslavement in the United States produced the "ungendering of blackness" as a "context for imagining gender as subject to rearrangement" (Snorton 2017, 57). In the early nineteenth century, this manufactured disjuncture between

Blackness and gendered humanity served as a gruesome justification for experimental gynecological surgeries, in which enslaved Black women were used as the "raw material for making the field of 'women's medicine'" (53). After the turn of the twentieth century, Black trans- and intersex life was "framed in atavistic terms" and defined against "white plastic potential"—which was accompanied by the systematic exclusion of young Black trans- people from accessing trans- therapeutic care (Gill-Peterson 2018, 27). In this and other regards, sex differentiation was continuous with projects of racial dominance (Schuller 2018). Racialized subordination therefore lives on, not only within the classifications directly relevant to trans- health but also in the very infrastructures of biomedical care more generally.

This summary provides only the most cursory analysis of a much deeper and more complex series of histories. However, it also forms a critical background for the discussion to which I now turn: the late twentieth-century birth and formalization of the trans- diagnosis.

Official Trans- Diagnoses

The prevailing trans- diagnosis from the late 1980s until the 2010s was Gender Identity Disorder, having been revised from its prior diagnostic life as Transsexualism.[11] Gender Identity Disorder appeared in both the psychiatric *Diagnostic and Statistical Manual* and the *International Classification of Diseases.* Scholars trace processes of breakdown and revision through social movement pressure, crises of authority, epistemological shifts, access, depathologization, and transnational legibility.[12] With some exceptions, these have focused rather squarely on specific diagnoses. I suggest that panning out to examine adjacent and work-around classifications—within the broader classificatory infrastructures of medicine more generally—enables a richer understanding of how classifications work in practice, a critical question for scholars of classification in the field of science and technology studies (STS).[13]

The *DSM* and the *ICD* have been home to the most salient diagnostic classifications for trans- health in the United States, Argentina, and other locales. Both classificatory systems play a large role in fostering a shared vocabulary for psychiatric and medical conditions and for determining conditions of care coverage. In recent years, the trans- diagnosis has become markedly less important for Argentines seeking trans- therapeutics, given the antidiagnostic provisions of the Gender Identity Law. Nevertheless, Argentine activists remain concerned about the diffuse effects of diagnoses in trans- politics more broadly.

As I alluded to at the outset of the chapter, the trans- diagnosis entered the *ICD* in 1975 and was formalized in 1979. In 1980, it was included in the *DSM.* Since that time, the trans- diagnosis has moved between these classificatory systems itinerantly, shifting in name, content, and placement within each nosological system and iteration. Figure 1 on the following pages charts how the trans- diagnosis has shifted in each of these systems over time.

The *DSM* and *ICD* operate at different scales and in distinct ways, but they have long swapped and shared trans- diagnoses. The *DSM* is published by the U.S.-based American Psychiatric Association, but it circulates well beyond these bounds. In fact, its diagnoses compose most of the mental-health chapter of the World Health Organization's *ICD,* the diagnostic system used in most of the world. However, Trans-sexualism in the *ICD-9* predated the first appearance of Transsexualism in the *DSM-III.* In the 1987 publication of the *DSM-IV,* the diagnosis morphed into Gender Identity Disorder. The *ICD* adopted the same nominal change in 1992. In 2013, the *DSM* developed a new diagnostic classification of Gender Dysphoria, and in 2019 the *ICD-11* adopted Gender Incongruence—both of which advocates claimed as "depathologized diagnoses."[14]

As Figure 1 makes apparent, the trans- diagnosis has migrated between chapters and itinerantly shifted in descriptive content, essential features, and differential diagnoses (APA 1980, 1987, 1994, 2000, 2013; WHO 1975, 1992, 2004, 2019). Its diagnostic neighbors have also changed, with adjacent diagnoses including, over the years, paraphilias, disruptive disorders, and sexual dysfunction disorders.[15]

Across these revisions and migrations, we can track the movement of the trans- diagnosis in the *DSM* from paraphilias to youthful

Source	Classifications and Subtypes	Chapter	Neighbor Classifications
DSM-III (1980)	**Gender Identity Disorders**	Psychosexual Disorders	Paraphilias (e.g., Fetishism, Transvestism, Zoophilia, Pedophilia); psychosexual dysfunctions (Inhibited Sexual Desire, Inhibited Sexual Excitement, Premature Ejaculation); other psychosexual disorders (e.g., Ego-Dystonic Homosexuality)
	302.5 Transsexualism		
	302.60 Gender Identity Disorder of Childhood		
	302.85 Atypical Gender Identity Disorder		
DSM-III-R (1987)	**Gender Identity Disorders**	Disorders Usually First Evident in Infancy, Childhood, or Adolescence	Disruptive behavior disorders; anxiety disorders of childhood or adolescence; eating disorders; tic disorders; elimination disorders; speech disorders
	302.60 Gender Identity Disorder of Childhood		
	302.5 Transsexualism		
	302.85 Gender Identity Disorder of Adolescence or Adulthood, Nontranssexual Type (GIDAANT)		
	302.85 Gender Identity Disorder Not Otherwise Specified		
DSM-IV (1994)	**Gender Identity Disorders**	Sexual and Gender Identity Disorders	Sexual dysfunctions (e.g., sexual desire disorders, sexual arousal disorders, orgasmic disorders), paraphilias (e.g., Exhibitionism, Fetishism, Pedophilia, Transvestic Fetishism)
	302.6 Gender Identity Disorder in Children		
	302.85 Gender Identity Disorder in Adolescents and Adults		
	302.6 Gender Identity Disorder Not Otherwise Specified		
DSM-IV TR (2000)	**Gender Identity Disorders**	Sexual and Gender Identity Disorders	Sexual dysfunctions (e.g., sexual desire disorders, sexual arousal disorders, orgasmic disorders), paraphilias (e.g., Exhibitionism, Fetishism, Pedophilia, Transvestic Fetishism)
	302.6 Gender Identity Disorder in Children		
	302.85 Gender Identity Disorder in Adolescents or Adults		
	302.6 Gender Identity Disorder Not Otherwise Specified		
DSM-5 (2013)	302.85 (F64.9) Gender Dysphoria	Gender Dysphoria	No others, only diagnosis in chapter

(continued on next page)

Source	Classifications and Subtypes	Chapter	Neighbor Classifications
***ICD-9* (1979)**	302.5 Trans-sexualism (Excludes 302.3 Transvestism)	Mental Disorders, (under heading "302 Sexual Deviations and Disorders")	Homosexuality; Zoophilia; Pedophilia; Transvestism; disorders of psychosexual identity; Psychosexual Dysfunction
	302.50 With Unspecified Sexual History		
	302.51 With Asexual History		
	302.52 With Homosexual History		
	302.53 With Heterosexual History		
***ICD-10* (1992)**	F64 Gender Identity Disorders	Mental and Behavioral Disorders	Habit and impulse disorders; enduring personality changes; specific personality disorders; disorders of sexual preference; psychological and behavioral disorders associated with sexual development and orientation
	F64.0 Transsexualism		
	F64.1 Dual-Role Transvestism		
	F64.2 Gender Identity Disorder of Childhood		
	F64.8 Other Gender Identity Disorder		
	F64.9 Gender Identity Disorder, Unspecified		
***ICD-11* (2019)**	Gender Incongruence	Conditions Related to Sexual Health	Sexual dysfunctions; sexual pain disorders; changes in male genital anatomy; changes in female genital anatomy; paraphilic disorders; adrenogenital disorders; predominantly sexually transmitted infections

Figure 1. Medical Classifications and Trans- Diagnoses

disruptive behavior and back, until it settles in a presumptively depathologized form in its very own neighbor-free chapter. The trans- diagnosis takes a similar but distinct U-turn in the *ICD,* from psychosexual identity disorders to habit and personality disorders, and back to a catchall collection of sexual dysfunctions, paraphilias, STIs, and genital changes. However, in its last stop, it exits the chapter titled "Mental and Behavioral Disorders." Instead, it enters a whole new chapter—despite some (especially Global North) activists' insistence on the separation between sex and gender—the depathologized version of the trans- diagnosis is enfolded into a chapter on sexual health and illness. In the next section, I follow how activists, advocates, and providers worked on diagnostic schema, conceptual framings, and care practices to materialize what they called "depathologization" in practice.

Revising Classification, Revising Care

The Depathologized Diagnoses

The changes that these revisions enacted were not in name only. The depathologized diagnoses in the *DSM* and *ICD* also involved revised diagnostic criteria, which veered away from the language of "disorder." For example, the *DSM*'s Gender Identity Disorder (GID) had focused on the longevity and intensity of sustained cross-gender identification. In contrast, Gender Dysphoria focused on the *distress* produced by the relational conflicts that arise with respect to nonnormative gender identification, experience, or comportment. As New York–based advocate Amanda commented during an interview (January 23, 2016), trans- therapeutic care "helps people . . . live healthier, happier lives. I see it [as] consistent with any other form of health care that helps you resolve distress, anxiety, depression." Amanda and others thus celebrated the turn to a distress-based model. Even among the most ardent supporters of diagnostic revision, pragmatic concerns about utility tempered celebrations. They found the new iterations of the trans- diagnosis to be promising bridges to care. However, they wondered about the strength of these bridges and whether they would work well for everyone seeking trans- therapeutic care.

Gender Dysphoria was the *DSM*'s answer to activists' demand for a nonpathologizing bridge to care.[16] The APA described it as a "new diagnostic class . . . [that] reflects a change in conceptualization of the disorder's defining features" (Regier, Kuhl, and Kupfer 2013). As Amanda said during our interview (January 23, 2016), "I like Gender Dysphoria. . . . [It's] acknowledging a situational experience. It's acknowledging a symptom and it's not pathologizing in the same way." Its utility was as important to Amanda as this conceptual reframing: "I think diagnosis is important. . . . [It] is a tool that helps people get things they need, and [it's] legitimizing."

The shift to Gender Dysphoria was part of a broader set of revisions to the *DSM-5*. The lead-up to this process began in 2006 through the appointment of a *DSM-5* Task Force. By 2008, thirteen work groups had formed that corresponded with each of the *DSM-IV* groupings. Psychologist Kenneth Zucker chaired the Work Group on Sexual and Gender Identity Disorders. This was a somewhat controversial choice, given his reputation among activists to be a proponent of what they called "conversion therapy," or therapy for youth that discouraged the development of trans- identities. Other members included Peggy Cohen-Kettenis, Jack Drescher, Heino Meyer-Bahlburg, and Friedemann Pfäfflin.[17] Activists and advocates submitted public comments on the draft diagnosis. Kelley Winters (2011), a trans- woman and head of GID Reform Advocates, urged trans- people to submit feedback to draft diagnoses to "clarify that nonconformity to birth-assigned roles and being victims of societal prejudice are not, in themselves, mental pathology." Another group, called Professionals Concerned with Gender Diagnoses in the DSM, expressed similar apprehension. Comprising trans- and nontrans- providers, the group asserted, "If the diagnosis remains, it must reflect a non-pathologizing, trans-positive health approach" (Professionals Concerned with Gender Diagnoses in the DSM 2010).

Taking some of this feedback into account, the work group made several changes to the final version of the *DSM* diagnosis, including incorporating an "exit clause" that Winters and others had proposed. Gender Dysphoria would only diagnose a temporary condition prior to trans- people's need for trans- therapeutics and would provide a bridge to care coverage (assuming its availability). Unlike Gender Identity Disorder, it would not remain on a person's medical record in diagnostic perpetuity. Yet as my informants emphasized, the diagnostic revision did little to shift existing conventions of care, given that the diagnoses remained within the pages of the *DSM*. As New York–based nurse practitioner Miranda (interview, August 10, 2013) noted:

> It's still in the *DSM*, as far as a mental health. . . . The good news about that is it allows medical intervention, but I think that most proponents that I'm aware of would like it to be a medical diagnosis so we can get away from the stigmatization of mental illness, and pathology. I mean, I think it's good, it's better. But I just hate the *DSM* really. I hate all of it. I don't think it's useful. And yeah, maybe I'm, like, throwing out the baby with the bath water, but it doesn't have to be the only way that we do things.

Providers, activists, and advocates alike regarded the Gender Dysphoria diagnosis as a somewhat tense compromise between old guard defenders of GID and those who sought to depathologize trans- health care but retain its bridging function (discussed in chapter 4).[18] Nevertheless, most of the providers and many of the activists and advocates with whom I spoke thought that it at least potentially improved nonstigmatizing access to care, at least in the United States.

Not everyone agreed. For example, trans- attorney Chase Strangio (2012) and trans- physician R. Nick Gorton (2013) thought that the turn to Gender Dysphoria would intensify barriers to trans- therapeutic care for people in situations of confinement, such as prisons, jails, psychiatric institutions, and immigration detention. Medical neglect is common in such institutions, and basic care can be difficult to access, let alone trans- therapeutic care. For trans- people who are in prison, Eighth Amendment legal claims—which define the failure to provide adequate health care as "cruel and unusual punishment"—have been a primary means of access to trans- therapeutic care. Gorton and Strangio were skeptical that a framework of "distress" would establish an effective basis for legal claims in these cases. Other activists and advocates were unconvinced that "distress" and "disorder" were all that different, or that gender-based "distress" could be isolated from other distressing conditions of poverty, racism, ableism, and state violence.[19]

For depathologization activists who worked on a transnational scale, the *DSM* revision signaled more of a tempest in a teapot than a sea change. They saw the *DSM* as a provincial system masquerading as a universal one. Some informants, like Buenos Aires–based transnational advocate Antonio (interview, July 25, 2015), viewed the preoccupation with revising the *DSM* as revealing "U.S. psychiatric imperialism." The APA's biomedical paradigm—reflected in large part by the diagnostically driven *DSM*—differs from the psychodynamic model that dominates Argentine mental health.[20] This was why transnationally focused depathologization activists focused on the *ICD,* and why they sought to remove the trans- diagnosis from its mental-health chapter altogether. Indeed, this effort to move the trans- diagnosis from the purview of psychiatry to that of medicine was a very compelling tactic for activists, advocates, and providers who promoted depathologization.

For example, I interviewed Beth (July 25, 2013), a New York–based nurse practitioner, in an East Village café. She longed for a way to diagnose patients without what she called the "stigma" of a psychiatric diagnosis. She described this as a solely "medical diagnosis"—correcting herself after having initially called it a "neutral diagnosis." Like Talia, the nurse practitioner mentioned in the last chapter who felt uncomfortable using a psychiatric diagnosis, Beth's desire for a medical diagnosis was in part jurisdictional. As anthropologist Eric Plemons (2010) points out, trans- therapeutics have the awkward distinction of ostensibly naming a condition of the psyche while enacting interventions on the physical body.[21] Beth was also expressing a political desire. She wanted to practice what she described as "trans-affirmative" care, and in her mind, this was inconsistent with diagnosing patients with a psychiatric disorder.

When we spoke, Beth was unaware of the work that transnational depathologization activists were undertaking in revising *ICD* diagnoses but was pleased to learn of it. The *ICD* revision was as lengthy and consequential a process as the *DSM* revision—and was accompanied by a greater global reach. The *ICD* is the most widely used diagnostic classificatory schema in the world, and most national health systems use it to structure health financing. It is revised in full roughly every decade. For the *ICD-11* revision, WHO staff convened a number of professional working groups, including a Working Group on the Classification of Sexual Disorders and Sexual Health. This comprised physicians, psychiatrists, and some nonmedically trained advocates from across the globe.[22] The work group also incorporated experts from the WHO Department of Mental Health and Substance Use as well as the WHO Department of Sexual and Reproductive Health and Research. The group was tasked with reviewing evidence and revising classifications, descriptions, and guidelines for conditions in the *ICD-10* chapter on mental and behavioral disorders relevant to sexual behavior, dysfunction, and orientation, as well as gender identity (Krueger et al. 2017; Epstein 2021).

Paralleling the *DSM*'s reframing, the group found the *ICD*'s trans- diagnosis that was up for revision to be desperately outdated. Several members proposed that it was necessary to

> abandon the psychopathological model of transgender people based on 1940s conceptualizations of sexual deviance and to move towards a model that is (1) more reflective of current scientific evidence and best practices; (2) more responsive to the needs, experience, and human rights of this vulnerable population; and (3) more supportive of the provision of accessible and high-quality healthcare services. (Drescher, Cohen-Kettenis, and Winter 2012, 575)

To materialize this effort, the group eventually proposed a new classification called Gender Incongruence.

First, though, they undertook a lengthy process of research and revision. This began with literature reviews, which was followed by a diagnostic proposal within a beta phase. This opened the draft diagnosis to public comments.[23] Advocates, activists, providers, and others gave feedback on the new proposed classification of Gender Incongruence and its potential site of placement within the *ICD*'s schema.[24] Transnational activist and advocacy groups like Global Action for Trans Equality, or GATE (which I discussed in chapter 1), as well as Stop Trans Pathologization (STP), Transgender Europe, the International Lesbian, Gay, Bisexual, Trans and Intersex Association, and others submitted comments and published press releases to support depathologization as a critical framework for the *ICD*'s revisions. While many among these groups remained skeptical about diagnostic classifications, they certainly preferred the medical diagnosis to the psychiatric one. After public comments and international field-testing, the group finalized a proposed diagnosis and placement in a chapter on sexual health. The new classificatory proposals were passed by the World Health Assembly in 2019.

Of the people with whom I spoke in New York, only two were aware of the proposed changes to the *ICD*. In Argentina, by contrast, those with whom I spoke were broadly familiar with the process—although the *ICD* would have little pragmatic effect following the Gender Identity Law's restructuring of trans- therapeutic care to hinge on self-perceived need rather than diagnosis.[25] Antonio, the Buenos Aires–based activist and advocate I mentioned before, had long-standing connections with providers and policymakers and served as an outside adviser to the WHO working group. He described feeling ambivalent about diagnosis in general but recognized that health infrastructures outside of Argentina usually required a diagnosis for coverage. In an interview (July 25, 2015) at my apartment in Buenos Aires, he explained why he was working to develop a diagnosis in the *ICD*:

> I think there should be a mention. I [would rather] not, but if there is no mention, that would mean that only the people that have money or only the people who are living in Argentina at this time can have access to the right to transition-based health.

Antonio viewed the process of the *DSM*'s diagnostic revisions with some measure of exasperation. In addition to asserting that North American infrastructures of care ought not determine how trans- therapeutics take shape worldwide, he also felt that the example of the Gender Identity Law's antidiagnostic coverage provisions were a more compelling blueprint for infrastructural change:

> I, myself, am not a nationalist or patriot . . . but I also take into account that I live in a country in the [Global] South where we speak Spanish. So I value a lot the things that happen here

and I get very disappointed when those things are completely ignored in the North.

But despite his ambivalence about diagnostic work in general, his frustration with epistemic imperialism incited him to advocate for revision of the trans- diagnosis in the *ICD*.

In this sense, Antonio's position revealed an analysis consistent with transnational feminisms, which view gendered difference as inseparable from the dynamics of imperialism, racial capitalism, neocolonialism, and the forces of globalization. In these reflections, he emphasized how notions of global peripherality play out in trans- health discourse. Rather than orient to Global North paradigms of diagnostic depathologization, he insisted instead on pursuing more capacious political projects that could confront the way pathologization takes different shapes across specific regions throughout the world, with differential effects for gender/sex nonnormative people. As I discuss in chapter 6, Antonio was also concerned about Global North philanthropic forces in directing Global South movement-building. In Inderpal Grewal and Caren Kaplan's (1994, 7) terms, Antonio attuned to the "effects of mobile capital as well as the multiple subjectivities that replace the European unitary subject." In so doing, he recognized the *ICD* revision as one site through which to intervene not only in the varying forms that trans- pathologization takes but also in Global North social movement hegemony.

Activists and advocates worked to develop some of the language and concepts that became key to the *ICD* revision in less direct ways. As I touched on in chapter 1, GATE was one of the organizations that anticipated the arrival of the *ICD* revision and tried to lay the groundwork for a less pathologizing and more useful diagnosis for its constituents. To this effect, GATE held an international gathering in The Hague in 2011. Convening a group of multidisciplinary experts—most of them trans- —they strove to provide early recommendations to the WHO as they anticipated the *ICD* revision. As mentioned before, their proposed Starfish Model intricately detailed multiple codes, groupings, and chapters that could be tailored to localized needs. The proposal was named "the Starfish Model" for the capacity of its parts to exist in separation. They contrasted the Starfish Model with what they termed a "Spider Model," in which a central and singular classificatory diagnosis would be expected to work as a diagnostic bridge across a multitude of health-care systems. In the report, authors wrote:

> At the Experts' Meeting the starfish was used as a metaphoric model that could give answer[s] to differentiated possibilities in terms [of] access to health care, including its coverage. In this sense, combining different chapters, blocks and codes (the starfish's legs) could exponentially increase trans* people['s] opportunities of accessing health care under very different circumstances without recurring to a single and potentially repathologizing diagnosis (a Spider Model). (GATE 2011, 10)

The Starfish Model suggested several different strategies for use in differing infrastructures of care, each of which might have different regulations related to health-care financing, subsidy, or reimbursement. In addition to the Z-code (or visit code) model discussed in chapter 1, they also suggested the possibility of using *ICD* codes associated with endocrine disorders or genitourinary disorders.

In addition to advocating for diagnostic heterogeneity, GATE advocates also insisted on the multiplicity of transness. Refusing the umbrella of *transgender,* they used *trans** with an asterisk. In their 2011 report on the Experts' Meeting, they wrote:

> GATE uses the term trans* to name those people who identify themselves in a different gender than that assigned to them at birth and/or those people who feel they have to, prefer to or choose to present themselves differently to the expectations associated with the gender role assigned to them at birth—whether by clothing, accessories, cosmetics or body modification. [It] encompasses many different and culturally specific experiences of embodiment, identity and expression. The asterisk aims to make its open-ended character explicit. (GATE 2011, 7)

In making this claim, they joined STP and other groups in arguing for a radical heterogeneity of trans- subjectivity, in addition to the decentering of "transgender politics" as such (also paralleling feminism's decentering in transnational feminist thought).

While the Starfish Model was not ultimately adopted, the language of depathologization, multiplicity, and care access found its way into the *ICD*'s reclassification. In what follows, the WHO (n.d.) website includes a brief about the new classification:

> This reflects current knowledge that trans-related and gender diverse identities are not conditions of mental ill-health, and classifying them as such can cause enormous stigma. Inclusion of gender incongruence in the *ICD* should ensure transgender people's access to gender-affirming health care, as well as adequate health insurance coverage for such services.

The working group members thus summoned the language of "diversity" and "stigma" in the updated classification and incorporated activists' and advocates' positions on the need for it to serve a primarily bridging function to better facilitate care coverage. As in the *DSM* revision—though through a different set of approaches—participants in the *ICD* revision incorporated activists' and advocates' perspectives to frame transness as a benign variation rather than an individual pathology. Further, each revision conceptualized this benign variation as becoming salient within the milieu of a social environment that involved threats to well-being that might be mitigated through therapeutic care.

In this sense, the official trans- diagnoses at the center of depathologization campaigns are of much import to trans- health practice. However, these often take center stage and obscure other classifications that also come into play in the practices of trans- health. For example, while some supportive providers waited for these depathologized diagnoses to become available in practice (or made sense of how to use them), they found other means of establishing bridges to care coverage.

Bridging Care with Work-Arounds

I interviewed Roberto in his office in a health clinic in New York in the summer of 2013. A nurse practitioner in New York, he described how the clinic where he worked had developed a work-around to insulate patients from the "stigma" of a mental-health diagnosis while helping them obtain coverage for hormones (interview, July 29, 2013).[26] As I discussed briefly in the previous chapter, the clinic had adopted the policy of using Endocrine Disorder, Not Otherwise Specified—an *ICD* code but not a *DSM* one—as a diagnosis for trans- patients needing coverage for hormones. When we spoke, he was concerned that insurance companies were beginning to catch on:

> AUTHOR: Are there any problems with that, with people's insurance and gender markers?
>
> ROBERTO: There hasn't been any yet but there's a concern there will be. I guess they're changing the . . . codes soon and they're worried that is going to be a problem. I think [with] Endocrine Disorder, Not Otherwise Specified, you don't have to attach a sex to it like [with] Gender Identity Disorder. I have started getting more denials. Some insurance companies are asking for prior authorization for hormones, and they ask flat out if it's for hormone therapy or cross-gender hormone therapy or something along those lines, which treats Gender Identity Disorder, and if you say "yeah," they deny it.

I also interviewed Tina (interview, August 8, 2013), a nurse at the same clinic. She commented:

> TINA: My understanding is that we use Endocrine Disorder because it's very vague and does not "out" somebody as being trans-, and there's more likelihood that insurance will cover the labs, visit, and medication.
>
> AUTHOR: What are your thoughts on [using] Endocrine Disorder?
>
> TINA: It's slightly dishonest. . . . But I get why it's done because

> again, it's pragmatic, but duplicitous, yes. But you sometimes have to be duplicitous, and it's better than Gender Dysphoria, which is so "mental health-y" and gross.

Tina was more concerned with the ethics of this work-around,[27] though she felt it was ultimately justified.

Another New York–based provider (field notes, July 25, 2013) mentioned to me during an ethnographic observation that the classification did not seem dishonest to her at all. She reasoned that trans- people did indeed have Endocrine Disorder, given that their bodies produce the "wrong hormone." As she saw it, the diagnostic criteria formally included for an Endocrine Disorder diagnosis had simply not yet caught up with the biological discoveries of trans- embodiment. In this assertion, she joined an increasing number of trans-supportive providers, advocates, and activists who strove to redefine gender nonnormativity as a biological phenomenon. To support their claims, some providers drew on research on "trans- brains," "trans- genes," and other hypothesized anatomical, hormonal, or molecular structures or functions that seek to identify biological indicators for transness (e.g., Case and Ramachandran 2012; Hare et al. 2009; Zubiaurre-Elorza et al. 2013).[28]

Regardless of whether providers regarded unofficial diagnoses such as Endocrine Disorder to be a shrewd work-around or an incipient scientific reality, it was clear that this diagnostic classification was doing some heavy lifting for trans- health provision among New York–based providers. Some saw this as an explicit bid to protect patients from the stigma of psychiatric diagnosis, while others were most interested in supporting patients by evading the potentially exclusionary effects of official trans- diagnoses. In each case, the primary focus for providers was on the outcomes for care coverage that Endocrine Disorder could bring about—especially when they were frustrated about the racialized and classed disparities that Medicaid exclusions brought about for poor trans- patients. Figure 2 shows a list of the nonpsychiatric diagnostic classifications that New York–based providers with whom I spoke used in their daily practice. This is no doubt an incomplete list, and one that fluctuates depending on conditions of bureaucratic

<table>
<tr><td>ICD-9 (1975)</td><td>259.9 Endocrine Disorder Not Otherwise Specified</td><td rowspan="2">Endocrine, Nutritional, and/or Metabolic Disorders</td><td rowspan="2">Disorders of the thyroid; disorders of the pancreas; disorders of the pituitary gland; disorders of the adrenal gland; disorders of the gonads</td></tr>
<tr><td>ICD-10 (1990)</td><td>E34.9 Endocrine Disorder, Unspecified</td></tr>
</table>

Figure 2. Nonpsychiatric Biomedical Classifications as Work-Arounds for Trans- Diagnoses

scrutiny, terms of reimbursement, and consensus on the part of providers.

Providers mobilized work-around diagnoses like Endocrine Disorder as a means of caring well for their trans- patients when medical systems imposed what they regarded as discriminatory or unfair roadblocks. This was only one among many work-arounds related to medical records and billing that they used to care for trans- patients. However, they were also implicated within a much larger patchwork of administrative and institutional work-arounds. This had to do with the fact that institutions ranging from the Department of Motor Vehicles to the Department of State to the Social Security Administration required medical providers' approval for gender reclassification—often using drastically different, sometimes conflicting, and often shifting criteria.[29] As such, providers were often pulled into the quagmire of navigating transness amid the incongruities of institutions and bureaucracies.

Alongside the ever-changing bureaucratic landscape, the late 1990s and early 2000s saw increasing scrutiny on the part of state officials when it came to trans- people (though it began long before and has not yet ceased) (e.g., Currah and Moore 2009; Spade 2015; Currah 2022). As part of this intensification, poor trans- Medicaid recipients in New York had their benefits for hormone prescriptions abruptly cut off in the early 2000s. Health care has been a primary site for disruptions in care coverage and benefits for trans- people, and poor people, people with disabilities, and people of color have borne the brunt of these. As such, health-care providers have often been in the position of using work-arounds to partially insulate patients from changes that have had profoundly negative lived effects. This was why, after Medicaid started rejecting coverage for hormones for trans- people, some supportive providers instead diagnosed patients with Endocrine Disorder to ensure continuity of care. They recognized that poor patients—most of whom could not conceivably afford the costs of paying for hormone prescriptions out of pocket—would be likely to turn to informal markets for hormones for the care they needed. They saw this as potentially dangerous and certainly unjust. As such, trans- health providers worked to "buffer the impact of the U.S. health insurance system on transgender people and help secure the payment for care" (Van Eijk 2017, 593).

It is likely that Endocrine Disorder became a go-to unofficial diagnosis for New York–based providers seeking to provide trans- patients with a bridge to care for a simple reason: it worked. At least during the period in which Roberto was working in 2013, the use of an Endocrine Disorder diagnosis enabled providers to prescribe hormones and circumvent coverage exclusions. As Roberto noted, this was likely only a temporary fix until administrators caught on. Furthermore, this diagnosis was useless for accessing surgeries, often the costliest parts of trans- therapeutic care.

Endocrine Disorder diagnoses thus worked as a conditional and temporary bridge to care. Other diagnostic classifications, however, became relevant in their capacity to *obstruct* access to care. Sonya, a New York–based nurse practitioner (interview, August 7, 2013), described how some of her patients—particularly poor transwomen of color, as well as some trans- men of color—came to her after having had a difficult time accessing trans- therapeutics elsewhere. At times, she said, this had to do with what she saw as the racist tendency to diagnose people with other forms of "disruptive" mental illness and to refuse or delay trans- therapeutic treatment. Sonya thought these providers diagnosed patients with "comorbidities" in an obstructionist way that required them to limit or defer trans- therapeutic care. In what might be understood as biomedical intersectionality, Sonya identified this intensified paternalism as profoundly racialized. I take up these dynamics in more detail in chapter 5's discussion of medical gatekeeping. Having interviewed mostly providers who saw themselves as particularly supportive to trans- people, I heard only secondhand about the use of obstructionist comorbidities in clinical practice. Nevertheless, the providers with whom I spoke were aware of people being denied trans- therapeutic care based on body weight and HIV status, in addition to mental health.[30]

Not Just Diagnoses: Classification and Care Infrastructures

I began this chapter with Clarissa's reflections about being able to diagnose her trans- patients with an illness but not being able to enter their lived gender in a medical record. This has since changed. However, when we spoke in 2013, it troubled her immensely and she had taken steps to address it. For example, she told me she had contacted the electronic medical charting vendor that her clinic worked with to confront this technical and, in her mind, ethical conundrum. As she explained, "I have been inquiring . . . 'Do you just have to ask this company to give you another button? . . . Has this company not invented this button? . . . What is the story on this?'" (interview, July 25, 2013).

Clarissa wanted to be able to designate that a patient was trans- so she could facilitate their access to high-quality care in whatever realm in which this was required. However, she realized that she could not necessarily anticipate whether providers would understand what she hoped to communicate to them and whether this information would improve or negatively affect the care they received. As it turned out, soon after our interview, sex and gender charting options in many organizations became far more capacious—though they have not necessarily enacted the changes that Clarissa hoped for.[31] Still, her consternation about medical records demonstrates the importance of engaging classification beyond the frame of diagnostics.

Within trans- health, it is not only *diagnostic* classifications that are subject to the expressed needs of trans- health activists but also a series of other classificatory infrastructures that prevent biomedicine from caring well for trans- people. Infrastructures related to health-care financing are perhaps the most directly relevant here. Nevertheless, the questions advanced by political formations advocating for trans- health also implicate many other infrastructures—particularly those that track sex classification, including state bureaucracies, public benefits systems, infrastructures of migration and confinement, and so on. Indeed, classificatory breakdown happens differently depending on when, where, why, and how people seek trans- therapeutic care, and this leads to marked variation in the solutions that people propose to address these breakdowns. Depathologization activism attends to some aspects of these ranging and geographically dispersed classificatory breakdowns, but in many regards it has been too focused a project to take a more sweeping account of classificatory barriers to care. In the final section below, I discuss some of these limitations through the refractions of unruliness: first, as a political claim advanced by depathologization activists and advocates; second, as a means of thinking about pathologization; and last, as a political orientation offering a different horizon for depathologization (and presaging discussions of coalitional depathologization in subsequent chapters).

The Unruly Terms of Depathologization

Over the past few years of the brief life of the trans- diagnosis, activists, advocates, and providers coordinated—albeit in uneven ways—to change biomedicine's stories about trans- people. They also worked to address the ranging ways diagnosis matters to care access across varying institutional and geographic infrastructures. In undertaking this revision work, activists and advocates especially emphasized multiplicity and heterogeneity. They described radical proliferations in perspective, politics, and subject position that T. Benjamin Singer (2006) terms "the transgender sublime." For Antonio and other transnationally engaged activists, this unruly sublimity might be described as "transnational transfeminism." The unruliness on which they insisted proved both frictional and generative to the classificatory logic of biomedical and psychiatric nosology.[32]

Even as they made a case for the unruly multiplicity of transness and its resistance to diagnostic containment, they still insisted on the importance of a diagnosis. Activists and advocates—as well as some supportive providers—were wholly uninterested in pinning transsness down to a contained set of meanings. Instead, they wished to maintain a diagnostic code as a bridge (where it was needed, in any case) to many different financial infrastructures of care coverage. While wealthy trans- people could afford care out of pocket, diagnostic frameworks often posed sharply stratified barriers to care for low- or even moderate-income trans- people.

For most activists and advocates, the particular affront of the psychiatric diagnosis was the raison d'être for depathologization campaigns. In characterizing this frustration, *stigma* was a widely used term to refer to trans- pathologization. However, the framework of "stigma," in Erving Goffman's (1986) terms, directs concerns to the "spoiled identity" of transness. Depathologization campaigns worked to supplant this "spoiled identity" with a revised notion of transness as not only heterogeneous but also healthy and desired. It is difficult to argue with the appeal of this shift. However, the use of "stigma" as a sense-making lens "side-lines questions about where stigma is produced, by whom and for what purposes" (Tyler and Slater 2018). In other words, the focus on stigma problematizes the social response to an identity rather than the pathologizing conditions that produce positions of subordination.

As such, disposing of pathologizing diagnoses did not dissipate the pathologizing sedimentations of racialized poverty, disability, or criminalization. These entangled forms of pathologization, too, are unruly and uncontained. Depathologization activism fell far short of confronting the interwoven pathologizing paradigms of white supremacy, anti-Blackness, colonial knowledge, racialized immiseration, eugenic ableism, criminalization of public space, and other modes of domination and authority—despite trans- pathologization's imbrications within these. While these unruly pathologizations share complex and interwoven historical legacies, their effects are scarcely relegated to the past. As Sonya's observations about biomedical intersectionality, Strangio's and Gorton's reflections on imprisonment, and Antonio's assertions about psychiatric imperialism made clear, diagnoses worked differently across racialized class, region, disability, and criminalization. Diagnoses stuck to people differently depending on who they were, where they were, and how they were oriented to the people and systems who diagnosed them. In this sense, classifications—including supposedly depathologized ones—were themselves sometimes stratifying tools that reproduced different forms of pathologization. Depathologization activism was ill-equipped to confront these stratifications, focused as it was on stigma and the singularity of transness.

These twin foci of stigma and the singularity of transness have produced some strange political dynamics within depathologization activism. For example, trans- people and people with disabilities (groups that are far from mutually exclusive) have been similarly pathologized for their failures to conform to racialized norms of work productivity, among other things (Irving 2008; Awkward-Rich 2022). However, the vehemence with which depathologization activists disavow mental debility reproduces similar currents of ableism. For example, one of the Argentine trans- activists with whom I spoke—who also had disabilities—described an awkward moment with another trans- activist at a public presentation on depathologization for an international group of health officials (field notes, August 20, 2013). He explained that she took the mic, passionately claiming to the officials that she was not ill but was rather a human being. The person with whom I spoke described laughing at this comment, since in addition to disavowing kinship with people with disabilities, this activist had also effectively declared him to be inhuman.

This brings us back to Beth's hope for a "medical" diagnosis rather than a psychiatric one. She corrected herself after describing this as a "neutral" diagnosis. However, this desire for political neutrality in the shift away from psychiatry and toward a "solely medical" diagnosis is shared by depathologization activists. Yet, as this chapter and the remainder of the book make clear, biomedicine has *never* been politically neutral—including in its present manifestations. Biomedicine, with or without psychiatry, is stratified and stratifying in its distributive politics, racializing forces, and techniques of population management.[33] The unruliness of pathologizing histories and forces shows up in biomedicine's contemporary power to establish norms, as well as in its establishment of thresholds of acceptable suffering (among other things). As such, an apolitical biomedicine is a patent impossibility. This does not negate the profound significance of the changes that depathologization has brought about, but it serves as an important reminder that the stakes of pathologization and depathologization far transcend the field of psychiatry and the status of the psychiatric diagnosis.

Depathologization activism converged temporally with the emergence of social movements like Marea Verde (Green Tide) feminism in Argentina, multisited Occupy movements, and other diffuse movements that confronted the unruliness of pathologization alongside political economies of debt and immiseration (Pis Diez 2019; Pickerill and Krinsky 2012). These "unruly politics," as Akshay Khanna and colleagues (2013, 14) name them, marshal "power from transgressing . . . the rules of the political game." Unruly political formations—scattered and diffuse as they were—encountered critiques that their plethora of political messages meant that they did not know what they stood for. What these critiques missed was that protesters were simply taking a very different approach to refusing the unruly and interwoven tendrils of pathologization and immiseration.

Rather than take a sweeping approach to pathologization, the activists, advocates, and supportive providers I discuss here trained their focus on classificatory revision. The shrewdness and success of their endeavors should not be underestimated. Providers and professional organizations—even far-reaching international bodies like the WHO—shifted their language, integrated activist knowledge, and oriented to the guidance of activists and advocates. They effectively shifted the biomedical gaze from pathological individuals to the broad social environments of *distress* or incongruence. Furthermore, the question of supposed truth related to classification took a back seat to issues of access—certainly among activists and advocates, but also among many providers. In the *DSM* and *ICD*, this materialized in revisions to diagnostic descriptions and classificatory placements. In the Gender Identity Law, it led to the legal abrogation of diagnostic power when it came to trans- therapeutics.

However, these interventions also required working within the structuring constraints of biomedical practice. As such, depathologization activism has been limited by this pragmatic obligation to focus too squarely on the singularity of transness in its work, and as a result it has missed opportunities to engage more synthetically and historically with the enduring and disparate effects of pathologization. "Unruly politics," in contrast, involve "a refusal . . . to speak in [the] language . . . defined by those in power" and "the insistence on the use of another language" (Khanna et al. 2013, 13). What might an unruly politics of depathologization look like? How might it orient differently to the limits of diagnostic depathologization, and what limits might it encounter in its unruliness? How might it assert trans- therapeutic care as part of demands for "everything for everyone" in the register of Occupy claims? Or wanting ourselves alive and debt-free, in the terms of Green Tide activists? In subsequent chapters, especially chapter 6, I discuss coalitional depathologization activists as a group that attempted to take up these questions.

In the Introduction, I quoted Stuart Hall's (1997) comment about words as a medium for power. Relatedly, classifications also are a medium of power and resistance. Even as they convey, they also enact, enable, and restrict. Classifications mean things, but they also do things. This book focuses on practices—activist practices, practices of care provision, and research practices. When depathologization debates focus on stigma, they often treat diagnoses as abstracted from their broader webs of pathologization, practice, power, and stratification. The proponents of depathologization with whom I spoke *were* concerned with what diagnoses could enact in their insistence on the bridge to coverage. However, destigmatized bridges worked better for some people than others.

Mark, a New York–based advocate, commented on this during an interview (January 15, 2016). He observed stratification as taking place not only in access but also in people's level of concern about stigmatization in the first place:

> I think no matter what [medicine] says, the same people are always going to *have* access and the same people are always *not* going to have access. [And] the same people are going to critique the fact that they're stigmatized, and that's [the] power structure we're working within. . . . I think we're just

> approaching it in the wrong way and building [the wrong] bridges where we could be building really strong, exciting alliances.

Mark did not look upon biomedicine as a productive site through which to make liberatory claims. Instead, he thought that a more generative intervention involved working within existing narratives to "redistribute better opportunities for survival." His interests in building "strong exciting alliances" aligned with the coalition-focused efforts that I describe in the following chapters of this book.

The antagonizing paradigms of pathologization that were established and elaborated throughout the twentieth century were not birthed with the advent of clinical transsexuality.[34] As such, we cannot expect that these currents will vanish with the decommissioning of a specific diagnosis. Proponents of depathologization accomplished a great deal in their rebuke of trans- pathologization. However, pathologization is a multiheaded hydra, and diagnostic revision falls far short of slaying the dragon.

3 Epidemiological Rage

Population, Biography, and State Responsibility in Trans- Health Activism

> The State is the main violator of the rights of travestis, by act or omission.
>
> —Lohana Berkins, "Travestis: Una identidad política"

In Buenos Aires in 2015, I attended the opening of an art exhibit called *Furia Travesti.* Loosely translated, this activist rallying cry means "travesti rage" or "fury." About a hundred people filled the Tierra Violeta community center in Buenos Aires where the show was held. Travesti artist Florencia Agustina Guimaraes García was showing photos from her collection—some of her own and others from her trove of vintage Polaroids and prints of travesti life in Buenos Aires over the past decades. As attendees milled about and gazed at Guimaraes's images, she entered the space and walked toward a sound system set up in a corner of the gallery. Dressed in black, her face obscured by a mourning veil, she took the microphone. "I am death!" she said quietly. She repeated this until the crowd fell silent and gathered around her. She spoke with a palpable urgency. "I follow you wherever you go," she continued. "I follow you as you walk and work on the streets. I follow you everywhere. Enough!" She began to shout. "Enough with the murders, enough with the travesticides! Enough with lives cut short too soon, like Laura Moyano's! Enough!"[1]

Moyano, a thirty-five-year-old travesti from Córdoba (in central Argentina, about 450 miles from Buenos Aires) had been killed two weeks prior. Widespread protests followed demanding "Not one more!" and "No more travesticides."[2] These slogans fit within a broader Ni Una Menos feminist movement, which has mobilized against gendered violence in and beyond Buenos Aires since 2015 (Friedman and Tabbush 2016). Increasingly, Ni Una Menos activists have turned to state complicity to frame violence, carrying banners that proclaim, "The State Is Responsible" (or the "State Is at Fault"). Guimaraes later described *travesticidio social,* or "social travesticide" in an interview: "We are condemned . . . to a string of violence that is reflected in our life statistics, with an average of 35 years . . . [and] we believe that society and the State are responsible for our lives being so short" (Máximo 2016). In these gestures, activists attributed responsibility for travesti and trans- violence to regulatory and economic violence rather than primarily ascribing it to individualized expressions of transphobia or dangerous life choices.[3]

The State Is at Fault

In this chapter, I analyze how trans- health activists in Buenos Aires produced what I call "epidemiological biographies." Looking to published community studies, laws, bibliometric data, and ethnographic observations, I analyze how these epidemiological biographies—which paired biographical narratives with statistical data—produced new ways of engaging what counts as trans- health. I examine how Argentine activists drew empirical attention to state violence and criminalization in their use of statistics to make claims for collective access to health. In chapter 4, I discuss how New York–based activists and advocates also used epidemiological biographies to shift thinking about trans- health, drawing largely on risk prevention and economic viability. Both approaches contrast with behavioral models of population health that emphasize individual conduct and the relative neutrality of state authorities and medical experts.

One of the most striking aspects of Argentine epidemiological biographies was the effectiveness with which they redefined root causes of foreshortened life to bring about new ways of thinking publicly about trans- health. Highlighting the uneven effects of state violence, activists used numbers as a tactical approach to enact their goals of resource redistribution and anticriminalization. These conceptual interventions had sustained material effects. For example, the 2014 "Expectativas" (or "Expectations") media campaign in Buenos Aires mobilized activist researchers' statistical reframings of health endangerment. Foregrounding the shortness of trans- and especially travesti lives, the campaign also referred obliquely to "expectativas de vida"—one translation of "life expectancy." Drawing on activist research, the campaign identified thirty-five as the average trans- life expectancy. The passage of the nation's 2012 Gender Identity Law just prior to the campaign was also shaped by activism that drew on language of life expectancy—or the likelihood of death in aggregate form—to make distributive claims for health-care access and other resources, as well as claims about state responsibility for violence.

In what follows, I show how activists selectively adopted quantification to make state violence more broadly apparent and win certain political demands. I then describe this work as statistical collectivization, or collective political action that refigures dominant modes of statistical aggregation. Activists' focus on statistical strategies pivoted from the formal rights-focused claims of trans- citizenship, emphasizing instead material relief and insulation from state violence. I conclude by arguing that the statistical turns I describe produced contradictory effects. At one level, they obscured some of the differential conditions of imperilment that gender nonnormative people experience. At another, they directed attention to the markedly racialized, sexualized, classed, and gendered forms of subjugation that materialize in transnational landscapes of trans- health.[4]

As it traces trans- health's shift from "individual" to "population," this chapter also shows how activist research portended population-health researchers' intensifying attention on health and state violence. In the wake of seemingly unending racialized police violence and political repression (particularly but not only in the United States), the public claim that state violence is a health crisis is gaining traction. This has required a broad reconsideration of what *health* signifies—and this chapter suggests that social movements have played a key role in these revisions. Comparisons between populations (including but not limited to trans- populations) have been key to making claims about state violence with respect to differential and collective health. However, the very notion of population raises questions about quantification and power, as such forms of rationalization are often associated with dynamics of state control and state racism. This chapter argues that in their work to reframe population health, activists redrew what political scientist James Scott (1999, 2) calls "state maps of legibility." Rather than mobilizing metrics in the service of state control, Argentine activist researchers instead used statistics to lay bare the nonneutrality and violence of state administration and security apparatuses.[5]

Trans- in Epidemiology

The aggregate health of populations is the purview of epidemiology, which tracks the occurrence, frequency, and distribution of health and illness using statistical methods. According to David Kindig and Greg Stoddart (2003, 381), *population health* can be defined as "the health outcomes of a group of individuals, including the distribution of such outcomes within the group." The objects of concern within this field are aggregate health outcomes, the "social determinants" that shape group-level patterns in health, and the interventions that mediate these aggregate outcomes and group-level patterns. Population-health research centers on comparative risk factors, and its proposed interventions strive to minimize group-differentiated risks to negative health outcomes.[6]

However, epidemiological methods often fail to capture the complexity of health inequities and other salient conditions of life and marginalization (Breilh 2008; Shim 2014). The subfield of social epidemiology comparatively analyzes "health disparities" to foreground these conditions (Kawachi, Subramanian, and Almeida-Filho 2002). Collective health (*salud colectiva*) movements in Argentina have also pressed for explicitly structural analyses of health (Logroño 2019). Social epidemiologists describe "fundamental causes" as "upstream" factors affecting health, such as institutionalized racism and poverty (Link and Phelan 1995). Some researchers draw on concepts like "structural violence" to design research, but they struggle to adhere to methodological expectations of the field to clearly infer direct causal relationships (Galtung 1969; Shim 2014). Health disparities research is increasingly central to national and transnational health research, policy, and medical practice (Farmer et al. 2013; Gourevitch et al. 2019). While social epidemiologists look to an expansive landscape of health determinants, few studies look specifically to the effects of state violence (Cooper and Fullilove 2016).[7]

Studies about trans- populations are few compared to other epidemiological subjects of concern. Nonetheless, attention to trans- population health has grown astronomically in the past two decades. Yet, some research foci remain better represented than others. Of the nearly 5,347 PubMed-indexed articles published between 2000 and 2019 with key terms *transgender* or *transsexual,* nearly 23.7 percent also included the key term *HIV,* while 6.7 percent included *violence,* and 0.2 percent included *criminalization.* LILACS, a Latin American and Caribbean database indexing mainly Spanish-language research, yielded 286 articles with key terms *transgénero, travesti,* or *transsexual,* of which 9.4 percent contain the key term *HIV.* In contrast, 3.1 percent contain the key term *violencia* and 0.7 percent include *criminalización* (see Table 1).

Much HIV-focused population-health research centers on health behavior models, which generally theorize social, institutional, and structural factors as influencing or constraining decisions about health (Baral et al. 2013). Some of these researchers attend carefully to the importance of "upstream" or "structural factors" in affecting relative health outcomes (Poteat et al. 2015).

Table 1. Trans- Health Research Publications 2000-2019

Keyword	PubMed	% Total	LILACS	% Total
Transgender or Transsexual*	5,347	100	286	100
& HIV	1,266	23.7	27	9.4
& Violence	359	6.7	9	3.1
& Criminalization	10	.18	2	.7

Quantity of research publications between 2000 and 2019 by keyword and indexing source. Bibliometric frequency data (PubMed and LILACS) (12/23/2019).

* *Travesti* also used as a search term in LILACS

However, the methodological foci of epidemiology—establishing robust causality and identifying "modifiable environmental factors" (Bonita, Beaglehole, and Kjellström 2006, xi)—tend to direct interventions toward behavioral change and policy intervention, even within an acknowledged milieu of structural violence. As such, their primary locus of proposed intervention tends to be individual conduct related to sexual health and communicable disease (Thompson and King 2015).

Some epidemiologists in trans- health have worked to address upstream conditions through policy recommendations, but these often rest on state or judicial arbitration or protection to enhance health outcomes (e.g., antidiscrimination laws). Epidemiological biographies strove to focus elsewhere in both their analysis and intervention: specifically, they looked to the directly causal dynamics of state violence, systematic immiseration, and criminalization as threats to the health of trans- people and travestis.

Estimating Institutional Violence

Guimaraes's performance at the *Furia Travesti* event, as well as her subsequent claims about social travesticide, drew directly on activist research on state and institutional violence. In fact, the mention of the age of thirty-five—the most well-traveled life expectancy estimate for travesti/transfeminine/trans- people—emerged in part from epidemiological biographies (Berkins and Fernández 2005; Berkins 2007a; Borgogno and REDLACTRANS 2009).[8] While many studies might aptly be described as epidemiological biographies, this chapter focuses most closely on three of these: *La gesta del nombre propio* (The struggle for one's own name; Berkins and Fernández 2005), its follow-up *Cumbia, copeteo, y lágrimas* (Cumbia, drinks, and tears; Berkins 2007a), and a related review publication that synthesized community-based studies in Latin America and the Caribbean (Borgogno and REDLACTRANS 2009). Additionally, I analyze the "Expectativas" campaign because it directly mobilized findings from these studies. *La gesta del nombre propio* (Berkins and Fernández 2005) was one of the earliest publications that I define as an "epidemiological biography," and it was the first I encountered that was undertaken largely by community-based researchers involved in feminist and travesti activism. It also explicitly theorizes and critiques police and state violence in its framing, where others simply include police violence as a variable (Berkins and Fernández 2005, 5–6). While this study and its follow-up (Berkins 2007a) were not necessarily representative of all epidemiological biographies in tone, their explicit politicized positioning reflects some of the implicit positions within other documents. In addition, each is highly representative in its synthesis of biography and quantification and in its emphasis on interventions centering material relief.

The numbers that activists generated were devastating. This provoked both anger and action on the part of some of those who were only recently encountering the profound effects of institutional violence on travesti and trans- lives. For example, the stark estimate of a thirty-five-year life expectancy stunned the creative director for the "Expectativas" campaign and guided his artistic focus: "The data on life expectancy for trans people were quite astonishing to me. For this reason, I looked for a campaign that would have the same impact" (Fundación Huésped 2014).[9]

The images in the "Expectativas" campaign aimed to visually translate the devastation articulated in the numbers. These were rendered from the shoulders up, directly facing the viewer (see Figure 3). In a split-image effect, the left side of the face invites a reading as masculine, while the right side offers cues of trans-femininity. The typically masculine name (Ariel) printed on the left shows only a date of birth. On the right is a feminine name (Alejandra), and under it is a set of dates indicating that for the presumptively transfeminine subject of the photo, death has arrived at thirty-five. Echoing the visual spectacle of before-and-after photographs of gender transition, the image seems designed to alarm a (nontrans-) viewer.

This was only one of several posters that appeared on signs around the city and on social media, each depicting different names and faces. However, each of the campaign's images followed the same visual script: the left side showed a masculine name, face, and birth date, and the right side showed a transfeminine face and name accompanied by a completed life span of thirty-five years. As in the other images associated with the campaign, Figure 3's caption claims that the life expectancy of trans- people in Argentina is thirty-five. However, the notable absence of transmasculine images from the campaign points to slippages between travesti life and gender nonnormativity more generally. In this campaign, the early death of the travesti poster child became the paradigmatic figure for trans- life in the nation—even as most travestis would not describe themselves as trans-, and even as life span estimates sprung from research conducted primarily among travestis and transfeminine people.

While the ad campaign took place in 2014, the data from which it drew dated back to the early 2000s, when travesti activists began incorporating statistical data-gathering within activist organizing. Many of these projects involved partnerships with academic researchers and foundations, but they were generally characterized by travesti or trans- leadership, coordination, or research teams. While formats ranged, many paired graphs and charts with photos or biographical narratives. Late travesti activist, researcher, and theorist Lohana Berkins led two of these studies with trans- and travesti collaborators, fellow activists, and academic researchers (Berkins and Fernández 2005; Berkins 2007a).

Berkins, who passed away in 2016, was an indomitable presence in travesti and feminist circles in Buenos Aires since the 1980s. In the 1990s, when the public surveillance of travestis remained at a fever pitch (despite the transition to democracy following the end of the Jorge Rafael Videla dictatorship in 1981), Berkins was a leader in anticriminalization movements. She worked with various organizations before founding the Association for the Fight for Transvestite and Transsexual Identity (Asociación Lucha por la Identidad Travesti-Transexual) in 1998. She was repeatedly jailed and estimates spending a cumulative nine years of her life locked up (Baird 2013). During the first decade of the 2000s, she was involved in transnational human rights campaigns and abortion access struggles along with trans- and travesti organizing. In 2008, she led the formation of a travesti textile cooperative, named after her late comrade, Nadia Echazú.[10] Berkins was deeply invested in coalitional politics, and she foregrounded her position as a communist, a feminist, and an Indigenous person from the provinces as much as she foregrounded being travesti. Along with Marlene

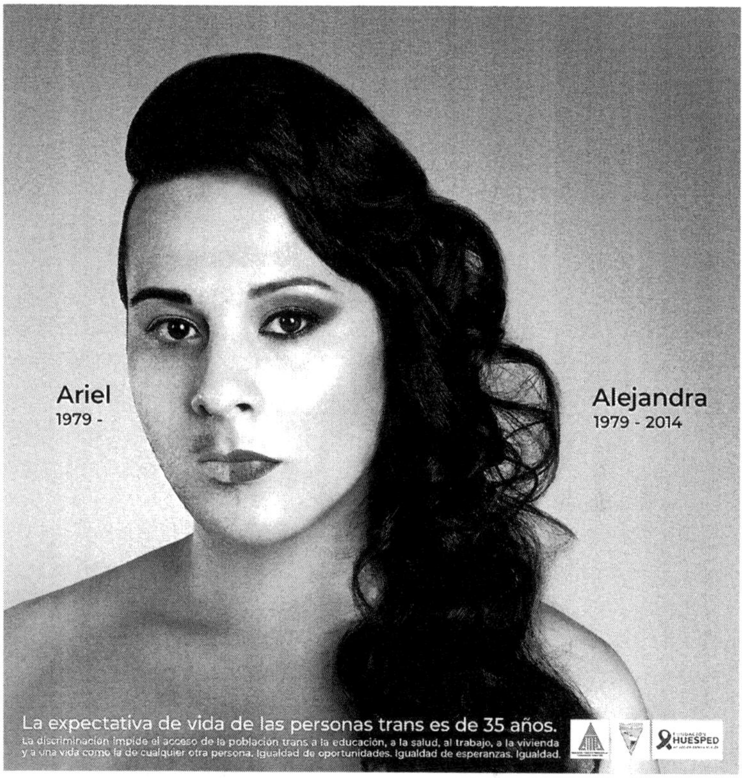
Ariel
1979 -
Alejandra
1979 - 2014
La expectativa de vida de las personas trans es de 35 años.
La discriminación impide el acceso de la población trans a la educación, a la salud, al trabajo, a la vivienda
y a una vida como la de cualquier otra persona. Igualdad de oportunidades. Igualdad de esperanzas. Igualdad.
FUNDACIÓN HUESPED

Figure 3. Poster from "Expectativas" Campaign (ATTTA, REDLACTRANS, and Fundación Huésped 2014).

Wayar (2018), Berkins (2007b) played a foundational role in theorizing travesti as a political position.

Berkins also maintained a close relationship with Josefina Fernández, an Argentine anthropologist who, up until her recent retirement, held a position at the University of Buenos Aires. Fernández authored a popular 2004 book about travesti identity entitled *Disobedient Bodies* (*Cuerpos Desobedientes*).[11] In this book, Fernández—who is not trans- or travesti—describes her initial connections with travesti groups being forged through feminist activism in the 1990s, during travestis' struggles against criminalization. Fernández co-coordinated research and publication of *La gesta del nombre propio* with Berkins, but Berkins was a sole coordinator for *Cumbia, copeteo, y lágrimas.* Indeed, in Berkins's (2007a, 9) introduction to the study, she expresses the desire for "travestis, transsexuals and transgender people [to] participate actively in the production of knowledge about our lives, needs and wants."[12] In each study, Fernández and Berkins worked with other institutionally affiliated and independent researchers—who also generally identified as activists—as well as with noninstitutionally affiliated travestis as community-based researchers.[13]

Research for both studies was financially supported by a Global North–based foundation. The first of these (Fernández and Berkins 2005) collected demographic information about "*travestis, transexuales,* [and] *transgéneros*" (excluding transmasculine people) from several locales within the capital province of Buenos Aires (including the city of Buenos Aires). The follow-up study (Berkins 2007a) used the same research design but also extended to cities across several other provinces (and included a small number of transmasculine participants). The focus on travesti and transfeminine participants was in large part shaped within the crucible of activism and advocacy of the late 1990s and early 2000s, in which travestis were organizing against highly public forms of harassment.[14]

Each research team gathered data from contacts that epidemiologists might call "nonrandom" samples. They reported results by locale. The small samples were not disaggregated by race or ethnicity, income, or other conventional epidemiological variables. Each study opened with an introduction, a collection of photographs, and lists of the names of travestis who had passed away. Graphical displays of data and interpretive analyses followed these.

Researchers surveyed respondents about education, earnings, housing, health, and violence, among other topics. Importantly, these explicitly included items about police harassment and violence. The first substantive results section in Berkins and Fernández (2005) is entitled "Travestismo and Police Violence." The chapter—attributed to Fernández (2005)—opens with quantitative results of the survey: eighty-six of one hundred travestis experienced police violence, followed by a distressing firsthand account from late travesti activist Nadia Echazú of being violently restrained and repeatedly struck by four police officers (Berkins and

Fernández 2005, 39). The chapter then draws on narratives of both travestis and police records to describe how municipal codes have been selectively mobilized to criminalize gender nonnormativity.

These were administrative regulations (not criminal ones) that delegated to police the power to regulate public life that extended beyond the national penal code. Installed during the Pedro Eugenio Aramburu dictatorship (which ousted President Perón in 1955), two of these articles affected travesti life most profoundly. One prohibited "those that publicly wear clothes of the opposite sex" while the other restricted sexual solicitation (which is not prohibited by the national penal code).[15] Following Buenos Aires's independence in 1997 as an autonomous district, these misdemeanor codes were replaced by a new municipal code. This shift revoked some of the power that police had formerly wielded to immediately arrest people for allegedly cross-dressing or sex work. After a brief drop-off in arrests, a conservative lobby pressed for increased criminalization, focusing in particular on travesti sex work. New provisions emphasized preventing "scandal" and disturbing public peace and were accompanied by arrests and fines (Berkins and Fernández 2005, 42–46). *La gesta del nombre propio* combines a detailed analysis of these regulatory shifts and their consequences, interweaving these with italicized firsthand reports by travestis who had been arrested, sexually abused, or beaten by police.

The imprecise charge of "disturbing the peace" or "public scandal" was used as a broad justification for harassment, arrest, and surveillance. As Berkins and Fernández (2005, 55) write, "to have a travesti identity, in the perspective of some representatives of the City of Buenos Aires, is synonymous with criminality." As discussed in this book's Introduction, Argentine travesti subjectivity is legible through racialized class and sexualized labor. These researchers make clear that travestis have also been made legible by being defined in their very existence as criminal. Given their subject position as migrants, Indigenous, Afro-descended, poor, and involved in sex work, criminalization was simultaneously racialized, classed, gendered, and sexualized.

The data that community-based researchers collected in both studies detailed ranging forms of police abuse or violence. As Figure 4 and Table 2 show, police abuse was a specific category of analysis in each study. In the earlier study (Figure 4), the vast majority of those surveyed (86 percent, as depicted in the pie chart) reported suffering police abuse. The accompanying bar chart below shows a breakdown of the types of abuse, including insults or jokes (experienced by 87.7 percent of those surveyed), physical aggression (72.8 percent), discrimination (68.8 percent), or sexual abuse (40.2 percent). The later study (Berkins 2007a) provided more detail (Table 2). In it, many reported being illegally detained. High numbers also reported being struck or being sexually abused, and many also reported insults or having bribes demanded of them. Some said that they were subjected to torture.

This emphasis on criminalization and the resulting state violence stands apart from dominant forms of epidemiological analysis. Both studies queried respondents about police violence within a section on violence (Berkins 2007a; Berkins and Fernández 2005). Here, data display enfolds state violence within statistics on violence more generally, reflecting an implicit claim to its non-exceptional status. In a section of *Cumbia, copeteo, y lágrimas,* Berkins (2007a, 126) summed up data on police abuse in a section called simply "Violencia" (Violence), emphasizing that those who serve in the role of "protector" are in fact primary among those who violate travestis' safety:

> What is the police? For one thing, the fact that state agencies continue to be systematic violators of human rights tells us that authoritarian practices and mentalities are still present today in the State, and have not been removed during democracy. Thus, the so-called "terrorist state" (which refers to that strange combination in which the one who guards the laws is the law's main violator), the state turned against society, continues to be a daily reality for a set of subordinate sectors.[16]

Significantly, this "set of subordinate sectors" includes travestis, transsexuals, and trans- people, among many others, using slang terms to describe other groups marginalized along lines of racialized class and targeted by police:

> Young thieves [pibes y pibas chorros], travestis, transsexuals, transgender people, slum dwellers [villeros y villeras], sex workers, people with dark skin [morochas y morochos], and migrants are subjected to a double violation of our citizenship and our integrity: the first, by being subjected to situations of violence; the second, by not being able to appeal to a higher authority, because those same authorities initiated the aggression.[17]

These groups were not mutually exclusive, of course—travestis were regularly interpellated as sex workers, slum dwellers, migrants, and thieves and were regularly racialized as nonwhite—regardless of what was indeed true about them. Yet, as this list indicates, researchers also recognized the interconnections between multiple forms of pathologization and criminalization. Finally, Berkins (2007a, 126) and her research team identified policing as a structural problem rather than one involving individual so-called bad actors:

> The information collected in this survey (as well as the work of other organizations that defend human rights) make it impossible to think of police abuses as individual problems that members of the force carry out. On the contrary, it is an institutional violence. This should not lead us to think that the police officer who hits us, mistreats us or assaults us is innocent; rather, they are the individual responsible for an act of greater responsibility that falls, ultimately, on a political decision.[18]

In this sense, they countered a liberal fantasy of state violence as a past relic of the dictatorial rule and instead posited policing as an ongoing source of racialized, classed, sexualized, and gendered institutional violence.[19] Acknowledging that travestis were not the sole targets of this violence, they still drew on graphs, charts, and stories to describe some of the particular effects of this violence.

The notion of institutional violence also frames health-care practice in each study (Gutiérrez 2005, 73; Berkins 2007a, 105–6). Biographical narratives describe specific instances of discrimination, neglect, or criminalization in the course of medical care

(Gutiérrez 2005, 71, 74–76). For example, in a chapter on health-care practices in the study authored by sociologist María Alicia Gutiérrez (2005), she reports on activist Diana Sacayán's reflections about travestis' frequent avoidance of hospitals and other formal sites of health care. Here, Sacayán describes the tendency for travestis to seek informal resources when ill or injured: "People don't go to the hospital because they know that the police might be involved. In this case, they go to the street to see how they can be cured" (80).[20] One of the photos included in the book depicts a travesti with long hair, reclining in a hospital bed, wearing nasal cannula, and speaking with a visitor sitting beside her. The caption dates and describes the photo: it is 2001, and the patient is HIV-positive and in a Buenos Aires hospital—in the male wing (Berkins and Fernández 2005, 27). Sacayán herself was no stranger to the abuse that took place in hospitals. In her chapter, Gutiérrez (2005, 87–91) includes Sacayán's complaints of discrimination in two public hospitals, including one in Buenos Aires. In one of these, Sacayán describes seeking a tuberculosis prophylactic and requesting that the doctor refer to her by her last name, as her masculine legal first name remained on her legal identification. The doctor did not respect this request, and when Sacayán protested, he commented that she could seek care elsewhere (87–88). Two years later, the Ministry of Health adopted formal policies dictating the use of self-identified name and gender, as well as placement within hospitals (Cutuli 2015, 300).

Authors link these dynamics not only to systematic marginalization but also to neoliberal restructuring of the health system. Since public-health decentralization following the 2001 economic crisis, Gutiérrez (2005, 72–73) asserts, "health is not considered a social good, but rather a commodity acquired through market mechanisms."[21] Authors present the data that follows in quantitative graphs about who regularly gets health care and discuss hospitals or clinics as sites where respondents encountered violence (Berkins 2007a, 171, 176; Berkins and Fernández 2005, 125, 130). These data are supported by narratives that point to the stratifying effects of hospitals adapting to austerity regimes. In *Cumbia, copeteo, y lágrimas,* travesti activist and theorist Marlene Wayar (2007, 49) describes how HIV-positive travestis are sent to "die on the streets."

"The hospital economy," she asserts, "doesn't support squandering its supplies, generic medication, beds, food, and overstrained and underpaid nursing care. We die on the streets while others bear HIV with a minimum of quality of life" (49).[22] In this account, HIV-positive people still cope with only a minimum of care in the dwindling distribution of publicly supported health care. Travestis, however, are expelled from accessing even this care minimum.

These modes of data presentation thus contest dominant epidemiological concepts of risk factors, which implicitly situate police, health-care providers, and other authoritative state and nonstate actors as protectors from rather than instigators of violence and endangerment. As such, researchers place responsibility on institutions and the state to make tangible changes to expand access to health and institutionalize decriminalization. In *Cumbia, copeteo, y lágrimas,* Berkins closes a section entitled "Nuestros Cuerpos, Nuestra Salud" (Our bodies, our health) with a demand for substantive change rather than a policy declaration: "As we have pointed out, the formal declamation of the right to adequate health care is not enough, it is necessary to develop policies that translate this into concrete possibilities for us here and now" (Berkins 2007a, 110).[23]

In addition to organizing data in a manner that emphasized the institutionalized causes of health disparities, researchers also requested that respondents name travesti and trans- friends who had died in the past five years, including cause and age at death. In the second study, the number of deaths recorded by respondents in each study were totaled, and average age at death was calculated (Berkins 2007a, 16; Berkins and Fernández 2005, 13). Results of these calculations showed that 9 percent died before the age of twenty-one, 43 percent died between twenty-two and thirty-one, and 33 percent between thirty-two and forty-one. Researchers took pains not to overreach methodologically, explaining that "even though these data cannot replace a census, they account for this current impossibility by doing something similar" (Berkins 2007a, 16). Figures 4 and 5 show two images from *La gesta del nombre propio,* exemplifying its combined approach to quantitative presentation and biographical narrative (Berkins and Fernández 2005). In addition to Figure 4's quantitative reporting,

Figure 5 contains a captioned photo of travesti activist Mónica León and several others holding a banner during a Pride march in the year 2000. The adjacent page is filled with several columns containing the names of travestis who passed away during the study. This list is one of nine such pages in the publication. Table 2 shows a somewhat more detailed display of data from the *Cumbia, copeteo, y lágrimas* study, which examines experiences of police abuse by region (Berkins 2007a). A subsequent regional study in Latin America and the Caribbean later presented an estimate of

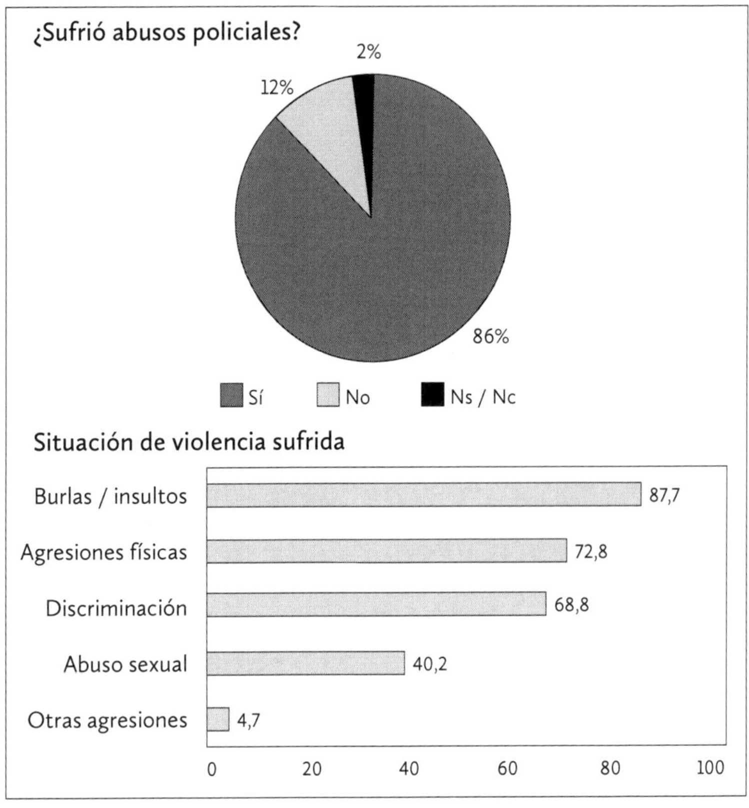

Figure 4. One of the data display pages from the first community-based study about experiences of police violence. The headings read, "Have you suffered abuse by police?" and "The situation of the violence you suffered." The bar graph lists mocking and insults, physical aggression, discrimination, sexual abuse, and other violations. From *La gesta del nombre propio* (Berkins and Fernández 2005, 129).

"average life expectancy of the trans community" (Borgogno and REDLACTRANS 2009). While also careful to stipulate methodological constraints, it offered an average figure of 35.5 to 41.25 years, attributing this to data from multiple community groups throughout the region (54).

Celeste
Abril
Micolosa
Daniela
Lourdes
Estrella
María José
Mariela
Karina Ferguson
Rosalinda
Cecilia
Romi
Vivi
Mary/Martin
Yiyi
Cristal

Rubi
Karen
Heidi
Cher
Andrea de Lugano
Marisa de Lugano
Daniela de Lugano
Stefanía de San Martín
Mónica de San Martín
Sasha
Carla Kustnier
Judith
La Rata
Silvana
Mariana
Barbi

Margarita
Jorgelina
Wendy
Jackeline
Princesa
Miriam
Yanina
Pamela
Andrea
Ángela
Flavia
Marcela
Agustina La Pedro
La Verde
Grisel
Giselle

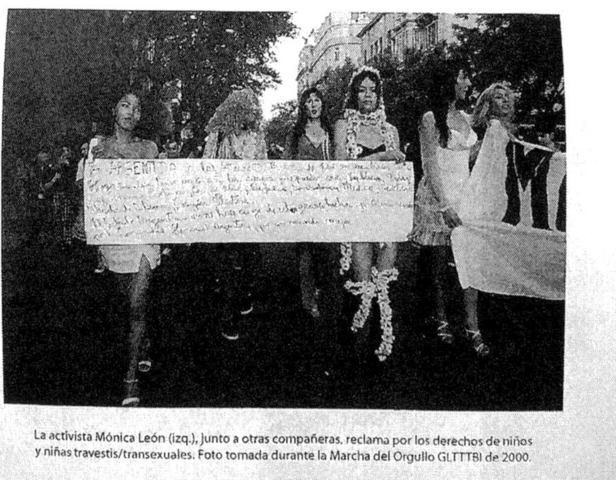
La activista Mónica León (izq.), junto a otras compañeras, reclama por los derechos de niños y niñas travestis/transexuales. Foto tomada durante la Marcha del Orgullo GLTTTBI de 2000.

Figure 5. The image shows two facing pages, one consisting of names of travestis who passed away during the course of the study and the other displaying a photograph of a street protest. From *La gesta del nombre propio* (Berkins and Fernández 2005, 29–30).

Table 2. Types of Police Abuse (Of total cases of people suffering abuses)

Type of abuse	Northwest	Central	South	Western interior	Total
Illegally detained	73.0%	97.0%	78.4%	86.4%	82.7%
Physically struck	49.4%	81.8%	45.9%	40.9%	57.9%
Sexually abused	53.9%	72.7%	21.6%	13.6%	50.0%
Bribe demanded	34.8%	16.7%	37.8%	27.3%	29.0%
Tortured	25.8%	7.6%	16.2%	13.6%	17.3%
Insulted	22.5%	1.5%	13.5%	27.3%	15.0%
Other type of abuse	22.5%	6.1%	51.4%	22.7%	22.4%
Total cases	89	66	37	22	214

This shows a sample data display about experiences of police violence in various regions throughout Argentina from the second community-based study. It lists responses by region and type of abuse. Reproduced from *Cumbia, copeteo, y lágrimas* (Berkins 2007a, 177) and translated from the original Spanish.

Despite these circumspect claims, an average figure of travesti and trans- life expectancy—namely, thirty-five—has since traveled. In addition to the "Expectativas" campaign, a report by the Inter-American Commission on Human Rights (OAS 2014, 3) mentions it, and it has circulated on the blogosphere and in the news media (La Información 2016; Magness 2018; O'Hagan 2018). While researchers had taken care not to overgeneralize their data, statistical conflations in interpretation appeared in media and policy interventions, largely through the variability in how populations were named. The 2012 Gender Identity Law, for example, referred to a disaggregated group of travestis, transexuales, and transgéneros, while the "Expectativas" campaign referred only to "*personas trans*"—trans- people—in its presentation of aggregate life expectancy (though ads showed only transfeminine subjects).[24]

The "Expectativas" campaign visually displayed these collapses in the split-image of the paradigmatically short-lived travesti. The paradoxical collapse of *travesti* into *personas trans* carried a series of implications about who was assumed to be at the center of policy interventions. It did so by focusing political attention almost exclusively on not only transfemininity but travesti subjectivity—which, as I have mentioned, is a racialized, criminalized, and classed position, as well as a sexualized/gendered one. This had the effect of foregrounding very particular forms of precarity and exposure to violence that were far from being shared by all Argentines who claimed transness. It is not *solely* femininity—and specifically, particular forms of racialized, classed, and sexualized femininity enacted by travestis—that became a target for state and interpersonal violence. For example, in 2021, a young Argentine trans- man named Tehuel de la Torre disappeared after what was supposed to be an interview for a restaurant job but seems to have been a trap. However, these forms of spectacularized violence most directly target travestis. The aggregations between travestis and other trans-identified people were nevertheless tactically useful in leveraging specific collective material changes. I return to the effects of these collapses in a discussion about statistical collectivization in the following pages.

While perhaps nonrepresentative, epidemiological biographies' claims about reduced life expectancy appeared to play a role in legislative debates leading up to the Gender Identity Law's passage. Before the congressional vote on the law, legislator Vilma Ibarra argued that "trans community members are generally people with the lowest life expectancies, and with the most difficulty completing schooling, and they are expelled, in general, from the labor sectors. They suffer enormous discrimination and social violence."[25] Ibarra's remarks not only highlighted the aggregated brevity of life as a concern, they also echoed epidemiological biographies' framing of structural and historical harm—though she did not emphasize state complicity or violence.

Since the passage of the Gender Identity Law, activist-driven legal strategies in Buenos Aires and throughout the nation have continued to build on this framing of criminalization and state violence as primary health risks. In 2018, Santa Fe, Argentina, passed a provincial law specifically extending an existing economic reparations program to travestis for political persecution during the military dictatorship (Caminos 2018). Travesti and trans- activists have been working on a national version of this bill since 2014, although it has not yet come up for a congressional vote. If passed, it would provide reparations for trans- people and travestis who have been targets of state violence both during and after the military dictatorship (Abogad*s por los Derechos Sexuales 2016; Conti 2016). The bill asserts that "trans people were—and in many cases continue to be—victims of a repressive state apparatus, both in times of dictatorship and in democracy" and directly cites an epidemiological biography as evidence (Conti 2016; Berkins 2007a). Quoting *Cumbia, copeteo, y lágrimas,* for example, the bill indicts what Berkins (2007a, 126) calls the "terrorist state" for enabling law enforcement to "criminalize trans identity" (Conti 2016).

Activist researchers' focus on state violence and criminalization as causal factors in reducing life chances has thus persisted in the popular imagination and regulatory domain in Argentina. Many of the community-based researchers who contributed to epidemiological biographies were directly affected by the conditions of criminalization and violence they represented. Their experiential insights led to a distinct means of thinking epidemiologically about the nonneutrality—indeed, often the *terror*—of actions undertaken though state formations of power. In utilizing inventive data-presentation techniques and asking different questions about health, they demonstrated how experts and authorities such as police, medical experts, and judges instigated state violence rather than protected certain travestis and trans- people from conditions of imperilment.

Social Movements and the Production of Population-Health Knowledge

Trans- and travesti activists entered a landscape of health and medicine already transformed by collective action on the part of social movements. As I discussed in chapter 1, trans- depathologization draws not only on efforts to depsychopathologize sexuality but also on other legacies of social movements that sought to refigure the power relations of science and medicine without surrendering access to vital aspects of health care. Some of these were specific to Argentine history in ways that contributed to their work to assert collective material demands over and above legal recognition.

Many trans- and travesti activists in Argentina lived through the prolonged period of the Videla dictatorship before the formal transition to democracy with Raúl Alfonsín's presidency in 1983.

The dictatorial state tracked the actions of travestis (as well as others they interpreted as nonnormative with regard to sex/gender), since Argentine fascism linked these subjectivities to political subversion (Rizki 2020). However, as trans- studies scholar Cole Rizki (2020) points out, police surveillance did not end with the transition to democracy. In fact, up until its dissolution in 1998, the Intelligence Office of the Buenos Aires Provincial Police continued surveilling emergent travesti political activity. As Rizki contends, the persistence of police violence in addition to ongoing political surveillance undermines a popular narrative that relegates state violence to history.

This echoes Berkins's (2007a) claims about the enduring violence of state security even after the end of the dictatorship and the Dirty War. For travesti activists, the disingenuousness of liberalism's claim to freedom led to a political skepticism. Rather than focusing on individual claims to formal recognition, travesti activists focused on collective forms of redress. Citing an interview between Berkins and Hebe de Bonafini, the president of the Madres de la Plaza de Mayo Association, Rizki (2020, 90) describes how Berkins in particular was inspired by the Madres' efforts to demand redress through a collective political force rather than on an individual basis. Indeed, quantification (and technoscience) have also proven crucial to the Madres and the Abuelas de la Plaza de Mayo to substantiate their political claims for redress and reparation.[26]

Epidemiological biographies framed questions of health in a manner similar to working-class health-based movements in Argentina. Popular health, or *salud popular,* took shape within and beyond existing Argentine movements, including among *piqueteros.* Piqueteros have gained recognition as a group of working-class Argentines that mobilized in the 1990s to resist President Carlos Menem's neoliberal policies. "Popular health" emerged as one way for this group to make claims on the state, despite being involved in informal labor markets that precluded their representation by trade unions. In her work on the development of popular-health movements, Argentine anthropologist Sol Logroño (2019) quotes an activist who explains that health is much more than "being sick." Instead, it is "something collective, that is not an individual disease process of a person but rather a collective social construction."[27] The authors of the epidemiological biographies I discuss here took a similar position, pointing out that health could be collectively constructed not only by addressing illness but also by attending to the institutionalized violence of policing and marginalization in health care, housing, and employment.

In making this case, the authors of epidemiological biographies drew on modes of quantification that evoke the techniques of "popular epidemiology" (Brown 1993), in which nonscientist political actors—including activists—use quantification and scientific authority to identify and solve health-related problems and provoke political action. Popular epidemiology identified "social structural factors" as direct and primary *causes* of ill health (18). In this sense, it presaged social epidemiology by transforming biography into population health. In the case of epidemiological biographies, however, data did not stand alone. Quantification was accompanied by emotionally charged images, stories, and long lists of comrades who had passed away.

Epidemiological biographies also filled a gap. When these epidemiological biographies were written, population-health research on trans- people and travestis—not to mention contemporary state violence—was far from robust. Community-based researchers thus circulated these studies in a milieu that Scott Frickel and colleagues (2010) and David J. Hess (2016) call "undone science." Even though standard population-health research methods might appear necessary to translate experience into epidemiological data, and data into action, there remain possibilities for persuasive claims-making irrespective of epidemiology's stringent requirements for attributing causality. The space left by undone science in both trans- health and state violence made room for the authors of these epidemiological biographies to circulate small-scale studies with significant effects on policy.

It was this explicit bridging—of collective and individual and of population quantification and emotionally charged narrative—that made epidemiological biographies a unique intervention. As they presented the multitude of barriers that interrupted the flourishing of travesti life, epidemiological biography authors linked individual health with broader political conditions (Nelson 2011). What was most salient, though, was their pointed contestation of what data mattered most in rendering an accurate epidemiological representation about health inclusive of state violence. In this regard, activist researchers issued correctives to dominant epidemiological paradigms by demonstrating the limits of population health, both in its methods and in its foci. Said otherwise, activist researchers highlighted epidemiological gaps and revealed them as part and parcel of the state violence and abandonment they worked to represent through their studies.

Such a move also reflects the phenomenon of "travar el saber" that Juliana Martínez and Salvador Vidal-Ortiz (2021) discuss in the realm of travesti-centered education. Escaping direct translation, this is a phrase that Berkins and others have used to "reconceptuali[ze] . . . knowledge-making and education through the centering of travesti experience and theorising" (669). As Martínez and Vidal-Ortiz point out, *travar el saber* is not precisely equivalent to "transing knowledge," although that might be one way to translate the phrase. Instead, they argue, it refers to a productive malfunction or obstruction that they term "jamming-as-intervention" (669). "By jamming the system," they write, "*travar* propitiates a necessary rebooting that is, at its core, regenerative" (669).[28] In this sense, travesti knowledge, life, and experience bring about dissonances in social systems that become apparent in their very presence and action within them. However, travesti theorizing rejects the view that their presence or existence is indeed the problem and instead proposes that these dissonances reveal "the system itself as problematic, as the issue that needs to be addressed" (669).

Taking this approach, the authors of the epidemiological biographies I discuss here are insistent in their focus on state violence and their assertion that this is a major problem for the health and well-being of travestis. In presenting data about police violence, they not only make this point but also underscore the troubling lack of data to track police violence after the transition to formal political democracy. Indeed, the authors of epidemiological biographies are among a broader group addressing the widespread inaction among many state actors in Argentina (and elsewhere) to aggregate population-based data on state violence. Community-based and journalistic research have taken the lead in generating these forms of accounting, which Morgan Currie and colleagues (2016) call "counter-data action."[29] Such work not only addresses knowledge gaps, it also contests the neutrality of official and expert data and reveals some of the mystifications of quantification (Bruno, Didier, and Vitale 2014). Some modes of counter-data action adopt a tone of impartiality, while others—like the epidemiological biographies I discuss here—draw on what Deborah B. Gould (2009, 230) calls collectively "channeled . . . grief-filled rage." Or perhaps in the case of these studies, *furia travesti.*

Population, Speculative Estimation, and Statistical Collectivization

Activists' turn to quantitative research came about only after years of efforts to air their grievances in other ways. Whether it was their turn to quantification, a shift in political tide, or other conditions that led to the material shifts they attained, it appeared that their embrace of the numerical opened up new avenues of claims-making. Yet, in their turn to the logics of population health—partial and ambivalent though they were—they also became enmeshed in the politics of aggregation in which population health must traffic. They undertook this project by enacting what I call "statistical collectivization." This refers to collective political action that intervenes in and reformulates dominant modes of statistical aggregation and conceptualization, often working to redefine a problem.

In my research, activists and advocates mobilized statistical collectivization to define bureaucratic and state violence as the most direct risks to travesti and trans- health. Such action contrasted with health behavioral models in epidemiology, which situate "upstream" factors as important and potentially causal, but in an analytic background that largely escapes scientific certainty or political intervention (Short and Mollborn 2015). The epidemiological biographies I examined instead framed criminalization and state violence as directly and primarily constitutive of negative health outcomes, whether "by act or omission" (Berkins 2007b). But to demonstrate negative health outcomes in the aggregate, population—or at least some sense of it—became a critical tool for leveraging empirical evidence and marshaling speculative estimation about the violent conditions for which states must take responsibility.

While certain population-health researchers are also centrally concerned with structural violence, few trouble the concept of "population" itself. However, critics contend that notions of population are central to subjugating political control. Similarly, scholars of feminist science studies and social studies of medicine caution that the concept of "population" is freighted with a eugenic logic that produces racialized hierarchies of social value. Trans- studies has also grappled with ambivalence about demography and population health, though the increasing emphasis on statistical analyses in "making transgender count" is reflected by growth in trans- population-health research (Currah and Stryker 2015). In this regard, social theorists view state violence not simply as a neglected variable of concern but rather as constitutive of the historical emergence of the concept of population itself.

For Michel Foucault (2003), for example, the advent of population as an object of knowledge and technique of governance was critical to formations of modern state power. In this regard, the mobilization of statistics—the science of the state—accompanies the enactment of state power and state racism (Scott 1999; Foucault 2003). It is through the figure of population that Foucauldian scholars assert that states administer aggregate forms of life by marking some as assets to sustain and others as drains to diminish or eliminate (Foucault 2003). Feminist science studies are also concerned with the biopolitical operations of population. For example, Michelle Murphy (2017) asserts that the concept of "population" cannot be disengaged from notions of surplus life, state racism, Malthusian theory, and their accompanying necropolitical ends.

In their work to statistically collectivize, community-based researchers also collapsed differences in subject position—including, for example, race and class. They also grouped a multitude of forms of transness and travesti identity into a singular sample, such that travesti femininity came to stand in for all "personas trans" (in the words of the "Expectativas" poster). As Sarah Lamble (2008, 36) points out in the context of primarily white-led community remembrance events for the mostly trans- women of color who have died as a result of violence, the universalizing reach of transness is part of what leads to a "narrative erasure of racialized violence." However, these researchers did *not* narratively subsume travesti identity into transness, nor were they necessarily in a position of privilege relative to the data and stories they presented. Rather, they adopted a tactic of statistical collapse to make a quantifiable case for material redress that they anticipated would benefit those who often bore the brunt of state exclusions.

Some trans- studies scholars share critiques of population as instrumental in defining people as legitimate or disposable—including within the broader social grouping of trans- people (Thompson and King 2015). For example, C. Riley Snorton and Jin Haritaworn (2013) describe how efforts for legal trans- inclusion turn on "value extraction" from the deaths of trans- women of color subjects. Such deaths, in their "nominal and numeric repetition," become "resources . . . for the articulation and visibility of a more privileged transgender subject" while eliding the differential racialized and classed conditions producing violence (71). "Trans necropolitics" thus sharpens lines between rights-worthy "recognizable" and disposable "subaltern" trans- subjects, resulting in conditional forms of admittance to citizenship and state security—often through selectively intensified police protection (74). Haritaworn, Adi Kuntsman, and Silvia Posocco (2013) call these dynamics "murderous inclusions." Other trans- studies scholars share these concerns but, despite serious misgivings, still identify population-health research as a site through which resources might be redirected toward marginalized people to enhance conditions of survival (Singer 2015; Thompson and King 2015). However, they remain concerned with the homogenizing gesture of population and the dangers of treating *transgender* as globally legible, particularly given the uneven material consequences of the erasures it performs (Dutta 2013; Thompson and King 2015; Singer 2006).

Social Travesticide and Redistributive Demands

The epidemiological biographies I studied did not generally prioritize citizenship rights in the form of antidiscrimination protections or securitization (in the mode of "murderous inclusions") but rather centered material relief. I argue that this shift was partly enabled by the refashioning work of statistical collectivization. This enacted a shift to state responsibility, partly by undertaking unconventional aggregative strategies.[30] Specifically, while epidemiological biographies glossed over questions of stratified population difference, their analysis incorporated state violence alongside nonstate violence, thus intervening in what activists saw as a fallacious separation between these.[31] Trans- rights claims have frequently relied on "respectability" claims that privilege whiteness and disavow sex work, blaming individual criminalized trans- subjects for the violence or poverty they experience (Aizura 2018, 91). Epidemiological biographies disrupted this narrative by framing state security forces as a source of violence and a danger to health and life, thus contesting the role of policing as protective and redirecting blame for perilous life conditions. I suggest that the shift to state responsibility thus led to an epidemiological and political refashioning of approaches to addressing trans- health.

I am suggesting that the intervention of these epidemiological biographies in 2005 and 2007 enabled the possibility for Guimaraes, a decade later, to make the claims she did about state responsibility and social travesticide. I am also suggesting that this intervention in part directed Argentine activists to prioritize demands for material access to publicly subsidized health care and to ease administrative processes for legal documentation change (Hollar 2018). These are the very domains that trans- legal scholar Dean Spade (2015, 15) calls "key administrative barriers to trans survival" that foster or delimit life chances.[32] The political focus on state responsibility emphasized concrete forms of access to means of survival over and above symbolic declarations of inclusion. Yet, even as Argentine activists intervened on these key barriers, the figure of the trans- population—along with its conceptual baggage—remained central.

These materially focused political objectives contrasted with a predominant parallel focus in United States–based trans- activism on antidiscrimination policies to mitigate health disparities. As I mentioned in the Introduction, trans- advocates have understandably focused on federal antidiscrimination provisions such as Rule 1557 of the Affordable Care Act to ensure broader access to care. However, substantial pressure on the Obama administration was required for it to explicitly assert gender identity as a protected category in Title IX antidiscrimination rules. In a far more aggressive register, the Trump administration endeavored to reverse this provision. Under the Biden administration, gender identity remains a protected status. However, a booming crescendo of state-level lawsuits are calling antidiscrimination provisions into question. Furthermore, even as Biden has appointed a trans- woman to the White House cabinet, he has flatly rejected proposals for universalizing health care through Medicaid for All. Even with antidiscrimination provisions in place, the difficulties associated with adjudicating and winning antidiscrimination claims have made these an unreliable form of protection. It was the paradox of appealing to justice at the hands of the primary violator of justice that led Berkins (2007a, 110) and her research team to reject the "formal declaration of the right to adequate health care" in favor of immediate material transformations and resource redistribution.[33]

It would appear that Argentine activists were able to advance their material demands to addressing barriers to survival through the techniques of quantification and narrative that they mobilized in epidemiological biographies. The notion of social travesticide rests on the explicit connections between bureaucratic and state violence, racialized and sexualized marginalization, and economic distribution that epidemiological biographies made. Such connections enabled activists to jam conventional logics by attributing responsibility for violence—even acts of violence by nonstate actors—to bureaucratic and state forces. Statistical collectivization thus redefined state security as violent and coercive rather than protective—and, in a sense, as infectious and transmissible to civilians in the form of masculinism, racialized misogyny, and transphobia. Furthermore, its explicit engagement with political economy found the Argentine state to be culpable for economic violence across both public and private sectors. Epidemiological biographies described travestis and trans- people as being historically and currently placed at risk within these dynamics and asserted that programs of redistribution and recompense were therefore an appropriate (if incomplete) intervention.

Activists drew on prior forms of activism to claim this as a "debt of democracy"—echoing one of the phrases used by the Madres de la Plaza de Mayo.[34] In this manner, statistical collectivization also articulated a failure of liberal citizenship and diverged from straightforward inclusionary claims. Rather than advancing travestis and trans- people as appropriate (and thus deserving) civil subjects, activists worked to compel state engagement based on entitlement to existence. While still mobilized through citizenship claims, these focused on entitlement to material relief rather than a symbolic normative value ascribed to state inclusion. Writing about activists in eastern India, Aniruddha Dutta (2013) describes a "*subversive re-fashioning* of normative political forms" that complicated straightforward citizenship claims and compelled action on the part of state actors. Extending Partha Chatterjee's (2004) work, Dutta (2013) suggests that Indian activists mobilized from both within and outside of civic domains, blurring lines between "deserving" civil subjects and "governed" populations. Similarly, the tactic of self-enumeration (Appadurai 2012) in epidemiological biographies catalyzed a powerful political bid irrespective of supposed deservingness. This was amplified by the use of bionarratives to vividly represent landscapes of bureaucratic, institutional, and state violence, which opened to demands for accountability and redress rather than securitization.

In their demands for decriminalization and concrete access to health care, the authors of epidemiological biographies made claims to health-care entitlement and decriminalization, and they certainly appealed directly to citizenship claims within this. In Berkins's (2007a, 126) description of state violence being inflicted on travestis, slum dwellers, and sex workers, those marginalized on the basis of racialized class experience a "double violation" ("doble violación") of rightful citizenship. However, the invocation of citizenship here is not a claim to respectability and desire for incorporation within the state. Rather, it is an assertion of the racialized, classed, gendered, and sexualized exclusions performed by the status of citizenship in the first instance. It is also an effort to lay bare the hypocrisy of postdictatorial Argentine statecraft in its claims to liberal democracy. From this grounding in the critique of citizenship, community-based researchers laid the empirical foundations not only to claim state redress but also to press for a radical reconsideration of regimes of accumulation and securitization.

Argentine activists used small-scale samples and nonstandard methods to represent the effects of harmful forces that dominant epidemiology could not readily demonstrate as causally valid. These forces—including violent policing, exclusion from labor, and racialized and sexualized violence—were made plain through both numbers and stories. Through such "militant mixed methods," activists enacted "counter-data action" to epidemiologically engage this nexus of "undone science" in trans- health and state violence (Currie et al. 2016; Frickel et al. 2010; Hess 2016).[35] In so doing, they persuasively asserted that state institutions instigated rather than arbitrated violence.

The travesti subjects of the studies I discuss were often subject to racialized violence and arrest, as well as systemic immiseration. But other trans- people are insulated from the most concentrated expressions of these dynamics: well resourced, transmasculine, and white trans- people might experience bureaucratic or state violence in far subtler terms. The epidemiological biographies I examined thus draw on what epidemiologists would call an "unrepresentative sample"—but the estimates the studies generated were extrapolated more generally. Often, publications emphasized that the estimate applied to trans- women, trans- women of color, or trans- women in the Americas (e.g., OAS 2014, 3), but they were rarely more specific.

Such aggregative slippages are meaningful and have often been a fulcrum for the "murderous inclusions" that Haritaworn, Kuntsman, and Posocco (2013) describe. Yet, in direct contrast to these dynamics, epidemiological biography data directed a political focus on those who were differentially exposed to perilous conditions. While murderous inclusions tend to expand state prosecutorial power to arbitrate antitrans- violence, these studies instead focused on labor conditions, bureaucratic and state violence, full access to health care, and other modes of material relief. In this manner, statistical collectivization contrasted with dominant trans- rights paradigms that center mainly on social tolerance and securitization. While the latter are largely divorced from political economic critiques of racialized immiseration, epidemiological biographies were direct in their economic analysis as expressed through both data and narrative. Ironically, the studies I examined enacted this thoroughly materialist politics in part by statistically eliding racialized and classed difference. Looking to the appendixes of each study, it is evident that researchers recorded some standard demographics, such as age, education level, and region in which people live. However, they made no distinctions between subgroups (travestis, transsexuals, and trans- people or between respondents on the basis of income), nor did they ask questions about race or immigration status. Further, researchers did not emphasize the predominance of transfemininity and travesti experiences, though this is certainly their narrative (and statistical) focus.

The travel of the age of thirty-five—made possible in part by Berkins and Fernández (2005) and Berkins (2007a)—may have been enabled by its very abstraction. However, the specific conditions of its emergence that epidemiological biographies carefully outlined have not necessarily traveled alongside this mobile estimate of life expectancy. Relatedly, trans- activists' more central intervention efforts to address the undone science of trans- population health—specifically in attributing causality to the effects of state and bureaucratic violence on community-wide health—has not been nearly as mobile. Nonetheless, I suggest that statistical collectivization has enacted tangible shifts in how activists and other stakeholders conceptualize trans- health and its primary objectives.

Statistical collectivization is a politicized demand for redress and a shift toward "social health" in which "therapeutic matters [are] inextricably articulated to social justice ones" (Nelson 2011, 10). This is the shift that travesti and trans- activists enacted by synthesizing population health and politicized analyses of structural inequity as crucial to conceptualizing trans- health. Moving from "individual" to "population health" has thus opened a field—though a narrow and somewhat perilous one—to foreground questions of state violence. Argentine epidemiological biographies produced persuasive evidentiary bases through which to engage data differently from dominant forms of epidemiological research.

Any methodological thinness stood less as a shortcoming and more as an indictment of epidemiological limits and attention. Through these means, activists diagnosed state and bureaucratic violence as first-order problems and fundamental causes of abbreviated life and compromised social health.

Many of the travesti and trans- researchers coordinating or taking part in such studies were directly affected by the dynamics they studied, and they often contributed their own biographical narratives to bolster quantitative evidence. Refusing behavioral explanations of abbreviated life, they instead faulted the Argentine state's generalized failure to foster material conditions for life—a claim that for some researchers opened into a broader racialized political economic critique. Further, in their focus on state agents and administrations as primary actors in imperiling trans- lives, they implicitly advanced a skeptical view of formal civil rights, favoring instead social and economic regulatory changes that they expected would address concrete conditions of life. As such, activist interventions skewed away from securitizing measures (e.g., more police protection, government-adjudicated antidiscrimination laws) and toward specific changes to regulations governing economic and goods distribution (e.g., health-care access, employment quotas, reparations). This constituted some degree of departure from the murderous inclusions of the struggles for trans- citizenship characterized by a cleaving of "deserving" from "undeserving" subjects.

In moving away from the formal civil rights claims that underpin many claims to trans- (as well as sexual and gendered) citizenship, the turn to a statistical lexicon advanced the key figure of *population*—inclusive of its Malthusian hauntings—to foreground structural dynamics that technologies of aggregation frequently obscure. Ironically, activists accomplished this in part by de-emphasizing differential insulation from violence and lack of access to goods, wealth, and state services. But the result was to direct attention *toward* markedly racialized, sexualized, classed, and gendered forms of subjugation. As Murphy (2017) nonetheless argues, it is precisely the deracialized and anonymized "quantity problem" of population that has justified the designation of "surplus" humans, as well as resulting regimes and infrastructures of immiseration and elimination. Statistical collectivization thus rests on and mobilizes tools of governance such as population to make distributive political claims in excess of liberal formal rights. In turning themselves into numbers to act politically, activists applied a dazzle camouflage to population.[36] Rather than mobilizing quantification as "state maps of legibility" (Scott 1999), they rendered legible the long-standing unaddressed concerns produced by sustained marginalization. However, even as activists opposed securitization and contested the legitimacy of state power, their claims remained within the space of regulatory distribution.

Trans- health's shift to population health is continuous with a more generalized turn outward from individual pathologies to broader collective conditions of life. It thus echoes shifts in biomedicine toward environment as a primary site of capacitation or limitation. However, rather than taking the form of distress as a condition of gendered interaction with a social environment, as discussed in chapter 2's analysis of diagnostic shifts, Argentine activists looked specifically to state institutions, security apparatuses, and laws as composing the "environment" in question. Within this milieu, they identified structural immiseration, racialized state violence, and misogynistic aggression as endemic to this environment. Such politicized research contesting state and bureaucratic violence found purchase in trans- health's turn outward—which also paralleled shifts within population health toward social or collective epidemiology and explicitly structural analyses of health.

Ruha Benjamin (2018, 56) riffs on W. E. B. Du Bois's (1903) famous question: "How does it feel to be a problem?" She instead posits, "How does it feel to be a . . . *population?* To be a racialized population, after all, is to be a stubborn *problem* and an insistent *people.*" In this insistence, she asks how we can "channel our tool-making prowess to artfully engender more just and equitable futures." Activists grappled with this question as they retooled population health as a basis for distributive claims. Statistical collectivization, in this instance, redirected trans- health away from behavior-based models and toward collective refusals of systemic harms. Their work raises pressing questions about the possibilities and limitations of quantification in politicized health research more generally.

In chapter 4, I discuss epidemiological biographies that New York activists and advocates also produced. Naming these *economized* epidemiological biographies, I show how they used these to bolster their successful efforts to eliminate a seventeen-year regulatory exclusion prohibiting Medicaid reimbursement for gender-affirming care. Like Buenos Aires–based activists, New York activists and advocates refashioned statistical data to foreground how racialized violence and structural poverty affect trans- health. However, they also drew on statistical speculations about the economic viability of reinstituting state coverage for gender-affirming care. Working with and against logics of austerity, activists used statistical collectivization and empirical biographies to contest the long-standing claims by state administrators and popular media that trans- therapeutics are too specialized, politicized, or expensive for public financing.

4 Saving Lives, Saving Money

Investing in Trans- Lives

> Healthcare for trans people is not "special" healthcare. It's just regular healthcare that non-trans people receive every day when they need it—but that is specifically denied to trans people.
>
> —Sylvia Rivera Law Project and GLAAD

> Funding transgender surgeries would have been a waste of taxpayer dollars. We're trying to cut back on Medicaid.
>
> —Marty Golden, New York State Senator, *New York Post*

> When the new [Medicaid] policy comes into effect, access to transition-related care could potentially save lives.
>
> —George Liam Steptoe, *NY City Lens*

On a winter day in downtown Manhattan in 2013, the New York State Department of Health hosted a population-health summit called "Making New York the Healthiest State: Achieving the Triple Aim." Presented by state health commissioner Nirav Shah, the event convened health-department workers, care providers, insurers, and other stakeholders to kick off New York State's four-year "Prevention Agenda" (Department of Health, New York State 2013). Governor Cuomo had entered office two years before and had promptly introduced a statewide initiative to save costs and improve outcomes in New York's Medicaid program. Commissioner Shah headed up this Medicaid Redesign Team (MRT) and touted the promise of "Achieving the Triple Aim" of care equity, prevention, and cost savings through a sustained review of quality measures, enrollee satisfaction and utilization data, and other measures. In addition to positioning himself as a vanguard population-health leader, Shah was a well-known figure among trans- activists and advocates. During his tenure, he and his staff had repeatedly dismissed, ignored, and resisted calls to lift a long-standing Medicaid exclusion preventing public coverage for trans- therapeutics.

The exclusion in question had been issued by New York State's Department of Health a decade and a half earlier, in 1998. It appeared in the state's social services regulations without a hearing and added a specific exclusion for state Medicaid payments for any surgical, hormonal, or psychological/psychiatric therapeutics related to what they called "gender reassignment" (Spade 2010). While many trans- Medicaid beneficiaries remained able to access coverage for hormones for the first few years after its implementation, this all changed in the early 2000s. Around that point, the Department of Health began flagging records with hormone prescriptions that were ostensibly "mismatched" with patient gender markers. Advocates at the Sylvia Rivera Law Project (SRLP)—a collective grassroots organizing project and legal agency for poor trans- people and trans- people of color—began to hear from clients that their hormone coverage was being cut off. Starting in about 2006, attorney advocates issued formal legal challenges to the provision, but after several years of unsuccessful courtroom battles, the exclusion remained in place.[1] Trans- communities and advocates were beginning to grow weary of the limitations of litigation efforts. Around 2012, a coalition of activists and advocates came together and decided to take the fight public.

While attorneys persisted in waging legal and regulatory challenges, advocates and grassroots activists mobilized a campaign to reframe public perceptions about trans- health and make demands on the Department of Health and other institutions. The campaign combined a multitude of tactics, including public education, petitioning, pressure on political officials, and direct-action campaigns. By the time the "Making New York the Healthiest State" population-health summit rolled around in late 2013, the group had honed their messaging. They framed the public provision of trans- therapeutics as a matter of care equity, prevention, and cost savings—objectives that aligned with the "Triple Aim" approach to health services that New York State population-health leaders were touting (Berwick, Nolan, and Whittington 2008; Department of Health, New York State 2013). Using quantitative techniques, activists and advocates asserted that public coverage for trans- therapeutics would lead to improved mental-health outcomes, a reduction in suicide rates, and an overall cost reduction for Medicaid.

As Commissioner Shah addressed summit attendees on that December day, a group of activists and advocates disrupted his presentation. They stood at the stage with a banner that read "Trans People Need Safe & Affordable Healthcare: Stop Discriminating, Shah" as they challenged him to commit to ending New York's discriminatory Medicaid provision. A few months later, activists and advocates staged a Valentine's Day action in front of the Department of Health building. With bundles of shiny red heart-shaped helium balloons in tow, upward of fifty protestors marched with signs and banners reading "Hey, Shah! Where's the Love? Trans people need safe & affordable healthcare now!" While he refused to acquiesce at that point, these and other actions made their mark. Less than two years later, the exclusion was formally lifted.

In this chapter, I discuss how New York activists and advocates adopted a strategy of statistical collectivization that overlapped with but also differed from the one undertaken by activist researchers in Buenos Aires. Specifically, I examine how they used quantification and population health to revise commonsense rhetorical claims about trans- therapeutics in their public form—much like activist researchers in Buenos Aires. However, in contrast with the approaches I outlined in chapter 3, I show how advocates and activists strove to frame new stories about imperilment in terms of prevailing state emphases on cost savings in health care. In addition to telling different stories about population-health risk, they also told different stories about *economic* risk to gain traction within United States austerity politics, even as they sharply contested the premise of trans- therapeutics as an unfair use of tax dollars. In what follows, I describe some of the epidemiological biographies that activists and advocates produced in New York—some of which, as I show, are more accurately described as "economized epidemiological biographies."

Working with and against logics of austerity, I show how activists and advocates astutely contested state administrators' and popular media's long-standing claims that trans- therapeutics are too specialized, too politicized, and too expensive for public financing. As they persuasively rejected these delegitimizing positions, they promised that broad access to trans- therapeutics could save money as it saved lives. Such a framing likely facilitated the victory that activists and advocates claimed in 2015 with the removal of the sixteen-year Medicaid exclusion. In so doing, however, they also placed both "risky subjects" (Patel 2017) and "economized life" (Murphy 2017) at the center of their political endeavors. This chapter explores the tensions between social movements' aspirations to enact redistributive claims and the specific tactics they are compelled to adopt in a political landscape so profoundly shaped by logics of austerity.

In what follows, I briefly discuss the methodological approaches of this chapter, which are not identical to those in chapter 3. Next, I describe the capaciousness of risk as a concept that enabled both financial shifts in health policy and forms of claims-making that worked in favor of trans- activists. Specifically, I show how activists and advocates contested the actuarial logics of state administrators who sought to exclude trans- therapeutics from public coverage by reframing trans- population health through revised economic assessments and projections. I follow this with close studies of several epidemiological biographies that circulated in and beyond New York, particularly as they turned to economization to make the medical, ethical, and economic case for trans- therapeutics. I then ethnographically describe the reversal of the exclusion in 2015, which culminated in both a celebration of the victory and consternation about the scarcity of trained surgeons qualified to deliver care. Finally, I conclude by engaging Geeta Patel's (2017) concerns about risk-pooling in activist claims-making and Michelle Murphy's (2017) apprehensions about "the economization of life," each of which argue for caution on the part of emancipatory projects in advancing tactics of aggregation. I end with these concerns *not* to suggest that activists and advocates were carrying the torch of neoliberalism or were unaware of the implications of their claims. To the contrary, I assert that activists and advocates carefully navigated narrow passageways of action to bring about material changes that addressed the racialized and immiserating conditions of certain forms of trans- life, even as they recognized that these actions could not enact the more sweeping changes they desired.

Methods

This chapter examines several examples of epidemiological biographies that circulated in and around New York from 2010 to 2014. I focus on materials produced as part of the coalition involved in the Medicaid access campaign during this time, as well as several community-based research studies leading up to the campaign's launch (GLAAD and Sylvia Rivera Law Project 2013a, 2013b, 2013c; Welfare Warriors Research Collaborative 2010; Sylvia Rivera Law Project 2014). As was the case in Buenos Aires, there were other examples of epidemiological biographies. The ones I analyze here best exemplify how New York activists and advocates adopted statistical collectivization to contest a central threat to public funding of trans- therapeutics (and care provision in general) in the United States: the figures of the scandalized taxpayer and the sparing public budget.

As I emphasized in the Introduction to this book, I do not consider this to be a strictly comparative study. As such, I am not making the argument that these epidemiological biographies were directly analogous to those that I analyzed in the previous chapter. Nevertheless, I am interested in the continuities and dissimilarities between the community-based studies that circulated in each study site. I observed how, in both sites, undone science made space for activists and advocates to make bold claims and stop state institutions from withholding resource allocation to poor trans- people. Because the Medicaid exclusion was lifted during the period of my study, I had the opportunity to hear direct reflections from activists and advocates about the campaign, its development, and its implications. This was not the case for most of the epidemiological biographies I analyzed in chapter 3. As such, this chapter contains more ethnographic data as well as primary source data and includes more background about the informal conversations that went into shaping the campaign.

The epidemiological biographies that I focus on in this chapter include the following: a participatory study by the Welfare Warriors Research Collaborative (2010) through Queers for Economic Justice called "A Fabulous Attitude: Low-Income LGBTGNC People Surviving and Thriving on Love, Shelter, and Knowledge"; a series of social media and videos produced by GLAAD in collaboration with the Sylvia Rivera Law Project, such as infographics entitled "Should Medicaid Cover Transgender Healthcare?" and "Everyone Needs Access to Safe, Reliable Healthcare" (Sylvia Rivera Law Project 2014), as well as a video series entitled "Healthcare for All," including "Give Trans People Access to the Care They Need" (GLAAD and Sylvia Rivera Law Project 2013a), "Healthcare Professional Calls for Care for All" (GLAAD and Sylvia Rivera Law Project 2013b), and "A Parent Calls for Healthcare for All" (GLAAD and Sylvia Rivera Law Project 2013c). In addition, I look to the fact sheet entitled "Eliminating the Medicaid Exclusion for Transition-Related Care in NYS: Good Public Health, the Right Thing to Do, and Ultimately a Cost-Saving Measure," produced by the Sylvia Rivera Law Project (2013), which set the stage for some of the assertions advanced in campaign materials. I focus on those resources that explicitly engaged Medicaid access (or, in the case of "A Fabulous Attitude," that directly preceded this work through its claims on welfare benefits).[2]

Much of the research that went into exposing the reactionary follies of the New York State Department of Health was undertaken by activists, attorneys, and other trans- advocates. Their labor often goes unrecognized, but it was critical in putting an end to the Medicaid trans- exclusion provision in New York State. The meticulous legal research that study participants and their colleagues undertook—often in close collaboration with activists—has been critical in grounding the insights I discuss in this chapter. I am grateful for the work they have done and for their generosity in sharing it with me.

Risk and Prevention: Repurposing the Triple Aim

The Birth of the Triple Aim

The Triple Aim currently is the dominant health-policy framework in the United States (Berwick, Nolan, and Whittington 2008). Developed just prior to the passage of the Affordable Care Act, it strives to balance individual health, population health, and cost containment through accountability and outcomes measures within health-care systems. The endeavor of the Triple Aim is to resolve the U.S. paradox of steep health-care expenditures and poor aggregate health outcomes. Sandra Tanenbaum (2017, 54) asserts that this is the latest in a series of progressively layered health-management strategies beginning with cost containment in the 1970s, adding quality improvement in the 1980s and 1990s, and eventually incorporating population health in the 2000s. As health-care systems have increasingly turned to population health as a requisite consideration, they have become more keenly attuned to the relevance of aggregate patient life beyond the clinic. Data-based population stratification has therefore become a cornerstone of health policy, and predictive analytics increasingly shape how health systems define and engage notions of both health and financial risk (Hogle 2019).

This shift in health-care management parallels the intensification and elaboration of austerity politics in the United States. Federal funds for public-health infrastructures in the United States have dwindled persistently over the last several decades, continuous with broader public divestments from social policies that characterize neoliberal economics (McKillop and Ilakkuvan 2019; Williams and Maruthappu 2013). Scholars and policymakers alike argue that this has left public-health infrastructures ill equipped to implement the kinds of effective population-health interventions that prevent "downstream" health problems—which has also made for sicker patients arriving into care (Welker-Hood 2014; Kennedy 2007). In the absence of robust public-health systems and social programs, responsibility for population-level health outcomes has come under the direct purview of hospitals, clinics, public systems like Medicaid and Medicare, and other care systems.

However, the entry of population health into health-care system management has transformed what kinds of populations and outcomes matter relative to financial risk. The emergent availability of big data for health systems has enabled the creation of new kinds of "at-risk" populations (Willse 2015; Hogle 2019). It has also produced new ways to track, manage, and anticipate the kinds of "investments" that ultimately produce cost savings for health systems. As Linda Hogle (2019, 569) argues, the shift to big data has brought about a boom in the market for predictive analytics to identify sites of investment in health-system interventions, despite the frequent opacity of the algorithms that data-analysis firms use in these analyses. Health systems may be taking new approaches to care provision in this milieu, such as considering patients' upstream determinants of health more closely. However, their interests generally extend only as far as interventions produce a return on investment or novel sites of capital accumulation (Willse 2015; Hogle 2019). In other words, health systems take on *economic* risk only for certain kinds of anticipated *health* risks.

Defining Risk

Risk is an expansive concept that spans fields. As a sociological keyword, it has signaled a broad social transformation to a "risk society" characterized by new forms and exposures to hazards (Beck 1992; Giddens 1990). Epidemiologists define *risk* as a function of aggregate probability over time that a person will experience a specific health-related outcome (Cole et al. 2015). Notions of risk have come to centrally characterize late twentieth- and early twenty-first-century economics, particularly through the elaboration of speculative investment (Machina and Viscusi 2014). For scholars of governmentality, risk comprises many "diverse forms of calculative rationality for governing the conduct of individuals, collectivities, and populations" (Dean 1998, 199). In each domain, risk mobilizes statistical techniques of aggregation to predict, manage, or intervene in uncertainty. And indeed, insurance and social-welfare systems weave together these strands of risk—economic, embodied, calculative, governing—into a logic of actuarial solidarity (Ewald 2020). As Mitchell Dean (1998, 25) writes, "Risk is a way—or rather, a set of different ways—of ordering reality, of rendering it into a calculable form." In his analyses of insurance as an "abstract technology," François Ewald (1991, 197) also emphasizes such processes of synthesis and assembly: "Insurance is an art of combining various elements of economic and social reality according to a set of specific rules." For Ewald in particular, collectivized risk is concretized in a financialized form of social solidarity through the proliferation of insurance technologies.

Building on the analyses of statistical collectivization in chapter 3, this chapter discusses how trans- activists and advocates developed new risk narratives to reorganize shared notions of reality. Activists in both study sites told new stories about risk. In so doing, they foregrounded the social and political dynamics they saw as being overlooked in old stories about risk. In chapter 3, I described how activist researchers in Buenos Aires contested causal narratives about health when it came to the racialized immiseration of travestis and trans- people in metropolitan Argentina. They revised notions of risk by defining state violence, among other things, as a primary health hazard or risk factor. New York–based activists and advocates also revised notions of risk. However, the latter group focused more squarely on *consequence* than on cause and integrated an explicitly economic dimension as they contested dominant stories of risk.

Specifically, trans- activists and advocates argued that the act of denying publicly funded trans- therapeutics to people who needed them would not only discriminate but also expose them to the risk of mental-health crisis and suicide. In addition to contravening the medical imperative to "first do no harm," activists and advocates also pointed to the likelihood that such outcomes would only increase direct and indirect costs for public-funding infrastructures. In so doing, they built the case for trans- therapeutics as a shared social good rather than an unjust taxpayer's burden or gratuitous public claim. In this way, they contested exclusion and advanced a forceful bid to expand solidarity. Their primary focus was on solidarity in its institutionalized form (as instantiated by insurance), but this was accompanied by an implicit invitation to rethink political solidarity through risk.[3] As they intervened in notions of risk and health outcomes, they advanced an understanding of trans- therapeutics as broadly enhancing aggregate life well beyond those trans- people who pursue it.

Advocates had long been working through regulatory and judicial avenues to argue that categorical denial of trans- therapeutics constituted discrimination based on diagnosis. This assertion remained central to the direct-action and social-media campaign that a coalition of activists and advocates undertook to overturn the Medicaid exclusion. As expressed in this chapter's epigraph, they defined *trans- health* as the "regular healthcare that non-trans people receive every day when they need it—but that is specifically denied to trans people" (GLAAD and Sylvia Rivera Law Project 2013a). Attorneys argued that nontrans- women regularly received Medicaid coverage for hormone-replacement therapy and nontrans- men were able to access "gender-confirming" surgeries for conditions such as gynecomastia.[4] However, judges and health officials consistently maintained that trans- therapeutics were different and that treatments were supposedly experimental and thus failed to meet eligibility standards.

Where arguments for antidiscrimination and care equity—the first of the "Triple Aims"—had failed, the Health Care for All! coalition of New York–based activists and advocates that led the Medicaid access campaign instead turned to the other two aims to build a case for coverage: population-level prevention and cost containment. The coalition's main objective was to foster conditions for survival among poor trans- people and trans- people of color. They saw broader access to health care, including but not limited to trans- therapeutics, as central to achieving this goal. Legal and judicial tactics were one route through which they sought to enact political change through state Medicaid systems. Yet, as grassroots activists and salaried attorneys came to grips with the repeated failures of these tactics, they turned to different forms of action and different narratives about health. Specifically, they mobilized direct actions and sought to transform public views about trans- therapeutics by telling new stories about the social risk of failing to provide access to these forms of care. Through these stories about social risk, they also proposed a notion of the social that required caring well for trans- people. In the vision they proposed, doing so would bolster rather than undermine health for all. Not only would this save money, they argued, but fighting racialized and classed transphobia in health care would strengthen the social fabric overall. The Medicaid access campaign was one of the primary vehicles through which these claims were advanced. In the following sections, I first discuss New York City's Medicaid politics and next draw on empirical accounts of how New York activists and advocates won the Medicaid victory in 2015—which included their mobilization of economized epidemiological biographies.

Cost and Controversy: Public Coverage for Trans- Therapeutics

In excluding Medicaid funding for trans- therapeutics, New York State administrators took a page from an older playbook. Moral and fiscal objections to trans- therapeutics—and indeed, to trans- people more generally—had been advanced throughout the 1980s in debates about public financing for so-called transsexual surgery in the United States. These culminated in the 1989 decision by the Department of Health and Human Services (DHHS) to exclude trans- therapeutic care from federal Medicare coverage. DHHS based this decision on a 1981 federally commissioned report that found care related to "sex reassignment of transsexuals" to be controversial, experimental, and expensive (DHHS 1981; C. Williams 2014). Several states followed suit, adding explicit exclusion clauses for trans- therapeutics.

As trans- historian Cristan Williams (2014) points out, the determination of "controversy" was based largely on a consultant report from Janice Raymond, the notoriously antitrans- author of the 1979 book *The Transsexual Empire.*[5] The fact that she was commissioned as a primary expert consultant on the government white paper would seem to indicate that the commissioning agency was seeking out a very particular outcome; Raymond was the proverbial fox guarding the henhouse. Her report was one of two that was leveraged to establish the "controversy" leg of the three-legged stool that led to the report's recommendations and later to the 1989 ban. This would last for thirty-three years, only to be reversed by the Department of Health and Human Services in 2014 (having persisted through the full first term of the Obama presidency, in addition to those of Presidents Bush, Clinton, and George W. Bush).[6]

Public and private insurance agencies mobilized some variation on the three-legged stool of trans- therapeutic exclusion throughout the 1990s and early 2000s (and beyond). It was precisely this combination of political antipathy, austerity, and manufactured scientific doubt that led to New York's Medicaid ban. This particular statewide exclusion was implemented in 1998, having been proposed the previous year. Administrators' reasons for imposing this exclusion at this time are not necessarily clear, given that discussions about it happened behind closed doors. The formal record shows that their ultimate findings rested on the "experimental" leg of the justificatory stool, as they categorically decided that such care was not medically necessary. The question of cost did not arise as a formal justification, at least at this point.

Yet the timing and politics of their scrutiny reveal a decision that was haunted by both austerity and antitrans- politics. Their decision arrived in the wake of the sweeping changes to public benefits programs in the United States in the late 1990s, specifically through the Personal Responsibility and Work Opportunity Reconciliation Act of 1996, passed during the Clinton administration. New York implemented these new federal regulations—widely recognized as representative of the austerity regimes introduced through late twentieth-century neoliberal economics—in its Welfare Reform Act of 1997.[7] This brought about a reconstruction of Medicaid's administrative relationship to other public benefits. In short, administrators were empowered by welfare reform to enact sweeping cost-cutting measures when it came to public benefits programs.

Welfare reform also concentrated laser scrutiny on state spending practices and the recipients of public benefits as a group. This enacted a new wave of moralizing criminalization when it came to the racialized politics of gender and sexuality (Cohen 1997; Young 2011; Roberts 1997).[8] In other words, welfare reform made administratively concrete a long-standing racialized hostility toward poor people, and this was enacted especially harshly on a wide swath of sexual and gender outsiders (Cohen 1997; Ferguson 2004). In the 1980s and 1990s, the rise of neoconservative politics that culminated in welfare reform drew on pathologizing discourses such as the Moynihan Report in their scapegoating of Black nonmarital and matriarchal relations (Ferguson 2004, 357). Welfare-reform measures specifically defined racialized nonheteropatriarchal gender and kinship as an urgent social problem enabled by welfare. Black women were targeted most maliciously and harshly in this concerted effort to dismantle the social safety net. Yet, many other expressions of sexual and gender nonnormativity were also implicated in these racist and racializing initiatives (Cohen 1997; Spade 2015). Poor trans- people and trans- people of color experienced the multiplicative effects of these intensifying austerity regimes, and the selective exclusion of public coverage for trans- therapeutics was but one expression of this phenomenon.

New York's Medicaid program was and remains the most expensive in the nation. Its relatively high cost is related to a series of factors, but most analysts attribute it in part to high service costs and more expansive eligibility requirements than those in other locales (Paradise and Kaiser Family Foundation 2015). New York is also unique in that it requires municipal contributions to support a large portion of Medicaid costs, rather than just state and federal contributions (as is the case in most other states). New York City contributes the lion's share of local Medicaid funding, placing the municipality in persistent tension with the state government. These political pressures, alongside rising Medicaid costs statewide and changes that accompanied the Affordable Care Act, were some of the driving forces behind the formation of Governor Cuomo's Medicaid Redesign Team.

New York City has long been blamed by the state for profligate spending on social services. Kim Phillips-Fein (2017, 5) writes that these fiscal difficulties have long been chalked up to "irresponsible altruism" of social democratic leaders. However, she argues that this story obscures the true conditions for the city's turn to austerity politics. Rather, federally subsidized suburbanization and white flight, racial hostility, concerted resistance from business, and regressive state taxation policies combined to produce a sharp decline in the city's tax base. This drop in revenue was exacerbated by dwindling support for federal poverty-relief programs under the Nixon administration.

By the time the Medicaid exclusion for trans- therapeutics was applied in the late 1990s and Cuomo initiated the Medicaid Redesign Team in 2011, the city's fiscal crisis of the 1970s was a distant memory. Nevertheless, the specter of "irresponsible altruism" had concretized into the story of the effectiveness of austerity politics in New York City and the grim terror of insuperable debt. Policies governing trans- therapeutics were one of the sites through which these dynamics were negotiated. Within this milieu, advocates and activists found that to win, they had to make their demands make economic sense.

Sparring with Austerity: The Campaign to Remove the Trans- Exclusion

In January 2016, I interviewed several of the advocates and activists who were involved in the legal fight to overturn the Medicaid exclusion. Among these were New York–based attorneys Valerie, Amanda, and Anya, all of whom had been directly involved in this protracted struggle. Governor Cuomo's office and the New York Department of Health had formally issued an amendment to authorize Medicaid coverage for trans- therapeutics in December 2014, reversing the sixteen-year exclusion.[9] Valerie explained that *Cruz v. Zucker*—a case that at the time we met was still being argued—had already provided a legal linchpin to overturn the exclusion.[10]

Cruz v. Zucker was a federal class-action lawsuit contesting the state ban, filed in 2014 on behalf of transgender Medicaid beneficiary Angela Cruz and an anonymous plaintiff by the Sylvia Rivera Law Project, Legal Aid, and the firm Willkie Farr & Gallagher. By this point, Commissioner Shah had resigned and had been replaced by his deputy, Howard Zucker. The court eventually decided in favor of the plaintiffs in July 2016. The Department of Health had first attempted to settle with the plaintiffs and then, in

December 2014, Cuomo quietly removed the blanket ban—instead imposing a long list of stipulations for excluded procedures and treatments. Many of these stipulations were reversed after the July 2016 decision in favor of the plaintiffs.

These events would seem to tell the story of several courageous lawyers and their clients—several of whom were trans- activists—winning a precedent-setting legal victory. Yet as Valerie, Anya, and Amanda all contended, the Department of Health's decision to lift the exclusion may have culminated in court, but it was in fact won through a sustained campaign of mass mobilization, targeted direct action, coalition-building, and political education. In what follows, I trace first the interwoven decade-long legal struggle and social-movement mobilization that led to Medicaid coverage for trans- therapeutics in New York. Within this, I focus in large part on how advocates and activists shifted the overall narrative about trans- health, its relevance to slow violence of austerity, and the imperative to define it as a public good.

From the Courtroom to Medicaid Reform

I interviewed Valerie as New York City was thawing after a record-setting blizzard. We met near her office at busy diner in uptown Manhattan, our conversation punctuated by coffee refills and patrons squeezing by between tightly packed tables. Among other client-based advocacy and health-access projects, Valerie had been working on the legal fight to end the Medicaid exclusion for about a decade. When we talked, she was part of a team of attorneys representing the plaintiffs in *Cruz v. Zucker.* Comparing her work on this case to her work in the early 2000s, she said:

> The world is a different place. [Before,] the state had no concern about appearing transphobic. I think [it has to do with] trans- people organizing and making noise about the fact that they exist and the oppression that people experience and . . . the noise that people [have] made in that time frame, just like the level of awareness about trans- people's lives . . . It made a huge political shift where then the state was like . . . "Yes this is important health care. We don't mean to be

> denying people healthcare." . . . I think that they didn't want to appear transphobic. (Interview, January 18, 2016)

In 2007, Valerie's colleagues had filed *Casillas v. Daines* on behalf of another trans- Medicaid beneficiary.[11] This federal class-action suit charged that Medicaid was discriminating against trans- clients based on diagnosis.[12] As Valerie explained, this case failed at the motion to dismiss phase—the first opportunity to stop it from going forward. In so doing, the court cited a regulation enabling states to put "appropriate limits on a service based on such criteria as medical necessity or utilization control."[13] In 2009, another plaintiff filed *Ravenwood v. Daines* on a similar basis and with a comparable result.[14]

I also interviewed Anya, an attorney and activist, at her office in Lower Manhattan in the winter of 2016. This was our second interview, after having spoken during the Medicaid access struggle in 2013. She had been involved in litigation and activism to remove the exclusion since the first case was filed. For this second interview, I sat on a couch next to her desk. Her walls were papered with political posters, including one from the "Where's the Love, Shah?" Valentine's Day protest. She explained that activists and advocates saw the dismissals of these cases as both a political setback and a grave indignity for poor trans- people in particular. According to Anya, up to that point, trans- organizations had mainly focused on changing administrative regulations under the radar and away from public scrutiny. After the Medicaid-related legal cases were dismissed out of hand, they took a different tack and began a broad-based organizing campaign. As she put it, "[At first,] we were quiet. And then, fuck no!" (interview, January 12, 2016).

Parallel to this broad-based community mobilization, advocates continued their efforts to seek legal recourse. This was propelled both by the profound need they saw and by a series of important regulatory changes. With respect to need, activists and advocates alike took note of the perils of being denied access to care. Amanda, another attorney involved in the Medicaid fight, did extensive direct service with poor trans- clients during this time. We met at a Brooklyn café, crowded with people retreating from the lingering snowstorm. She described her work with clients related to the Medicaid exclusion:

> It was just a huge problem. . . . Everyone . . . every client . . . was affected by it. People [were] buying medications on the street, hustling to get money for surgeries, and I can't overstate the significance of it. So we started thinking around 2012 of bringing a new case. (Interview, January 23, 2016)

A cascade of regulatory shifts also took place during this time. In 2010, the Affordable Care Act was passed, which included an antidiscrimination provision. After several years of consistent pressure, this provision was clarified to explicitly include gender identity, which became key in fighting exclusions for trans- therapeutics.[15] In 2014—the year that attorneys filed *Cruz v. Zucker*—the U.S. federal Medicare program dropped its thirty-three-year prohibition on coverage for gender-affirming care. In addition, Medicaid programs in other states began adding coverage for gender-affirming care and moved to prohibit blanket exclusions. As Valerie (interview, January 18, 2016) commented during our interview:

> I think the . . . month we filed [*Cruz v. Zucker*] was when [Laverne Cox] was on the cover of *Time*. We filed directly after that [Medicare] case won. [We] would have filed anyway, but the timing worked out that we were like, "We should do this. And we should do this right now. Medicare has removed their exclusion. Laverne is on the cover."

Indeed, attorneys cited these regulatory shifts in their arguments. Yet as Anya, Amanda, and Valerie all contended, the legal victory did not emerge in a vacuum. As Anya (interview, January 12, 2016) asserted, it had as much to do with the "public, political pressure" that activists put on Cuomo's administration and the Health Department. Amanda (interview, January 23, 2016) described how advocates' efforts in public mobilization also shaped their legal tactics: "We ended up taking this multiframed approach to the lawsuit [and] to the policy issue."

Amanda (interview, January 23, 2016) went on to describe a fact sheet that an SRLP intern had compiled from a public-health perspective, titled "Eliminating the Medicaid Exclusion for Transition-Related Care in NYS: Good Public Health, the Right Thing to Do, and Ultimately a Cost-Saving Measure":

> This advocacy document . . . held a lot of the evidence around trans- health care and cost-benefit analysis. So we had these . . . statistics that we could use. It was mostly qualitative, but it was stuff we could put together and use to argue a little bit better. We had these new legal theories.

The document distilled the messages and approaches of epidemiological biographies and accordingly mobilized a reconceptualization of risk. In addition, the fact sheet incorporated an economic rationale that strove to preemptively stymie the austerity arguments they were anticipating from public commentators on behalf of an allegedly skeptical taxpaying public. Epidemiological biographies and the shift in thinking they brought about thus not only shaped advocates' legal arguments; in Amanda's eyes, they brought about new modes of legal theorization.

In the wake of the legal losses of the late 2010s, mobilization efforts took the form of both grassroots organizing and political coalition-making. Anya described a series of town halls that took place in the Bronx, Brooklyn, Queens, and Manhattan. SRLP hired community-based organizers and shifted to a membership-based structure. Anya described community members' reactions to being rebuffed by both Shah and the federal court:

> People in our community . . . were like, "Oh *hell* no, we're *bringing* this!" . . . So then we had a series of town halls . . . [and] one thing that was clear was that people really wanted to sue, to litigate it again, and also go public. [They said,] "We want this to be our campaign and we're not being quiet." (Interview, January 12, 2016)

During the Medicaid campaign, SRLP members worked in organizational coalition with the TransJustice program of the Audre

Lorde Project, immigrant-justice group Make the Road New York, the Trans Women of Color Coalition, and others. Amplifying each other's work, activists and advocates defined the Medicaid exclusions as part of a deeper set of political exclusions and folded their health activism into a much broader political program (which I discuss as coalitional depathologization in chapter 6).[16]

On a legal level, broad-based legal coalitions also emerged in the wake of the defeat in court. As Anya mentioned:

> We were really sad, but one thing that came out of it was all of these poverty lawyers came out of the woodwork and were like, "We really want to help you with this. We have trans- clients who are poor, and we see them being denied health care. It's a crisis." (Interview, January 12, 2016)

Thus began in earnest the collaboration between trans- health advocates and a broader group of health and poverty lawyers to collectively intervene in restrictive regulations though nonlitigative means.[17] Trans- health advocates had already been working in coalition with other LGBTQ advocates—groups that Anya (interview, January 12, 2016) described as having a "more mainstream" orientation when compared with the approaches that she and her colleagues took. Nevertheless, as coalition members debated tactics, advocates came to reframe the ways they discussed trans- therapeutics from a legal standpoint. Specifically, they began articulating it not only in terms of medical necessity but also in terms of the individual and social cost of the repercussions of it being withheld.

Anya and others were in the middle of this reframing work when I first interviewed her in the summer of 2013. At that point, we met on the patio of a bar near her previous office in the Chelsea neighborhood on the West Side of Manhattan. Over the din of the summer crowd, she described how she and other attorneys and advocates had begun discussing the shared life hazards they were seeing among clients in terms of life costs: incarceration, homelessness, rates of HIV infection, and others. While she acknowledged the "data gap" that made it difficult to establish causation, she explained that the depth of their anecdotal experience working with clients provided powerful evidence (interview, July 30, 2013).

Further, activists who were directly affected by these conditions made these connections in their own lives and in their public activism. Anya's organization had been part of the "Welfare Justice" campaign that had just a few years before forced the New York Human Resources Administration to adopt formal provisions to protect against rampant racialized and classed transphobia. Through this work, beneficiaries of public benefits who were closest to the problems at hand had already been identifying public benefits systems as sites of cruelty, surveillance, coercion, and exclusion. Activists who were directly affected by these issues, as well as the advocates who worked with them, were therefore already telling persuasive stories about "administrative violence" (Spade 2015) as a primary risk to health, a significant barrier to thriving, and a source of slow violence.

A 2011 Institute of Medicine report on LGBT health disparities lent both language and traction to framing trans- therapeutic access in terms of health disparities. This publication, which was funded by the National Institutes of Health, called for expanded federal funding on matters related to LGBT health, acknowledging aggregate disparities in health among LGBT and non-LGBT people and asserting "significant gaps in our understanding of the health issues confronting LGBT people" (Institute of Medicine 2011). As was the case among Argentine activist researchers, this undone science afforded analysts more latitude in speculating about causal relation and drawing on small-scale and community-based studies. This affordance may also have been enhanced by the broader shift in health policy toward predictive analytics and risk speculation that was underway through the folding of population health into health-system management.

It was in this milieu that trans- health advocates began drawing on population-health research to investigate the relationships between upstream health risks, trans- therapeutics, and the broader effects on trans- populations. This was the point at which SRLP hired a public-health researcher as an intern to develop the fact sheet "Eliminating the Medicaid Exclusion for Transition-Related Care in NYS" as an advocacy tool. As mentioned previously, the document made a case for access to trans- therapeutics as a means of reducing or eliminating negative health outcomes by drawing on extant studies in population health. A three-page document with two full pages of scholarly references, the fact sheet took five main positions: (1) trans- therapeutics are medically necessary; (2) covering trans- therapeutics is affordable; (3) access to trans- therapeutics improves health and wellness; (4) access to trans- therapeutics minimizes negative health outcomes of self-medication; and (5) coverage for trans- therapeutics saves money for Medicaid. It established an evidentiary basis for these claims and asserted that coverage for trans- therapeutics "saves Medicaid money, because healthier patients are less expensive patients." This focus on prevention of negative health outcomes and associated cost savings became one of the centerpieces of coalition-based advocacy through the statewide Medicaid reform initiative. It also became a key feature of grassroots activism, which sought to cultivate public understanding of trans- health as a social good.

After his election in 2011, Governor Cuomo undertook a sweeping effort to modernize and streamline New York's Medicaid program. The work of the Medicaid Redesign Team and its Triple Aim sought to save Medicaid money while enhancing its capacity to save lives. Trans- health activists and advocates recognized this as a new, nonlitigative opportunity to address the Medicaid exclusion as part of the state's formal effort to improve the program's effectiveness. It also became a site through which to advance trans- therapeutics as a mode of health care that simultaneously comprised solid science, care equity, and collective social benefit through cost savings.

Among the MRT's subgroups, a Health Disparities Working Group was formed to "undertake measures to address health disparities based on race, ethnicity, gender, age, disability, sexual orientation and gender expression" (New York State Department of Health 2011). Several advocates submitted a proposal regarding trans- therapeutics for consideration to this working group, who in turn passed the proposal to the governor's team. As Anya and Amanda mentioned, advocates developed a proposal that marshaled evidence of medical necessity, long-term benefit, and cost effectiveness and drew on the language of health disparities to argue that the current exclusion exacerbated subpar health outcomes—which were also potentially costly to the program. Advocates thought this nonlitigative regulatory route to lift the exclusion might prove fruitful, particularly given what they thought were persuasive arguments about cost savings, but their hopes were soon dashed.

Claire, an advocate, activist, and media analyst who was involved in the public grassroots campaign, explained what happened next:

> [The MRT work] had all fallen apart, basically, after it was scooped by the *New York Post*. . . . One day there was a story in the *New York Post* saying that Cuomo is considering taxpayer dollars for "sex changes" and the next day you see that is completely off the table, like Cuomo . . . makes a statement saying, "I'm not doing that. We're not supporting that. That's off the table." So clearly that story had an impact. (Interview, January 14, 2016)

As Claire described it, the proposal to lift the exclusion and cover trans- therapeutics was leaked to a *New York Post* reporter, Carl Campanile, who wrote an article reporting that the Health Disparities Working Group was advising Cuomo to allow "taxpayers to foot the bill for transgender residents to get 'sexual-reassignment surgery'" (Campanile 2011a). Harkening back to myths of irresponsible altruism as detrimental to social solidarity, the reporter wrote, "New York's costliest-in-the-nation Medicaid program would cover the tab."

Valerie (interview, January 9, 2016) explained that this caused an uproar within the MRT and governor's office. While the process was supposed to be "transparent and public," the MRT and Cuomo's team were concerned with the negative press. Following this, Commissioner Shah met privately with some of the people involved in submitting the proposal. Soon thereafter, the proposal to lift the exclusion was pulled from consideration. Just two days after the initial *New York Post* story ran, the paper ran a second story by the same reporter stating that "the Cuomo administration killed a controversial proposal that would have required taxpayers to foot the bill for transgender patients to get sex-change surgery" under the salacious title "Cuomo Chops Off Sex-Change Funds" (Campanile 2011b).

Going Public with Trans- Health as a Public Good

Advocates and activists were disheartened to have yet another leverage point closed off to address the exclusion. Campanile's vindictive invocation of austerity politics came as a particular affront—not because such arguments were unfamiliar but because they so swiftly shut the door for advocates even to address such claims head-on. With both litigation and under-the-radar regulatory changes off the table, they decided that a grassroots organizing and education campaign could set the stage for different outcomes in a near future. Advocates and activists began to solidify a broader coalition for a public Medicaid fight, which involved using media to reframe the narrative. As Claire explained:

> So what was the other option? Was it to just continue to try to keep things under the radar as much as possible and be careful about who you talk to and that kind of thing, which is very hard, or was there another way of actually using the media this time? . . . So that was the way it started. . . . Could . . . a media plan . . . [be] possible or worth it, or would it be bad to say anything at all? . . . We decided that . . . it was just worth it to try just to see if it would work, so we decided to kind of plan out a campaign particularly around the media side of things. (Interview, January 14, 2016)

This organizational and grassroots coalition campaign crystalized in 2013. In its public-facing tactics, the Health Care for All! coalition enlisted the support of staff from GLAAD, a relatively mainstream LGBT media organization, to collaborate on a media campaign.[18] Graphic designers and content managers drew on research that advocates had presented in court and in the MRT proposal, including the fact sheet about overall Medicaid cost savings. This resulted in two infographics, which circulated alongside a link to a petition to Cuomo and Shah and three videos spotlighting stories from trans- and nontrans- activists, advocates, and providers. The video articulated the campaign's main messages: trans- therapeutics are simply standard care to which others already have access, exclusion from care imperils survival, and coverage is eminently affordable.

GLAAD's involvement meant that the coalition had access to media and messaging research. As Claire (interview, January 14, 2016) explained:

> When it came to health care, some of the messaging research had said that getting into the specifics of health care was not a good way to go. . . . [What worked] was . . . making people feel connected to the issue so that they weren't thinking about someone who wanted something special that they couldn't even relate to or imagine.

This was how the coalition navigated the risk of turning to a potentially unsympathetic public. With messaging information in hand, coalition members performed several revisions on the notion that trans- therapeutics were too specialized, too costly, and otherwise overly burdensome to nontrans- taxpayers. Without departing from their insistence that state violence, housing deprivation, and other conditions of marginalization and structural violence were primary harms, the coalition carefully crafted a message that could still play well to a broader public.

Key to this work was the coalition's effort to reframe notions of risk. These are most clearly illustrated by the infographics used in the campaign, as depicted in Figures 6 and 7. The first infographic (Figure 6) proclaims "Everyone needs access to safe, reliable healthcare." It goes on to draw on statistics to demonstrate disproportionate poverty and lack of health coverage among trans- people compared with the general population. The text narrates a set of claims about trans- therapeutic care accompanied by simple images (including a cheekily placed unicorn on a pill bottle to dispute the notion of trans- therapeutic care as "special" health care). The combined narrative and images suggest the positive effects of access to care (enhanced mental health and Medicaid savings),

EVERYONE NEEDS ACCESS TO SAFE, RELIABLE HEALTHCARE

MEDICAID PROVIDES CRUCIALLY NEEDED CARE TO LOW-INCOME PEOPLE ACROSS THE COUNTRY, INCLUDING NEW YORKERS. [1]

[2]

DID YOU KNOW?

- **15%** OF TRANSGENDER PEOPLE ARE LIVING IN POVERTY

COMPARED TO

- **4%** OF THE GENERAL POPULATION

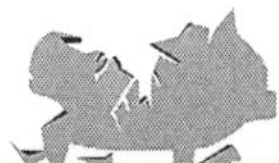

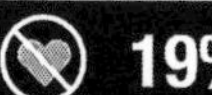

19% OF TRANSGENDER PEOPLE REPORT LACKING ANY FORM OF HEALTH INSURANCE, INCLUDING MEDICAID [3]

SELF-MEDICATION IS DANGEROUS

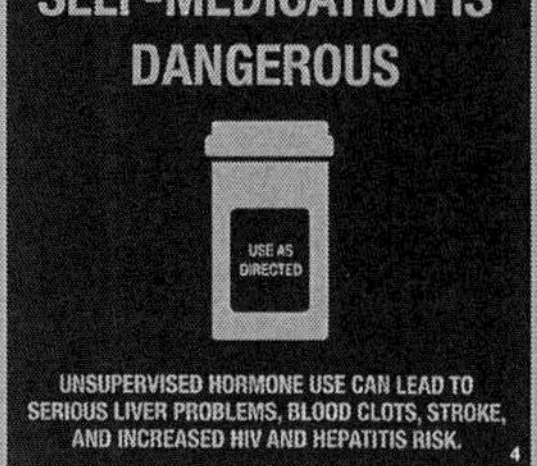

UNSUPERVISED HORMONE USE CAN LEAD TO SERIOUS LIVER PROBLEMS, BLOOD CLOTS, STROKE, AND INCREASED HIV AND HEPATITIS RISK. [4]

HEALTHCARE FOR TRANS PEOPLE IS NOT 'SPECIAL' CARE

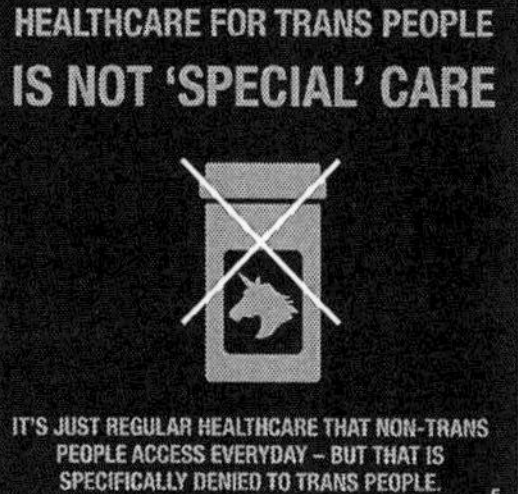

IT'S JUST REGULAR HEALTHCARE THAT NON-TRANS PEOPLE ACCESS EVERYDAY – BUT THAT IS SPECIFICALLY DENIED TO TRANS PEOPLE. [5]

COVERING THE HEALTH CARE NEEDS OF TRANS PEOPLE IS AFFORDABLE

MANY INSURANCE PROVIDERS COVER TRANS HEALTH NEEDS – WITHOUT RAISING PREMIUMS. [6]

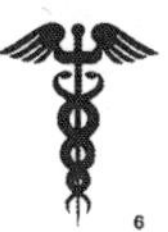

WHEN TRANS PEOPLE GET THE CARE THEY NEED

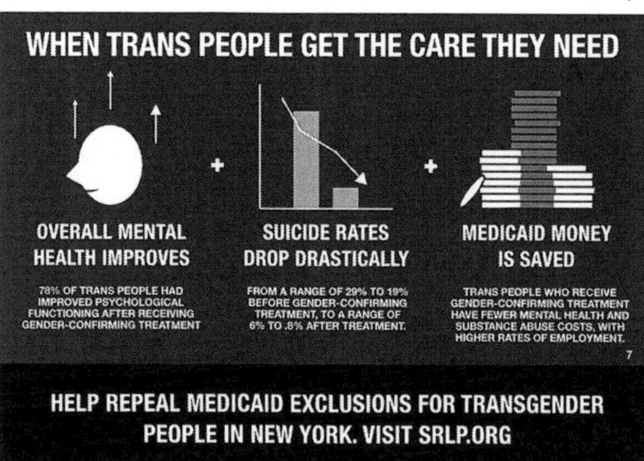

OVERALL MENTAL HEALTH IMPROVES

78% OF TRANS PEOPLE HAD IMPROVED PSYCHOLOGICAL FUNCTIONING AFTER RECEIVING GENDER-CONFIRMING TREATMENT

SUICIDE RATES DROP DRASTICALLY

FROM A RANGE OF 29% TO 19% BEFORE GENDER-CONFIRMING TREATMENT, TO A RANGE OF 6% TO .8% AFTER TREATMENT.

MEDICAID MONEY IS SAVED

TRANS PEOPLE WHO RECEIVE GENDER-CONFIRMING TREATMENT HAVE FEWER MENTAL HEALTH AND SUBSTANCE ABUSE COSTS, WITH HIGHER RATES OF EMPLOYMENT. [7]

HELP REPEAL MEDICAID EXCLUSIONS FOR TRANSGENDER PEOPLE IN NEW YORK. VISIT SRLP.ORG

glaad.org

SYLVIA RIVERA LAW PROJECT

1. American Psychological Association Council of Representatives "APA Policy Statement: Transgender, Gender Identity, & Gender Expression Non-Discrimination" http://www.apa.org/about/governance/council/policy/transgender.aspx.
2. National Center for Transgender Equality, National Gay and Lesbian Task Force "Injustice at Every Turn Executive Summary. A Report of the National Transgender Survey" transequality.org/PDFs/Executive_Summary.pdf
3. National Center for Transgender Equality, National Gay and Lesbian Task Force "National Transgender Survey Report on Health and Healthcare October 2010" transequality.org/PDFs/NTDSReportonHealth_final.pdf
4. National Center for Transgender Equality, National Gay and Lesbian Task Force, "Injustice at Every Turn Executive Summary. A Report of the National Transgender Survey" transequality.org/PDFs/Executive_Summary.pdf
5. National Center for Transgender Equality, National Gay and Lesbian Task Force, "Injustice at Every Turn Executive Summary. A Report of the National Transgender Survey" transequality.org/PDFs/Executive_Summary.pdf
6. Human Rights Campaign, "Transgender-inclusive benefits for Employees and Dependents" www.hrc.org/issues/workplace/benefits/transgender_inclusive_benefits.htm
7. National Center for Transgender Equality, National Gay and Lesbian Task Force "National Transgender Survey Report on Health and Healthcare October 2010" transequality.org/PDFs/NTDSReportonHealth_final.pdf

Figure 6. A poster produced by GLAAD and the Sylvia Rivera Law Project depicts an infographic showing the broad benefits of providing trans- health care. Infographic available at "End Healthcare Discrimination for Transgender People," GLAAD, https://www.glaad.org/healthcare.

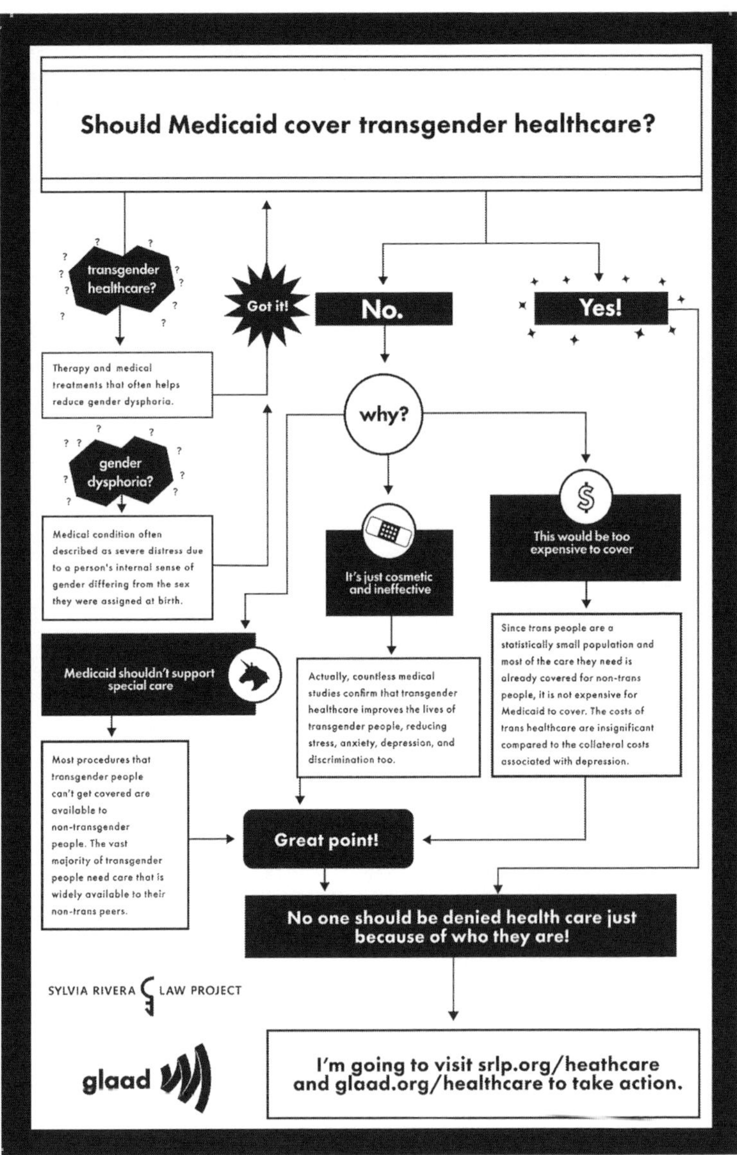

Figure 7. Another infographic from GLAAD and the Sylvia Rivera Law Project shows a decision flowchart titled "Should Medicaid Cover Transgender Healthcare?" Infographic available at "End Healthcare Discrimination for Transgender People," GLAAD, https://www.glaad.org/healthcare.

as well as the negative potential consequences associated with a lack of access (self-medication and suicide risk). The second infographic (Figure 7) represents a decision tree under the heading "Should Medicaid cover transgender healthcare?" Its varying paths guide readers through brief definitions of *transgender healthcare* (by which they mean "trans- therapeutics") and brief refutations of common positions that people were taking against coverage. All positions converge at a box that reads, "No one should be denied health care just because of who they are!" and then to a URL where a reader can take supportive action.

The infographics drew on small-scale and community-based studies about mental health, suicidality, and self-medication to draw an anticipatory conclusion that Medicaid coverage for trans- therapeutics would yield a net economic benefit, in addition to providing necessary care. Taken together, the infographics and video defended against the arguments leveled by health administrators and media spokespeople alike. They brought together concepts of medical necessity and equity, prevention of negative health outcomes, and cost savings—paralleling the Triple Aim that the Cuomo administration so proudly touted in its efforts to reform Medicaid. As they did so, they leveraged direct experience—although significantly less in depth than the epidemiological biographies discussed in chapter 3. However, even more than leveraging personal narratives, activists and advocates in a sense *biographized* economic conditions to tell a different story about money, public benefits, and social risk.

This angle of the media campaign was only part of the public fight. As the coalition grew, they started putting public pressure on the Cuomo administration through direct-action events. The protest at the population-health summit and the Valentine's Day event were only two among several direct actions that sought to expose the hypocrisy of excluding trans- therapeutics from Medicaid coverage and to pressure the Department of Health and the Cuomo administration to take action. SRLP and TransJustice started holding direct-action planning meetings for the Health Care for All! coalition. The tactics they discussed followed the approach of a "Welfare Justice" campaign that TransJustice, SRLP, and Queers for Economic Justice had won in 2010 to push New York's Human Resources Administration to adopt a policy addressing sustained transphobic discrimination against trans- people seeking benefits. As in the "Welfare Justice" campaign, the Health Care for All! direct-action planning meetings focused on organizing people who were directly affected by the Medicaid exclusion. Meetings involved town-hall-style discussions, trainings, and activities such as sign-making and screen printing. Experienced organizers trained new members in tactics of stakeholder identification, direct action, and media messaging, and organizational funds provided food and covered transportation costs.

The Prequel: Epidemiological Biographies by Queer and Trans- Welfare Warriors

Linking economic conditions to survival was not a new endeavor for these activists, some of whom had been involved in drafting "A Fabulous Attitude" (Welfare Warriors Research Collaborative 2010).[19] This document, which was exemplary of the small-scale, activist research in the epidemiological biography genre, served as a critical precursor to the public-facing Medicaid campaign. The study included poor LGBQ people as well as trans- and gender-nonconforming people and framed gender and sexuality as "class issues" that "affect . . . material conditions." I include a brief analysis of this document here as an epidemiological biography that set the stage for the analyses that later emerged in the work of the Health Care for All! coalition. I suggest that the Welfare Warriors Research Collaborative foregrounded questions of risk and survival in a manner similar to that of activist researchers in Buenos Aires, particularly in the ways they redefined *health risk.* The authors' conclusions in "A Fabulous Attitude" also formed the foundation for the Health Care for All! coalition's future work:

> Our lives are as explicitly shaped by class as anyone else's but because we are facing poverty, those shapes challenge us everyday—whether accessing public benefits, navigating homeless shelters, or just moving down the street, we consis-

> tently encounter threats to our survival. (Welfare Warriors Research Collaborative 2010, 2)

The self-published report qualitatively analyzed video-based oral histories and audio-recorded research meetings, in addition to analyzing quantitative survey data. A series of detailed graphs and charts disaggregated respondents' race or ethnicity and gender (among other factors).

Authors emphasized a need to focus on what they referred to as "the racialized and classed dimensions of homophobia and transphobia" (3). They criticized the conventional framing of queer and trans- issues as being "primarily in terms of sexuality, and to some extent gender in many political and research agendas, at the expense of intersectional approaches" (3). Further, they situated their work as a continuation of Black women's welfare-rights campaigns of the 1960s and 1970s and poor people's social movements more generally.[20] Grounding in these legacies, community-based researchers strove to shift "not only *what* is known about our communities, but also *how* what is known comes to be known" (7). In so doing, they sought to develop what they called "poverty knowledge," describing storytelling as a critical instrument through which such knowledge could be developed (7, 9–10).

Much like the epidemiological biographies described in chapter 3, the report drew on militant mixed methods to redefine major issues of concern for poor queer and trans- people in New York City. Like the Buenos Aires–based activist researchers, authors referenced concerns about stable housing, police, and institutional violence as primary risks to health and survival. While the Medicaid exclusion itself was not a focus in this study, participants referred to denials for Medicaid and other welfare benefits within the broader milieu of racial, economic, and gender injustice. Politicized action in response to these conditions was also a feature of the study. A section titled "Daily Resilience and Resistance" included a list of some of the actions that respondents described taking when confronted with violence, exclusion, and injustice. These included direct confrontation, use of media, community education, protest, and more (51–52). In the concluding section, "What Can This Knowledge Do?," authors referred to the successful "Welfare Justice" campaign as an example of how community-based "poverty knowledge" can be leveraged to shift conditions of survival—even if such projects fall short of transformative or system-level change.

This study formed the foundation for the coalition work that followed, within which activists scaled up poverty knowledge and identified institutional violence for queer and trans- people as being especially concentrated within public benefits systems. It also advanced the imperative that people who are closest to a problem are best positioned to both define it and determine solutions. However, there was a key difference between this document and both the "Eliminating the Medicaid Exclusion for Transition-Related Care in NYS" fact sheet and the Medicaid campaign infographics that emerged from Health Care for All! coalition work. The latter sources combined a statistical reframing of risk and endangerment with assertions about cost savings. Directly countering the austerity politics that Campanile (2011a, 2011b) and others played on, activists and advocates mobilized these to make a powerful bid for the social good of trans- therapeutics.

Biographizing Trans- Health Economics

The Health Care for All! coalition anticipated several potential audiences and developed messaging to engage groups on several fronts. In addition to continuing the familiar public struggles for medical necessity and access equity for trans- and nontrans- patients, they also waged a new battle over expenditure. Here, advocates and activists revised notions of economic risk to meet austerity proponents on their own turf. In other words, they proposed a scenario in which coverage for trans- therapeutics made for a more economically rational plan than noncoverage. They contested the economic storytelling of critics like Campanile who claimed that trans- care was an unreasonable burden for taxpayers and instead told new stories about how money *actually* works when it comes to care and prevention.

This is where the "Eliminating the Medicaid Exclusion for Transition-Related Care in NYS" fact sheet did some heavy lifting. It provided data-based arguments not only for medical necessity and population-health improvement, it also strongly emphasized cost savings. The arguments it advanced also aligned with the Triple Aims of care and became a cornerstone of the coalition's efforts to persuade the Cuomo administration and the N.Y. State Department of Health to revise the exclusionary regulation. Through its varying assertions, it claimed not only the legitimacy of trans- therapeutics but also that the state's sustained insistence on withholding them endangered trans- people, as well as public funds and the broader social fabric.

While the fact sheet itself was not consistent with the genre that I identified as an epidemiological biography in chapter 3, it did build on these revised notions of risk to advance a policy-ready framing to evade austerity arguments and redefine conventional notions of risk. The fact sheet was foundational to the development of the coalition's infographics, in addition to providing a key document for legal arguments. I assert that the fact sheet and infographics (as well as some elements of the video series)—which were each part of a suite of campaign resources—can be defined as economized epidemiological biographies. Rather than combining biographical narratives with quantitative data, these documents drew on established epidemiological data to tell a different story about *economic* as well as health risk.

In this sense, the "Eliminating the Medicaid Exclusion for Transition-Related Care in NYS" fact sheet and the resulting infographics rewrote the austerity script about the unwarranted or excessive expense of trans- therapeutics. Instead, proponents of public coverage for trans- therapeutics took the position of frugality and thriftiness. In Ewald's (1991, 197) terms, these documents reworked the "abstract technology" of "combining various elements of economic and social reality." Combining new stories about health risks (self-medication, negative mental-health outcomes, suicidality) and economic risks (investing in preventive care rather than costly acute outcomes), these economized epidemiological biographies made a strong claim for public coverage for trans- therapeutics.[21] In addition to framing these as medically and ethically sound, they asserted such coverage—*and* the elimination of transphobia in health care more generally—was a prudent financial investment and a broader social good. In so doing, they condemned the N.Y. State Department of Health for its poor economic decision-making, in addition to its callous selective abandonment of poor trans- people and trans- people of color.

"Health Care That Non-trans People Receive Every Day"

One of the three videos that the coalition produced for the Medicaid campaign—"Healthcare for All: Give Trans People Access to the Care They Need"—featured several New York–based trans- activists, advocates, and care providers (GLAAD and Sylvia Rivera Law Project 2013a). At two minutes long, it includes only sparse narrative. However, it echoes some of the major assertions of activists and advocates for access to public coverage for trans- therapeutics. For example, Tourmaline, an organizer and advocate at SRLP, asserts that every day, SRLP clients describe having "been denied the basic health care they need to survive." Commentators in the video ground this claim not only in the lack of coverage for trans- therapeutics but in well-established discriminatory denials of care for preventive and routine care. Finn Brigham, one of the health advocates interviewed, comments, "Transgender people, like all people, are healthier when they get the medical care they need." Maureen Ridge, Tourmaline's mother, also appears in the video. In her interview, she says, "Transgender care . . . isn't special care. It's the regular health care that non-transgender people count on every day when we need it." Egyptt, a coordinator at TransJustice, follows up, "I hope I am able to get safe and affordable health care options when I need them."

Two other brief videos feature interviews with two nontrans- advocates—one with Maureen Ridge as a parent of a trans- child (GLAAD and Sylvia Rivera Law Project 2013c) and one with Ronica Mukerjee as a health-care provider who works with trans- patients (GLAAD and Sylvia Rivera Law Project 2013b). In Ridge's video, she expands on the notion of trans- therapeutics as "the regular health care" that nontrans- people can easily access but that nontrans- people are discriminatorily denied. Specifically, Ridge explains that New York's Medicaid program provides coverage for estrogen for menopausal nontrans- women but excludes coverage for trans- people. "The very same care is needed," she asserts, "but the health care is denied to one group of women because they're transgender. When you think about it like that, it's just not right." She goes on to gesture toward the economic argument, describing her work with a large organization whose insurance shifted to adopt trans-inclusive coverage. "I know this is not a difficult thing to fix," she asserts. "All the fears that people had fell away as people learned it didn't change anything, except the insurance policy stopped excluding one group of people." Here, she implicitly describes how each of the Triple Aims—antidiscriminatory care equity, population-based preventive health, and cost containment—applies to trans- people seeking care.

In her video, Mukerjee—a nurse practitioner who had long worked with trans- patients—echoes the message that trans- therapeutics, as she asserts, "is not extra or special care." She also references Ridge's assertions that estrogen and progesterone are covered by Medicaid for postmenopausal nontrans- women but excluded from coverage for use by trans- women. About halfway through her narrative, Mukerjee refers to a series of statistics. Among these, she shares the high rate of self-reported suicide attempts among trans- people. This statistic—41 percent—originates from the 2011 National Transgender Discrimination Survey and has since taken on "a life of its own" (Tanis 2016).[22] Starkly contrasting with a 1.6 percent rate of suicide attempts among nontrans- people, the proliferating paths of 41 percent parallel the thirty-five-year life span estimates discussed in chapter 3. In the video, Mukerjee attributes the alarming comparative attempted suicide rate to "experiences of unemployment, low-income, [and] sexual and physical abuse in the home." Leveraging such population-level data, Mukerjee emphasizes the potential of trans- therapeutics to affect population-level health outcomes. In addition, this anticipatory work drew links between the causes and social consequences of exclusion from health in ways that implicated a broader public.

It is worth noting that suicide statistics have also been used by reactionaries such as so-called trans-exclusionary radical feminists (TERFs), alt-right groups, and others to further pathologize trans- people. Instead of taking these as a cause for alarm about the conditions with which trans- people contend, TERFs, right-wing politicians, and others link high suicide rates with mental unwellness or instability. Mukerjee and other trans- advocates who draw on these data to support enhanced care are unlikely to have anticipated this weaponization of data, and advocates' choice to discuss suicide rates was unlikely to have made a difference in how these data would be otherwise mobilized. Nevertheless, TERF and right-wing appropriation of these data reflects some of the limits of quantification, which can be appropriated to bolster a multitude of positions and actions. Of course, as Tanis (2016, 375) points out, a particularly disturbing element of right-wing and other groups' use of these statistics is their failure to "offer any mechanisms to lower this rate." The implied action is rather intensified resistance to trans- claims to care.

New York's eventual decision to lift the exclusion was likely related to a host of factors, but it remains noteworthy that state regulators' persistent refusals to do so ceased after the coalition's sustained grassroots and legal campaign. As Valerie (interview, January 16, 2016) noted, though, this victory did not necessarily solve all the problems of exclusion:

> This case is not about access. It's really about this regulation. Access to care is an entirely different animal. . . . People *do* have actual access to care that they didn't have before and that's wonderful. It feels really good when I hear about all the things that are happening, clinics that are being set up. . . . [But] the biggest complaint I hear from people is there aren't enough doctors. This law can do nothing about that. . . . You want to know what trans- people need right now? [Doctors are] what trans- people need. There are four of them in New York State doing [trans- health]. There are zero surgeons that do bottom surgeries, zero that take Medicaid. So that's a problem. There are not enough doctors.

These dynamics have begun to shift in more recent years, with major hospitals such as Mount Sinai having opened new comprehensive care and surgical programs for trans- people. As I mentioned in the Introduction, this had to do in large part with the growing infrastructures for robust reimbursement that enabled large health-care systems to see trans- health as good business (even after participating in its delegitimization for many years). Yet, given the stratified system of care and low Medicaid reimbursement rates, it remains likely that Medicaid recipients will have trouble accessing the care they want and need. Gaps between regulation and action are persistent features of legal advocacy worlds, but when it comes to care access, it is difficult to characterize a regulatory change as a victory until it indeed makes good on its promises.

In their epidemiological biographizing, activists and advocates in both New York and Buenos Aires shifted the focus on conditions of imperilment for trans- people and travestis from individual pathology to population health. However, they each took distinct approaches to this endeavor. For example, activists and advocates in New York who were part of the Health Care for All! coalition developed a fact sheet, infographics, and videos that focused on the economic soundness of publicly subsidized trans- therapeutics. The New York–based Welfare Warriors Research Collaborative's 2010 study had more of a resemblance to the Argentine community-based studies I discussed in chapter 3. It combined rich qualitative biographical data with small-scale survey data to redefine dangers for low-income and BIPOC queer and trans- people in New York. However, the 2010 "A Fabulous Attitude" report differed from Berkins and Fernández (2005) and Berkins (2007) in that it carefully disaggregated respondents on the basis of race, class, gender identity, sexuality, and a number of other factors. In addition, it focused on LGBT experiences more broadly, though trans-specific experiences in benefits offices received some specific attention.

There was some crossover among those who were part of the Welfare Warriors Research Collaborative and the Health Care for All! coalition, and these members brought their insights from the prior "Welfare Justice" campaign to their efforts to overturn the Medicaid exclusion. For example, each group defined risk and imperilment in a manner that was shaped by poverty knowledge. However, the messaging in the materials produced by the Health Care for All! coalition skewed toward a more popularly accepted premise: namely, that trans- therapeutics make economic as well as ethical sense to define as a social good. This may have been related to the image-sensitive orientation of GLAAD, the anticipation of a cynical public audience, or other factors. Regardless of their reasons for doing so, activists and advocates spent less time highlighting conditions of imperilment (although they still referred to them) and focused on the economic risk of failing to cover trans- therapeutics. In this manner, they relied on both *risk* and compatibility with austerity to argue for eliminating the Medicaid exclusion.

Medicaid Warriors: Navigating the Narrow Path to Coverage and Social Good

These economized epidemiological biographies made a powerful claim *against* austerity politics by demanding redistributive public investment in trans- health and aggregate life by removing the long-standing exclusion on trans- therapeutic coverage. Nevertheless, they did so by casting their lot *within* an actuarial logic that was ultimately compatible with a broader politics of austerity. The Health Care for All! coalition took a bold step in taking their fight public, given the racialized transphobia and antipoverty sentiments that enduringly shaped the political landscapes within which they navigated. As they made claims for the legitimacy of trans- therapeutics as a sound public investment and broadly beneficial social good, they also advanced arguments about the preciousness of trans- life—specifically, poor trans- life and Black and brown trans- life. Yet in doing so, their arguments were routed through regimes of risk-pooling, cost saving, and the broader "economization of life" or the production of differential (racialized, classed) human value through naturalized and sedimented regimes of quantification (Murphy 2017).[23]

The New York activists and advocates with whom I spoke did not place a great deal of emphasis on trans- people's collective contribution to economic productivity. However, they recognized this as a site of traction—perhaps one of the few that remained open in their efforts to achieve the minimal provision of basic and essential forms of care. Some even recognized New York regulators' political foot-dragging as being about something more or different than money, despite what Campanile and other critics implied. As Valerie (interview, January 16, 2016) commented:

> There are just not that many [trans-] people. So even if everybody got every imaginable surgery . . . it's just not that much money. Our Medicaid budget is so big. This is nothing. This is not about money and the state doesn't say that it is. They've never made that argument in this case. Their arguments are more about necessity and . . . what they're required to do. It's about things you should defer.[24] . . . [They say,] "This is a totally reasonable limitation that we need to place in order to monitor how people . . . are getting care, appropriate care." As far as they're concerned, these are appropriate limitations.

Likewise, Murphy's (2017) analysis refers to the enmeshment of population and macroeconomy as accompanying the emergence and proliferation of neoliberal regimes—which, Murphy notes, are at once material, symbolic, and affective.[25] As Valerie implied, arguments against coverage for trans- therapeutics shape-shifted depending on where they originated or to whom they were directed. As discussed in chapter 2, some states did indeed make financial arguments related to limiting trans- therapeutics, in some cases leading to federally directed statewide audits. Nevertheless, Valerie echoes Murphy's claims that these restrictions are about something more—specifically, about what kinds of care, and *whose* care, may be recognized as necessary and who should make these decisions. Agencies' views on medical necessity had, up to this point, reinforced broader notions about what forms of racialized, classed, gendered, and abled aggregate life necessitate care. Much like Welfare Warriors of the 1960s and 1970s, New York–based activists and advocates were wise to the permeability between moral, economic, and technical arguments, and ultimately they recognized regulators' and journalists' shifting assertions as being about the legitimacy of trans- life.

Geeta Patel's (2017) concerns about the narrowing effects of risk-pooling and financialization in political action resonate with Murphy's. "Political economy," she writes, "has made it increasingly impossible to think about community, family, self, and care except through capital" (312). Her analysis focuses on *kinnara* (also called *hijras*) in West Bengal, as well as others in positions of precarity vis-à-vis neoliberalism in India more generally. She traces their efforts to marshal risk-pooled collectivity and actuarial forms of solidarity to protest the impossibility of stable life for most within neoliberal regimes. Acknowledging the narrowness of the political fields they navigate, she describes risk-pooling as "an estranged form of safeguarding and sharing care" (305). As activists in New York redefined risk and risk-pooling (much like activist researchers in Buenos Aires) and hitched these arguments to cost savings (which was unique among those in New York), they cast themselves—and the state economy—as being at risk of not being well cared for.

Against the varied operations of racialized transphobia, medical and employment discrimination, state abandonment and exclusion, and the resulting desperation that sets conditions for suicide, New York–based activists and advocates asserted a claim to both social belonging and financialized care for trans- people on Medicaid. In Patel's (2017, 280) terms, they assumed the position of "risky subjects"—specifically those who are "imbued with finance." Patel suggests that such claims inadvertently stabilize financialized relations and naturalize the inescapability of neoliberalism and instead proposes a "materially buttressed sustainability" (319). Such "sustainability compensation," she asserts, might manifest future forms of "life with pleasure at heart, and social, political, financial, and legal sustainability included as life ecology in those promises" (320).

If we are to follow Murphy (2017) and Patel (2017), we might recognize in New York advocates' and activists' economized forms of statistical collectivization a reification of economized life. Indeed, activists and advocates drew on notions of human capital to tell new stories about risk and anticipated social consequences—including their own risky encounters related to exclusion from care, as well as the social and economic risks of certain decisions about public funding. Within this, they identified trans- people as worth investing in and as having lives worth saving. However, few activists or advocates took these claims at face value. Instead, having tried and failed for a decade to attain these minimal provisions otherwise, they pivoted toward a set of arguments that could be heard and registered in the here and now of racial capitalism and neoliberalism. Few activists and advocates would have chosen this framing, but they certainly recognized it as a leverage point where few others were available and, just as importantly, as a means to enact a redistributive politics and invite solidarity in a period of extreme divestment from public programs.

These are the familiarly constrained landscapes of social transformation. As Karl Marx (1971, 245) famously declares, people "make their own history, but they do not make it as they please; they do not make it under self-selected circumstances, but under circumstances existing already, given and transmitted from the past." Activists and advocates may have gazed toward other and varied horizons of futurity: sustainability (Patel 2017), survivance and sovereignty (Kuhn 2021), abolition (Gilmore 2007; Critical Resistance and Incite! 2003), and others—and indeed, I take this horizon-focused orientation up in chapter 6. None of these future visions likely centered on the contracted, paltry, and brutally administratively violent forms of care we collectively call "welfare" or "social programs." In contrast, their broader political visions probably included forms of solidarity and mutual support that far exceeded the actuarial forms of solidarity that distribute *risk* rather than justice or other forms of lively sustenance. Yet in *this* historical moment, actuarial solidarity provided one means of asserting claims to life and care, however minimal and limited this might be. Similar to a politics of prison abolition, and in André Gorz's (1967) terms, New York activists and advocates threw their political weight behind the "non-reformist reform" of Medicaid access pending deeper redistributive or transformative endeavors.[26] In their redistributive efforts, the coalition's interventions were modest but aimed to cut a path for broader materially based political transformations.

Even as their political actions shrewdly navigated constraint and exceeded the bounds of human capital, New York activists and advocates still routed their political action through the "risky we" (Patel 2017, 312). In this vein, the cautions that Patel (2017) and Murphy (2017) issue about the dangers of economization and financialization serve as important considerations at a critical moment of trans- political development. Currently, companies such as Mastercard and Citibank are designating certain trans- people—generally marked as white, professional, or otherwise credit-worthy—as being entitled to use "True Names" on credit cards and accrue debt in an ever more financialized economy (White 2020).[27] In this register, the notion of "investment" in trans- life takes on an entirely different connotation. Indeed, such slippage is precisely the point of Murphy's (2017) and Patel's (2017) interventions—the conjoining and seemingly boundless elaboration of quantified techniques of population and economy are variable in their expressions, but they perpetually work to differentiate groups of investable and noninvestable forms of life. To subscribe to a politics of *investment* may do little to address the persistent forces of racialization, economic marginalization, and ableism that divide trans- people into groups of those who supposedly deserve to live and those who do not.

As activists and advocates navigate narrow straits to eke out conditions for trans- life to flourish—and not only trans- life, but poor trans- life and Black and brown trans- life—what is required to bring about these forms of life beyond the confines of embodied, political, and economic risk? The answers to these questions remain open, and guiding accounts are still emerging. Yet among our tasks as scholars of and participants in social movements, I suggest, is to tell stories such as the Medicaid access campaign in their fullness. Too often, social movements are flattened into supposed successes or failures, and too often they are given short shrift in the multifacetedness of their expressions, ambivalences, and varied articulations. Revising notions of hazard, danger, and risk were key tools for activists and advocates in Buenos Aires and New York—but the poverty knowledge they brought to bear on these revised accounts came with a strong cognizance that new stories take on a life of their own. Further, this new life does not always travel in anticipated directions. In a broader landscape of social-movement studies, we rarely pay sufficient attention to the internal, informal, and unarticulated forces that animate the campaigns and actions that make the news. We disregard these to our peril in comprehending a fuller account of how social movements imagine and work toward transformation while navigating constrained presents.

In chapter 5, I shift focus to activists' attempts to put care without pathology into practice through antigatekeeping activism and collective self-determination. This marks a conceptual shift in the book from collectivizing claims to transfeminist practices of care in the clinic. The thematic strands of collectivization and care are, of course, braided together. Nevertheless, chapter 5 emphasizes how activists and advocates worked with care providers to revise care relations in the space of the clinic by contesting medical gatekeeping and enacting consent-driven modes. As in this chapter, I continue to interrogate how activists worked to bridge constrained presents with potentially more capacious futures when it came to trans- health and politics.

5 Crashing the Gate

Consent-Driven Care and Self-Determination

When it passed in 2012, Argentina's Gender Identity Law authorized the most sweeping legal contestation to date against gatekeeping models in trans- health. This is most evident in its eleventh article, the "Right to Free Personal Development":

> All persons older than eighteen (18) years, according to Article 1 of the current law and with the aim of ensuring the holistic enjoyment of their health, will be able to access total and partial surgical interventions and/or comprehensive hormonal treatments to adjust their bodies, including their genitalia, to their self-perceived gender identity, without requiring any judicial or administrative authorization.[1]

The article goes on to state that "comprehensive hormonal treatment" and "total or partial reassignment surgery" will be accessible without any requirements except for "informed consent by the individual concerned."[2] Scholars and activists recognize this aspect of the law as providing the model for laws related to gender identity and "self-determination" in Denmark, Malta, Colombia, and Ireland, among others (Davy, Sørlie, and Suess Schwend 2018). There is pointed irony in some of these countries providing the template for bodily self-determination, given their restrictions on abortion. Malta is the only nation in the European Union that bans the practice altogether, and feminists in Ireland overturned a constitutional abortion ban in 2018 after a nearly four-decades-long struggle. Despite these paradoxes of autonomy, though, notions of (selectively applied) self-determination have increasingly entered the field of national law when it comes to trans- therapeutics.

The concept of self-determination, bodily autonomy, and the practice of informed consent as they appeared in the Gender Identity Law were based in part on their codification in the *Yogyakarta Principles* (Yogyakarta Principles 2007). Drafted by a group of advocates following a human-rights convergence in Indonesia in 2006, these applied international human-rights law to gender and sexuality. The authors describe sexual orientation and gender identity as "one of the most basic aspects of self-determination, dignity and freedom" (11). This group of advocates—which included Argentine trans- and intersex activist Mauro Cabral Grinspan—intended for the principles to guide international governing agencies like the United Nations and individual nation-states in law and policy-making efforts to enhance human rights regarding gender, sex, and sexuality (37).

The principles were expanded in 2017 to include additions focusing even more extensively on self-determination and informed consent, reflecting a growing interest in alternatives to medical gatekeeping in health care related to gender, sex, and sexuality. The same year, Global Action for Trans Equality (GATE) published a position paper entitled "Gender Is Not an Illness" that similarly asserted informed consent as a global requirement for nonpathologizing care (Kara 2017). In each of these documents, the provision of informed consent was not framed as unique to practices of trans- health. It also pertained to the ability to freely seek or *refuse* care more generally in matters of sex, sexuality, and gender. For example, the requirement of informed consent was intended also to prevent medical abuse in the form of supposed normalization therapies or eugenic practices, such as so-called conversion or reparative therapy (which aim to use psychotherapy to convert queer desire into straight desire and gender transgression into gender normativity), interventions for intersex conditions (which are often performed on infants or children), and sterilizing surgeries or procedures (whether for trans- or nontrans- people) (Kara 2017; Yogyakarta Principles 2017).

In this chapter, I return to the question of medical gatekeeping to analyze how activists used informed consent as a tactic to concretize claims for self-determination. Turning back to the notion of care without pathology that I developed in chapter 1, I examine how activists, advocates, and providers collaborated to enact care without pathology in practice. While this discussion is closely related to the concepts I outlined in chapter 1, this chapter focuses on the gulf between activists' aspirational politics and the limits of their enactment within the quotidian operations of concrete clinical sites. Specifically, I tell the story of how something as expansive as the activist concepts of "gender self-determination" and "trans-liberation" found material traction in the realm of bioethics and in the material form of clinical informed consent.

Drawing on the same data sources I used in chapter 1, I show how activists and advocates mobilized these concepts to contest hierarchical power dynamics and pathologizing ideologies within biomedicine. I also describe how practices of informed consent and notions of autonomy became objects of shared concern and mutual commitment for activists, advocates, and providers. In so doing, I consider the following questions: How did activists understand and articulate *self-determination* in their work to intervene in dominant gatekeeping models in trans- health? How did activists and providers bridge very different positions and objectives through informed consent? Finally, what are the implications of this work for health activism and biomedicine writ large?

In what follows, I will first describe what I mean by *consent-driven care* and how it works in practice. I will then discuss how informed consent arose in biomedical practice, emphasizing its roots in bioethical claims to autonomous action and examining philosophical debates about agency and the consenting subject. Next, I will describe activist claims to collective self-determination and its parallels and divergences with bioethical notions of autonomy. I will then show how informed consent became what Susan Leigh Star and James R. Griesemer (1989) call a "boundary object" that enabled "cooperation without consensus" (Star 1993)—which ultimately resulted in what I call a "tempered revolt." Finally, I will discuss the opportunities and limits presented by consent-driven care as a transfeminist and emancipatory approach to trans- health care and a materialization of care without pathology in care relations more generally.

Consent-Driven Care in Trans- Health

Recent History of Laws and Protocols

Article 11 in the Gender Identity Law displaced a gatekeeping model of care in trans- health by defining informed consent as the sole eligibility requirement for accessing trans- therapeutics. This did away with the need for travestis and trans- people to be diagnosed with a mental illness or to be forced to undergo mental-health care that they found unnecessary. Just as importantly, it shifted the locus of decision-making from the provider to the person who sought care. Consent-driven care in trans- health has thus challenged gatekeeping models in two key manners: by refusing coercive forms of care and pathologization and by contesting biomedical power in decision-making about care.

I name this "consent-driven care." Most stakeholders discuss this model as an informed-consent approach to care. The reason for this perhaps subtle distinction is to emphasize that informed-consent processes are already part and parcel of most contemporary forms of biomedical care. Even the most stringent forms of gatekeeping in trans- health still involve processes of informed consent prior to the provision of therapeutics. As a model, however, consent-driven care is intended to replace the protracted processes of surveillance involved in the gatekeeping model of trans- therapeutic care. Even though gatekeeping approaches still dominate, consent-driven care offers an alternative to what critics identify as the exceptionally stringent medical paternalism that characterizes trans- therapeutic gatekeeping.[3]

Various clinics in the United States—especially those that have historically served trans- or lesbian, gay, bisexual, and queer people—have gradually adopted clinic- or system-wide guidelines implementing consent-driven care.[4] For example, Callen-Lorde, an LGBTQ health clinic in New York City, has formally organized the provision of hormone prescription and care through this approach for more than two decades. Certain providers informally provided consent-driven care even prior to that. Clinic-based consent-driven protocols (at least for hormone provision) have since become common, though they are far from standard. During the early 2000s, though, such approaches were quite unusual, since providers understood them to contravene the World Professional Association for Transgender Health's (WPATH) care standards. Tom Waddell Health Center (currently Tom Waddell Urban Health Clinic) in San Francisco is known to be among the first clinics in the United States to regularly offer consent-driven hormone provision in a primary-health-care setting, followed soon after by Callen-Lorde.[5]

After utilizing these protocols clinic-wide for several years, clinic providers at Tom Waddell Health Center began publicly sharing their guidelines in 2001 (Tom Waddell Health Center 2001). Callen-Lorde Community Health Center (2000) providers published their guidelines the prior year. Activists, advocates, and providers shared these widely through formal and informal networks, including a growing number of conferences and digital listservs organized around trans- health. These guidelines facilitated transnational exchanges about how clinics and health systems were grappling with activists' demands of depathologization.

Tom Waddell providers had many reasons for developing consent-driven protocols. Among these was a shared desire to mitigate the negative effects of barriers that poor patients encountered as they navigated steep and costly requirements for accessing trans- therapeutics within a gatekeeping-driven system—especially protracted psychotherapy, which was often not covered by insurance.[6] As a public health clinic that served many poor and unhoused people, their patients often ran into the automatic exclusions that Medi-Cal (California's Medicaid program) exercised prior to the judicial decision ending this policy in 2001. Having launched a trans- clinic day in 1993 (Transgender Tuesdays), clinic providers were familiar with the double bind of steep eligibility requirements and delegitimizing denials of coverage. They were also familiar with emerging activist demands to end gatekeeping and depathologize trans- therapeutics. Director and physician Barry Zevin, who also directed homeless health care for the San Francisco Department of Public Health, described taking a "harm reduction" approach in the clinic's consent-driven model of care. In a 2002 interview, Zevin described three reasons why the clinic moved away from WPATH's (then the Harry Benjamin International Gender Dysphoria Association) gatekeeping model: first, the approach "undermines patient autonomy"; second, the standards "discriminate against poor people"; and third, standards have been "oriented more toward protecting physicians and surgeons than toward providing the best possible treatment for patients" (Health Care for the Homeless Clinicians' Network 2002, 3–4). As such, early clinic-wide efforts to lessen gatekeeping requirements and provide hormone prescriptions without stringent eligibility or psychotherapy requirements simultaneously addressed biomedical power and economic stratification.

Enacting Care without Pathology in Practice

How does consent-driven care actually work in the clinic? It depends on the varying standards and protocols that govern its operation. At its most basic, informed consent involves a process in which providers and patients discuss expectations of care. These conversations generally cover what procedures or treatments are involved, what desired effects or side effects might accompany these, possible concerns or dangers, and a shared plan about what actions will follow. When it comes to consent-driven care, these processes replace previous modes of establishing eligibility through extended psychotherapy, clinical letters of support, and a mental-health diagnosis from a therapist. Beyond this, processes of informed consent range greatly. Many clinic-wide protocols in the United States, for example, require that patients complete a "psychosocial intake interview" and provider visit before receiving a prescription for hormones (Tom Waddell Health Center 2013). Most clinic-based protocols in the United States also specifically stipulate that providers should assess patients' ability to provide informed consent.

Unlike in Argentina, the turn to consent-driven care in the United States has not necessarily meant circumventing diagnosis altogether, since diagnostic codes generally remain necessary for insurance reimbursement. However, it has meant that primary-care providers rather than psychotherapists are those who provide this diagnosis, which eliminates the requirement to seek sustained or undesired psychotherapeutic care. While some providers employ the *Diagnostic and Statistical Manual*–based diagnosis as an enabling formality, others use Endocrine Disorder as a less pathologizing work-around as part of consent-driven protocol standards (as discussed in chapter 2). In general, reimbursement schemas play a prominent role in structuring the extent to which consent-driven care is possible, particularly when it comes to requirements for therapists' letters of support authorizing care (as discussed in chapter 1). For example, Medicaid reimbursement regulations in New York State enable coverage for "cross-sex hormones" so long as a "qualified medical professional"—including a primary-care provider—ascertains medical necessity. Reimbursement requirements for so-called gender-reassignment surgery, in contrast, are more stringent and require two letters from psychotherapists, a "well-documented case of gender dysphoria," and authorization of having lived "for 12 months in a gender role congruent with the individual's gender identity."[7] Given their enmeshment in insurance policies and regulations, biomedical practice guidelines are thus limited in their flexibility to implement consent-driven care beyond the practice of prescribing hormones.

As part of their updated consent-driven care protocol for hormone provision, Callen-Lorde Community Health Center included a sample informed-consent form (Callen-Lorde Community Health Center 2014, 24–25). At this clinic and in other sites with established consent-driven care protocols, forms make up only part of a full protocol guiding expectations of care utilization and provision. The sample form nevertheless provides a sense of the clinical expectations of informed-consent processes for people requesting hormone prescriptions. It resembles many of the medical forms with which many of us are intimately familiar. The two-page form includes a space for a patient's name, date of birth, and medical record number, followed by a long series of bulleted lists of "potential adverse effects," blurbs about the limits of scientific knowledge about long-term health outcomes, and a statement that "side-effects from hormones are irreversible and can cause death" (24). The final provision of the form states that patients have reviewed and understood risks and benefits, received physician education and support about treatment and community resources, and have had ample opportunity to discuss medical expectations with the care team. Financial considerations and insurance coverage are not explicitly named, and the focus is mainly on the physiological effects of hormones on bodily structures and systems. In form, it resembles a contract—and indeed, it is one. As is the case in informed processes in general, the signed form not only scripts collaborative decision-making, it also mitigates physician responsibility in potential malpractice claims.[8]

Such clinic-wide forms and accompanying protocols have generally been developed among clinical interdisciplinary teams and have drawn on empirical data from scientific literature, professional standards and guidelines, and input from advocacy groups, patient groups, or community advisers. Talia (interview, August 3, 2013), the New York–based provider I discussed in chapter 1, described her work on a team that developed informed-consent protocols at a clinic where she had previously worked:

> So we rewrote the entire protocol of how you access hormones to be an informed-consent model instead of the old WPATH way. . . . The original intention was to have an optional educational group first, so people really know their choices . . . [and so that] they could pursue transition whatever way they wanted. . . . The whole purpose of that protocol was to make sure people had factual, high-quality, evidence-based information upon which to make their decision and that they had the cognitive ability to make a decision. Which most people do if they're already consenting for their medical care for everything else, they should be able to do this.

The team that Talia worked with first developed this as a pilot program and implemented it clinic-wide about a decade after informed-consent protocols had been circulating. For her, informed consent offered a way for providers "to hear solutions from people." She commented:

> It's also really a harm-reduction thing, really being like, "What do you need and what is the way to meet those needs?" instead of "Oh, I think you need this and here's how I'm going to meet that for you" without asking first. So *agency*, I believe that's where it needs to go. I don't know if we've seen a lot of that.[9]

When we spoke, Talia had regularly been attending and presenting at conferences about medical education around trans- health, including informed-consent protocols. She described the shortcomings of trans- health care as originating in large part with providers' orientation to care:

> You will get way different information if you're showing interest in somebody than if you're just like okay check, check, going down a checklist. If you're having a conversation with somebody and you care about them, that comes across . . . and they're going to open up to you and be more honest with you and they are going to tell you things that ultimately will affect their health. . . . If you're hostile, then clearly you're going to not give good care to someone. . . . Health care is collaborative. The person receiving the health care that they need is obviously an incredibly important part of the equation.

In her capacity as a trainer and presenter, Talia emphasized this collaborative approach to care as fundamental to consent-driven approaches. Alongside other health-care providers who were particularly sympathetic to trans- activists' demands, she was interested in seeing consent-driven care being taken up as broadly as possible within trans- health.

Argentina's shift from gatekeeping to consent-driven care, at least in a formal sense, arrived swiftly and through a sweeping federal law, rather than gradually through clinic-specific policies. The Gender Identity Law formally defined consent-driven care as the nation's standard in the provision of all trans- therapeutics, including for surgeries. It also removed any requirement for demonstrating "authentic" trans- identity to be eligible for care or for legal gender reclassification. Such requirements in Argentina had previously been highly restrictive. For example, among other anachronistic conditions, they had legally mandated a proclamation of heterosexuality to qualify for trans- therapeutics and required sterilizing surgeries to be eligible for gender reclassification on identity documents (Cabral and Viturro 2006).[10] The Gender Identity Law dispensed with this gatekeeping approach in part by asserting a right to identity and bodily autonomy (Litardo 2013).[11]

In developing and drafting the law, Martín De Mauro Rucovsky (2019, 224) asserts, activists (including himself) conceptually foregrounded bodily autonomy to assemble a "social and political toolbox . . . associated with the dejudicialization, depathologization, decriminalization, and destigmatization of diverse trans bodies and subjectivities." By *dejudicialization,* De Mauro Rucovsky and others refer to the removal of trans- and travesti legitimacy from the whims of the court system.

Joaquín, the Buenos Aires–based advocate I discussed in chapter 1, explained how Comunidad Homosexual Argentina, one of the organizations in the Frente de Liberación Homosexual, came to foreground the importance of informed consent and autonomy as central to these organizing tenets of the Gender Identity Law. At first, he said, the (largely queer and nontrans-) lawyers who were involved were mainly focused on easing restrictions for reclassifying sex/gender on legal documents. In sustained discussions with travesti and trans- collaborators, it became clear that legal tactics would be insufficient if they contested only judicial authority to authorize gender, since this could not be separated from biomedical processes of pathologization. As he said during our interview:

> But in this process we realized that [people had to say] that there was something wrong about you or something ill about you. [We had] to question the authority of the judge because it was something that was naturalized, that was normal to have them question the person that you were. . . . [Or] some doctor or some public officer. So those were structures that were there, and nobody questioned them before and we [in the Frente] started to do that. (Interview, August 3, 2015)

It is worth noting that other members of the Frente *had* been questioning these structures for more than two decades. Nevertheless, the Frente's legal strategy was certainly distinctively sweeping in its imperative to push simultaneously for changes in judicial, legal, and biomedical domains. To this end, informed consent became a means of gaining sufficient medical legitimacy and legibility in these efforts while simultaneously insisting on trans- and travesti autonomy in care.

As the federal law replaced the professional guidelines issued by WPATH, however, expectations of how to enact consent-driven care remained confusing to some providers in the absence of specific guidance. The three-year delay in the regulation of the Gender Identity Law meant that on a national level, implementation of consent-driven care was left up to individual providers and clinics—and in concrete terms, this often meant that clinical care proceeded as if the law did not exist.

Adán, a Buenos Aires–based physician, confirmed that the law did not necessarily do what it promised—at least not initially. I spoke with him in a public health clinic on the city's outskirts, where he staffed a *consultorio inclusivo,* or focused clinic that provided care specifically for travesti, trans-, and other marginalized patients (which I will discuss in more detail in chapter 6). He talked about the difficulty of bringing into clinical practice a "law that you have as a utopia" and commented that "actually doing that is a lot of work." While he routinely used consent-driven models, he described hearing other doctors say that they would keep referring patients to psychiatrists, regardless of what the law said.

Three years after the law's passage, the Ministry of Health published a guide for health-care teams, which includes a combination of technical care guidelines, social science analysis of sex/gender systems, discussions of human rights, and abstract recommendations about how to address power relations in clinical interactions. It discusses processes of informed consent in abstract terms and emphasizes the importance of flexibility and attentiveness to power in clinical interviews. An excerpt from the guide about clinical interviews states:

> Within the framework of any consultation between health providers and patients, there are relations of power and knowledge at play that have been valued unevenly and asymmetrically. The challenge is to make the consultation a meeting that allows for the joint construction of knowledge. The objective is to create a space that recognizes the care resources of each person. In this sense, it is necessary to take into account the various experiences and practices that many trans- people have developed in relation to embodiment

> in the face of their historical expulsion from the health system. . . . The uniqueness of each person means that each consultation is different. For this reason, the exchange should not be thought of as a space made up of fixed and unchanging moments, but rather as sufficiently flexible in a way that enables a care relationship to develop between the health-care team and patients without determining it. These variable instances are articulated based on connection and communication and are based on the demands and needs of each person. (Programa Nacional de Salud Sexual y Procreación Responsable 2015)[12]

This language emphasizes exchange, connection, and mutuality—precisely the modes of horizontal relation that care without pathology strives for. In this sense, it echoes the desires and demands of activists agitating for a transfeminist politics of care, in which health-care providers would be not gatekeepers but rather supportive collaborators with specialized skills and tools.[13]

However, the sample informed-consent document published in the appendix of the guide is somewhat sparse. This one-page document includes spaces for basic patient information and a signature line asserting that a "dialogue and exchange" took place during which patient and provider discussed risks, benefits, and possible complications (Programa Nacional de Salud Sexual y Procreación Responsable 2015). Like the Callen-Lorde form, it is more or less a contract—but one that contains even fewer specifics. As Joaquín (interview, August 3, 2015) commented:

> It was funny because . . . they published these guidelines and . . . regarding human rights, everyone makes guidelines and guidebooks, and no one is doing any mandatory training. No protocols. It's just guidelines and they take the picture and have a big smile but that doesn't change anything.

The very need for flexibility that the guide's authors emphasize in their recommendations about consultations may have prompted the development of a relatively open-ended sample consent form. Yet, as Joaquín pointed out, this lack of standardization and mandatory training might have led to providers disregarding the terms of the law, particularly among those who were unaccustomed or resistant to implementing consent-driven forms of trans- therapeutic care.

Consent-driven care was one way for activists to operationalize autonomy and enact their objectives of "dejudicialization, depathologization, decriminalization, and destigmatization." In clinical practice, consent-driven care models in trans- therapeutics were facilitated by a normative understanding in medical ethics that care should proceed at least somewhat collaboratively and certainly noncoercively. Advocates, activists, and certain providers expanded on this understanding of collaborative care relations to encourage open, narrative, nonpathologizing, and flexible approaches to care consultation. In this way, actors within these social worlds established collaborative consent-driven care as a commonsense consensus position. Yet among advocates, activists, and providers, shifts toward collaboration and consent-driven care involved differing commitments and desires.

For those who were active in transnational human-rights networks, such as the *Yogyakarta Principles* developers or GATE advocates, consent-driven care was a means of extending the apparatus of international law into a global politics of sex, gender, and sexuality.[14] Among the providers with whom I spoke (who were not necessarily characteristic of others in their profession), consent-driven care produced opportunities for building trust and communication in foregrounding patient autonomy. They spoke less frequently, however, about their role in assessing capacity for consent or the function of informed-consent processes in offering them legal protection against malpractice claims. Activists wished to level power relations between trans- people and care providers and thus shift dynamics of trans- therapeutic care provision from a *vertical* to a *lateral* relation of care.

Some collectives I studied sought to intervene directly in vertical relations of care through the introduction of consent-driven care. Informed Consent for Access to Trans Health Care, or ICATH (n.d.), the provider network comprising primarily trans- activist providers that I described in chapter 1, developed templates for patient self-advocacy to enact this shift. In addition to sample guidelines for providers that they included on their website, ICATH also made available sample letters for trans- people to preemptively send to their providers requesting care provision through a consent-driven model. The text of this sample letter follows:

> Dear Provider:
>
> Thank you for working with me. As my provider you are in the position to offer me medical care that can support me to express my gender physically. I am writing this letter to request that you follow the standards of care outlined for this medication or procedure and allow us to use informed consent. I am aware of the following in regards to this gender affirming care and expect to discuss this with you in our appointment:
> Potential social consequences
> Potential occupational consequences
> Potential effects on familial relationships
> Potential financial costs
> Potential impacts on mental and physical health
> I am informed on the psychosocial impacts of this medical procedure and/or medication and am able to make an informed decision.
>
> Sincerely,
> [Blank]
> (ICATH, August 31, 2016)

This invitation for trans- people to enroll providers in consent-driven care worked to reverse the prevailing conventions of biomedical care in which providers led discussions and established care plans. Such an invitation is consistent with notions of "lay expertise" in which biomedicalized subjects assert authorizing knowledge by navigating language and concepts familiar to biomedicine (Epstein 1996; J. Singh 2016). Through this process of enrollment, activists and advocates worked not only to contribute to clinical protocols but also to correct the foundational pathologizing errors of biomedical knowledge that had shaped prior care relations. In addition, they sought to introduce the relevance of cost and debt as issues central to clinical interactions.

The extent to which ICATH's guidelines were taken up—

whether by those providing or seeking care—remains somewhat unclear, given the group's relatively small web presence and circulation compared to more well-known care protocols and guidelines. Nevertheless, these sample documents usefully demonstrate how advocates found ways to bridge the language and requirements of clinical care provision with the desires and demands of those seeking care. They also reveal some of the specific (and even mundane) ways that patient autonomy could be enacted in the clinic through dynamics of care relation and agenda-setting on the part of people pursuing (rather than providing) care. These positions were also emphasized in the rhetoric they expressed on their website. These are best summed up in two stickers that the group circulated that claimed, "We Are Who We Say We Are: Free Trans Health Care on Demand Now" and "Autonomy and Self-Determination for All Trans People Now." Notably, the matters of concern and conversation that were advanced in ICATH's sample letter diverged somewhat from those centered in clinical informed-consent documents, such as the one published by Callen-Lorde or by the Argentine Ministry of Health—particularly in its inclusion of a prompt about questions of financial consequence.

The development of consent-driven care in hormone provision has marked a paradigmatic shift away from the gatekeeping models of transsexual medicine and has become an aspirational model for activists, advocates, and some providers in trans- health. Mounting critiques of gatekeeping and increasing support for consent-driven models led to the seventh version of the WPATH (2011) guidelines mentioning the compatibility of consent-driven care with its care standards for the first time in its history.[15] In practice, the actual uptake of consent-driven care has been dependent on both infrastructure and clinical willingness to abide by its tenets. In the United States, the need for public and other forms of insurance reimbursement have set limits on the reach of consent-driven care. Insurance guidelines have often required the use of psychiatric diagnoses, even if requirements to undergo psychotherapy and obtain authorizing letters have been relaxed in some cases. In addition, the practice of consent-driven care has raised questions about how providers assess capacity to issue consent and the reintroduction of medical paternalism in the process.

Darryl was one of the people I interviewed who spoke to these clinical tensions (interview, July 29, 2013). I interviewed this New York–based nurse practitioner during his lunch break in a clinic office. He described one of the few incidents in which he had decided against prescribing hormones to a patient without requiring psychotherapy first. The clinic at which he worked used a consent-driven care protocol and did not generally require patients to seek psychotherapy relevant to gender expression if they did not wish to do so. However, Darryl was concerned that this particular patient was in need of psychiatric care:

> I really thought they had symptoms of psychosis during our visit, and I didn't feel comfortable. The biggest thing was . . . "I don't think you're getting the appropriate psychiatric care that you need" [and] my way into . . . getting them to see someone was that "I can't give you hormones unless you see this person to make sure you can give full consent legally." It was kind of like dangling the carrot kind of thing. It sounds horrible to say. That person didn't come back, but I don't know what happened. They really needed psychiatric care. I'm not sure what's going on with them but in seeing them, I was like, "There's no way I'm going to just give you hormones right now."

In sharing this, Darryl shifted in his seat and averted his gaze. In his words and gestures, he communicated a troubled ambivalence about his position in making decisions on the patient's behalf. However, Darryl's assessment of his patient's mental health was issued as a self-evident reason why informed consent would be an impossibility without further intervention. While he appeared uncomfortable with the coerciveness involved in "dangling the carrot," he understood this to be in his patient's best interest.

Yet his efforts to lure this patient into psychiatric treatment prior to prescribing hormones may just as likely have resulted in their seeking other means of access. There is a long history of trans- people and travestis seeking do-it-yourself body modification, including the informal use of hormones—whether to circumvent pathologizing or lengthy clinical interactions or to find more affordable options in the absence of care coverage. As

Michelle O'Brien (2013) points out, informally procured hormones are the norm in situations of formal exclusion from care, but U.S. drug-war-era criminalization of syringes and illicit pharmaceuticals combines with historically sedimented pathologization to disproportionately target those who are forced into these economies. Still, these become the most viable options for many in situations of clinical pathologization.

In spite of these tendencies (or perhaps in the hopes of repairing them), activists, advocates, and providers who were part of the study often saw consent-driven models as facilitating trust and developing respectful relationships of support—or even as moving toward leveling the sharp and stratified hierarchies of care provision.[16] Psychologist Sarah Schulz (2018, 85), an advocate of consent-driven models, writes that providing care through the "lens of the diagnostic model . . . focuses on 'treating the disorder' and deemphasizes the importance of the therapeutic relationship." In the realm of trans- health practice, consent-driven protocols have become synonymous with *autonomy*—a concept that resonated with providers, advocates, and activists alike, albeit in very different ways. The following sections describe the relevance of autonomy for providers, advocates, and activists. A full understanding of how each social world oriented to the concept necessitates a brief and nonexhaustive examination of bioethics and the ethical philosophies that underlie it. This digression into theories of autonomy and agency are key to understanding the flexibility in these concepts that enabled developments in consent-driven care that I have outlined in this section.

Autonomy in the Clinic: Bioethics and the Subjectivity of Consent

In chapter 1, I discussed Anya's (interview, January 12, 2016) understanding of depathologized care, or care without pathology, as involving "having autonomy in the way that you choose the health care that you want or don't want." This is a crucial question for trans- people (among many others). The capacity to refuse the care you *do not* want is also key to other concerns related to health, including for intersex movements and resistance to forced sterilization. It is also relevant to David Valentine's (2012) "theory of non-transsexuality," which posits that the naturalization of *not* being trans- obscures the agency that people regularly exercise as "non-transsexuals."

Questions about what kinds of care patients can choose or refuse—as well as who has the capacity to make these decisions—are also central to clinical bioethics and associated practices of informed consent. While definitions range, bioethicists understand informed consent as "the core notion that decisions about the medical care a person will receive, if any, are to be made in a collaborative manner between patient and physician" (Applebaum, Lidz, and Meisel 1987, 12). As a guiding ethical touchstone for clinical research and medicine, informed consent emerged from the internationally recognized medical guidelines established by the Declaration of Helsinki in 1964. These were initially established in the wake of World War II following the Nuremburg trials to ensure ethical soundness in clinical research after the devastating abuses that Nazi doctors and scientists inflicted on subjects of research.[17] Informed-consent guidelines were soon extended to clinical care practice and have been expanded and updated since their original implementation.

Respect for autonomy is the core ethical principle orienting informed-consent guidelines. Medical ethicists, who often span philosophy, law, and clinical medical practice, range in their definitions of *autonomy*.[18] Across varying interpretations, bioethicists generally agree that informed consent is key to enacting autonomy and collaboration and providing a counterbalance to medical paternalism or coercion. Turning to the Greek origin of the term, Tom L. Beauchamp and James F. Childress (2001, 57–58) explain its original meaning as "self-rule or self-governance of independent city-states." Currently, the concept "has been extended to individuals and has acquired meanings as diverse as self-governance, liberty rights, privacy, individual choice, freedom of the will, causing one's own behavior, and being one's own person" (58). Despite this conceptual elasticity, bioethicists tend to focus squarely on individual action and choice: *personal* rather than collective autonomy. Sharing a vocabulary with the moral philosophy of the European Enlightenment, bioethics thus asserts the importance of personal self-rule, freedom from others' control, and the capacity to act with agency. Informed-consent processes serve as the observable means of assuring that the decisions people make to undertake care are indeed their own and are not coerced or compelled.

In Argentina and Latin America more broadly, debates on matters of bioethics often center on Catholicism. As Florencia Luna and Arleen L. F. Salles (2006, 9) assert, the "link between the Church and bioethics in Latin America is so tight that serious public discussion of some controversial bioethical issues is often hindered." Luna and Salles advocate for a secular, philosophically grounded approach that can counter the persistent classed and racialized paternalism of medical practice. In Argentina, informed consent was not legally required until the congressional passage of the Patients' Rights Act in 2009.[19] According to Martín Hevia and Daniela Schnidrig (2014), this was made possible by two primary elements in Argentine constitutional law: the constitutional right to health and the shift to autonomy and human rights as governing principles in the wake of the last dictatorship. The legal requirement of informed consent combined with Catholic-inflected bioethics has resulted in controversies around euthanasia, abortion, assisted reproduction, and other practices.[20] As such, debates about who is entitled to act as a consenting subject and under what conditions also remain fraught.[21]

In fact, questions about who has the capacity to grant informed consent and under what conditions remain a prickly terrain for debate within bioethics well beyond Argentina, including in the United States. For example, some critics denounce the "empty ethics" (Corrigan 2003) of informed-consent processes that overlook dynamics by which coercion and power are expressed in clinical relations of care (Holloway 2011). Trans- health activists, advocates, and certain providers have enthusiastically embraced informed consent as a powerful means of asserting autonomy and countering autocratic and paternalistic medical provision. Nevertheless, its promises are constrained in practice, particularly as consent processes involve providers assessing patients' capacity or ability to provide consent. Disability studies scholars have cautioned against the sometimes-false promise of consent when it may be so easily and unceremoniously revoked for people who do not fit ableist norms. For example, disability studies scholars Eli Clare (2017) and Alison Kafer (2013) each describe how concerns of consent seem to vanish when it comes to people with disabilities. As Clare writes, "being seen as intellectually, cognitively, or developmentally disabled is dangerous because intelligence and verbal communication are entrenched markers of personhood" (157). Since mental incapacity is often routed through race as well as gender and sexual nonnormativity, this exclusion from personhood and agency becomes a flexible eugenic tool.[22]

Some trans- and feminist studies scholars are also raising questions about the limits of consent as a definitive assurance of bodily autonomy. For example, sociologist stef shuster (2019) found that providers in the United States who provided trans- therapeutics at times questioned whether their trans- patients were prepared to act as fully consenting subjects.[23] Providers' concerns about their patients' mental unwellness (or, as Beans Velocci [2021] suggests, their concerns about controversy and legal ramifications) might result in their decision that a patient is not up to the task of providing consent. In this manner, the claim that certain people seeking trans- therapeutics may have diminished capacity becomes a pretense for rebuffing challenges to biomedical authority while technically adhering to the requirements of informed-consent processes.[24] Finally, as Kristina Gupta (2019) suggests, consent can only guarantee so much in circumstances of profound inequity.

Social scientists of medicine have long argued that certain patient narratives are highly legible to providers while others remain alien or incomprehensible.[25] Such legibility in the realm of bioethics (and philosophical ethics in general) often requires that the narratives and actions of consenting subjects are recognizable as "hegemonic agency" (Bierria 2014, 137). As the late Argentine decolonial philosopher María Lugones (2003, 210–11) asserts, such a notion of agency relies on an actor's intentions comporting with "social, political, and economic institutions that back him up" and not challenging institutional legitimacy. For Lugones, the promise of individual agency—fictional as it is—favors the "subject who makes public sense to others" (216).[26] As such, the constraining and subjugating forces of hegemony misrecognize or inhibit the actions of those who do not make "public sense" (216). As I discussed in chapters 1 and 2, the racialized criminalization of gender nonnormativity frequently precludes all but perhaps the most normatively aligned (and thus also white, abled, and class-ascendant) forms of gender variance to be institutionally recognized.

This is not to say that people who are excluded from recognition as hegemonic agents do not undertake meaningful and persuasive action. As Lugones (2003, 218) asserts, the actions of "active subjects" (as she terms marginalized people who fail or refuse to abide by dominant institutional logics) continually highlight how hegemonic "worlds of sense" fail to account for the breadth and multiplicity of life. In the situation of trans- health, activists continually highlighted these failures of sense-making in varied confrontations with care providers, interventions in laws and policies, and forms of cultural production. They did so by exposing the multitude of forces enacting the stratified erasures of travestis' and trans- people's claim to life—whether in the form of gender-reclassification regulations, insurance exclusions, or criminalization. Crucially, this "emancipatory sense making" (217) is a *collective* rather than an individual endeavor; its capacity to make apparent the limits of hegemonic social worlds depends on its multiplicity.

Indeed, this pivot from *individual* to social, relational, or collective forms of autonomy has long been key to feminist correctives to bioethics (Sherwin 1992). Yet, simply to rewrite autonomy as a collective rather than an individual endeavor remains insufficient to the task of resisting and reckoning with institutionally backed positions. As Hil Malatino (2019) describes in his discussion of biomedical interventions in intersex and trans- embodiments, this turn to collectively attuned decision-making is fraught even in circumstances of ostensible medical autonomy. Given the uneven forms of public violence and marginalization that discipline the people who are perceived as gender/sex nonnormative, he writes, "Could we understand decision making that takes place within this milieu as an instance not of willed, autonomous self-making but instead as consent compromised by conditions of coercion?" (116).[27] Coercion, in this regard, is also collective, socially diffuse, and institutionalized. Its dispersed force encompasses the cumulative material effects of racialized pathologization, expressed through biomedical and other forms of cultural and political knowledge.

In conversation with Lugones's work on active subjectivity, Black feminist philosopher Alisa Bierria (2014) discusses the counterhegemonic forms of agency that Black women and other women of color exercise in the midst of state violence. Among these are forms of "transformative agency," which challenge structural "conditions that facilitate the displacement of some agents and the distortion of their actions" (139). She also elaborates forms of resistant agency that she calls "insurgent agency." These instead "manipulate and maneuver [structural] conditions to achieve ends that are structured as unachievable" (139). While these still unfold "within the violent constraints of power," she writes, they "have the potential to corrode elements of structural domination" (139). These differing forms of counterhegemonic agency might either confront dominant structures and dynamics of power head-on or through the gradual production of distinct structures of meaning and action. I suggest that activist visions of depathologization assert a transformative agency while activist-initiated operationalization of consent-driven protocols for care-seeking subjects strives (sometimes unsuccessfully) to enact insurgent forms of agentic action.

In the next section, I consider how these varying modes of agency—hegemonic, transformative, and insurgent—were at play as trans- health activists elaborated and enacted what they called "self-determination." Activist accounts of self-determination propelled demands for consent-driven regimes of care and, as I will discuss below, were often narrated as demands for autonomy. Yet, self-determination in this sense departed markedly from notions of personal autonomy and individual intentionality that structure bioethics—and also departed from the ostensible neutrality of the field of medicine. As trans- studies scholar Eric Stanley (2014, 90) points out, self-determination presents a pointed challenge to the negation of a collective entitlement to selfhood, including the negation enacted in the circulation of hegemonic biomedical knowledge. In this sense, some trans- activists draw on a heterogeneous concept of collective self-determination that borrows from anti-imperialism, Indigenous sovereignty, and working-class collective action.

Self-Determination

In the film *Criminal Queers* (Vargas and Stanley 2015), radical queer and trans- protagonists lead an insurrection against the "multiple ways our hearts, genders, and desires are confined." During the film, the protagonists and their accomplices work to free a comrade from prison. In the course of this endeavor, several characters drop from the top of a building a bright orange banner that reads "Gender Self Determination" (Figure 8). In the inaugural keyword issue of *TSQ*, Stanley (2014, 90–91) describes gender self-determination as "open[ing] up space for multiple embodiments and their expressions by collectivizing the struggle against both interpersonal and state violence." This is mobilized cinematically in the film as a malleable and unruly desire, anchored in an

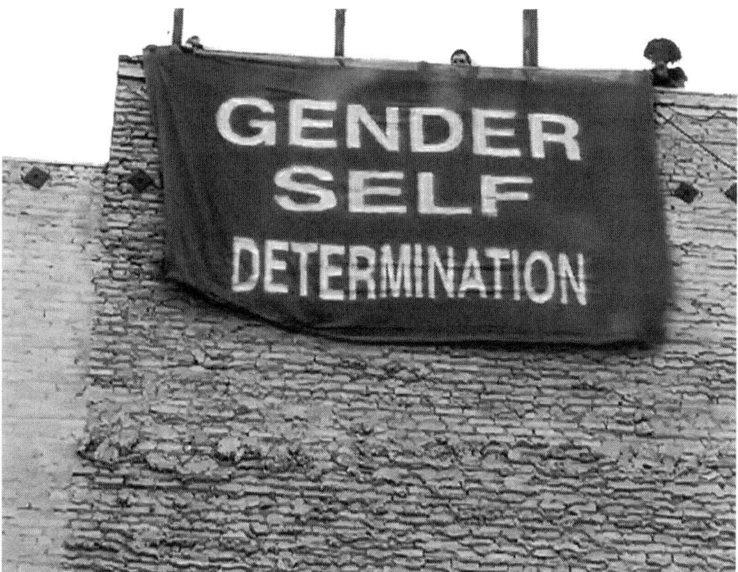

Figure 8. Still from *Criminal Queers* (Vargas and Stanley 2015). The image shows characters in the film dropping a large banner proclaiming "Gender Self Determination" over the edge of a brick building.

expansive field of political possibility and through resistant action to violence and state power. It is also ineluctably collective.

Gender self-determination (or *autodeterminación*) has become a central claim from trans- activists across geographic sites through activist cultural production, political claims, protest chants, and organizational objectives. In this study, claims to gender self-determination were often expansive and frequently accompanied by claims to bodily autonomy. Some of these echoed the expansive claims of coalitional depathologization activists and mobilized self-determination as an antidote to pathologization and racialized criminalization. Even in its more circumscribed form, activist demands for self-determination drew explicit connections between access to trans- therapeutics, freedom from coercive biomedical/psychiatric intervention, and the eradication of the eugenic practices structuring hegemonic forms of biomedical practice. In other words, gender self-determination conjured up transfeminist notions of care: relations of interaction, support, and collaboration that are collective, lateral, anti-immiserating, and founded on the presumptive multiplicity of expertise and critique of its hegemonic forms.

In the activist-generated resources I examined, this transfeminist articulation of self-determination also mobilized a collective critique of "criminalizing forms of gendering" instantiated by systemic immiseration (Welfare Warriors Research Collaborative 2010, 39). In one of the epidemiological biographies that I discussed in chapter 4, participatory action research collective Welfare Warriors Research Collaborative from New York asserted:

> Autonomy and self determination over our bodies is vital for low-income queer and trans people and is constantly threatened by the institutions we access for basic needs such as food, safe housing or shelter, unemployment benefits, and wellness services. . . . But our community members are not victims; rather, we are decision-makers when it comes to our lives. While facing the violence of poverty, isolation, ablism and reproductive injustice, our very survival is an act of resistance and a sign of the depths of our resilience. (47–50)

For these activist researchers, self-determination and autonomy were not only about what decisions people should be able to make about their bodies. They were also about *resisting* the ways that racialized economic distribution, austerity politics, state services, and the punitive and eugenic politics of poverty in the United States perpetually restricted people's ability to make such decisions. Such positions were similarly conveyed in a poster by Roan Boucher depicting New York–based trans- activists Sylvia Rivera and Marsha P. Johnson, with Rivera holding up a sign that reads "Gender Self-Determination" (see Figure 9).[28]

This attentiveness to distribution, broadly speaking, as a matter of transfeminist care was key to activists' understandings of autonomy and self-determination.[29] For coalitional depathologization proponents, distribution related explicitly to racialized political economy. As I discussed in chapter 3, the organizing that preceded and followed the Gender Identity Law in Argentina led to broad, multiprovince and federal efforts to enact quota laws that would formally require public-sector employers to hire travestis and trans- people, as well as to sustained efforts to develop policies for the provision of formal state reparations.[30] Similarly, in chapter 4, I discussed how advocates framed Medicaid exclusions as a matter of racialized and classed exclusion and offered up a distributive transfeminist approach to expanding care infrastructures. In the lead-up to the passage of the Gender Identity Law, Mauro Cabral Grinspan (2010) published an op-ed in the popular Buenos Aires weekly paper *Página 12* titled "Autodeterminación y libertad"—"Self-Determination and Freedom." In it, he positions depathologization as an intervention that must occur at both an economic and an epistemological level. All of these political endeavors presumed an inseparability of immiseration, racialized marginalization, and institutionalized pathologization when it came to trans- and travesti life. Such attention to distributive politics and the fruitful interventions of transfeminist care were also seeded in large part through trans- and travesti movements to claim public space and resist state violence in the 1990s and 2000s, primarily in Buenos Aires but also in New York.

For other activists, distribution and political economy formed an implicit backdrop to self-determination claims, even if these

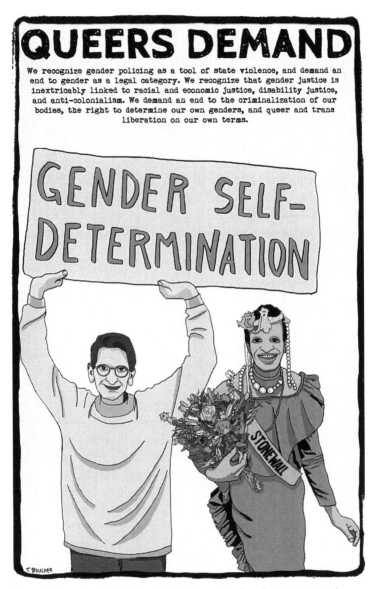

Figure 9. A poster by U.S.-based artist Roan Boucher depicts New York activists and founders of the STAR House Sylvia Rivera and Marsha P. Johnson in a stylized line drawing. The text reads: "Queers Demand: We recognize gender policing as a tool of state violence, and demand an end to gender as a legal category. We recognize that gender justice is inextricably linked to racial and economic justice, disability justice, and anti-colonialism. We demand an end to the criminalization of our bodies, the right to determine our own genders, and queer and trans liberation on our own terms." Roan Boucher, *Queers Demand Gender Self-Determination,* 2012, digital media.

were not as overt as those advanced by proponents of coalitional depathologization. These claims often focused on the uneven distribution of a capacity for undertaking actions that are, in Lugones's (2003) terms, illegible to hegemonic "worlds of sense." For example, Argentine artist Tirre Grillo's 2018 rendition of trans-masculine subjects as the "owners of our own bodies" asserted that trans- people should be able to choose names and pronouns, whether or not to pursue hormones or surgeries, with whom to have sex or not, and whether or not to give birth (see Figure 10). In examples such as this one, access to trans- therapeutics—in a financial as well as a technical sense—were present in political claims to self-determination, even in the absence of broader claims about labor and other material life conditions.

The meanings of self-determination range as broadly as those of autonomy, and the concepts are cotravelers. As Raymond Williams (1983, 183) points out, self-determination's antiquated origins are in seventeenth-century philosophical debates on personal liberty and free will. As in the case of autonomy, the connotations of self-determination span individual and collective domains of signification. However, as Swiss historian Jörg Fisch (2015, 22) notes, early use of the term *self-determination* (unlike *autonomy*) focused on individual conduct. Only later did it become a collective claim through its uptake in decolonization processes and twentieth-century international politics, particularly through the framework of international human-rights law. This shift in emphasis from personal agency to popular sovereignty was key in its mobilization as a salient geopolitical principle endorsing both national independence and international diplomacy.

Yet questions about who the "self" of self-determination is have been at the center of pointed debates about the terms of sovereignty and infringement on formal rights of self-determination (Fisch 2015).[31] Legally speaking, rights to self-determination are adjudicated in international courts—which set the standards by which international systems of governance are expected to abide but are not bound and have little recourse to enforcement (Mustafa 1971). Nevertheless, as Zubeida Mustafa (1971) points out, the principle has been invoked both within and between nations to address issues of foreign domination (i.e., colonialism) and sovereignty.[32] In its abstract form, principles of self-determination

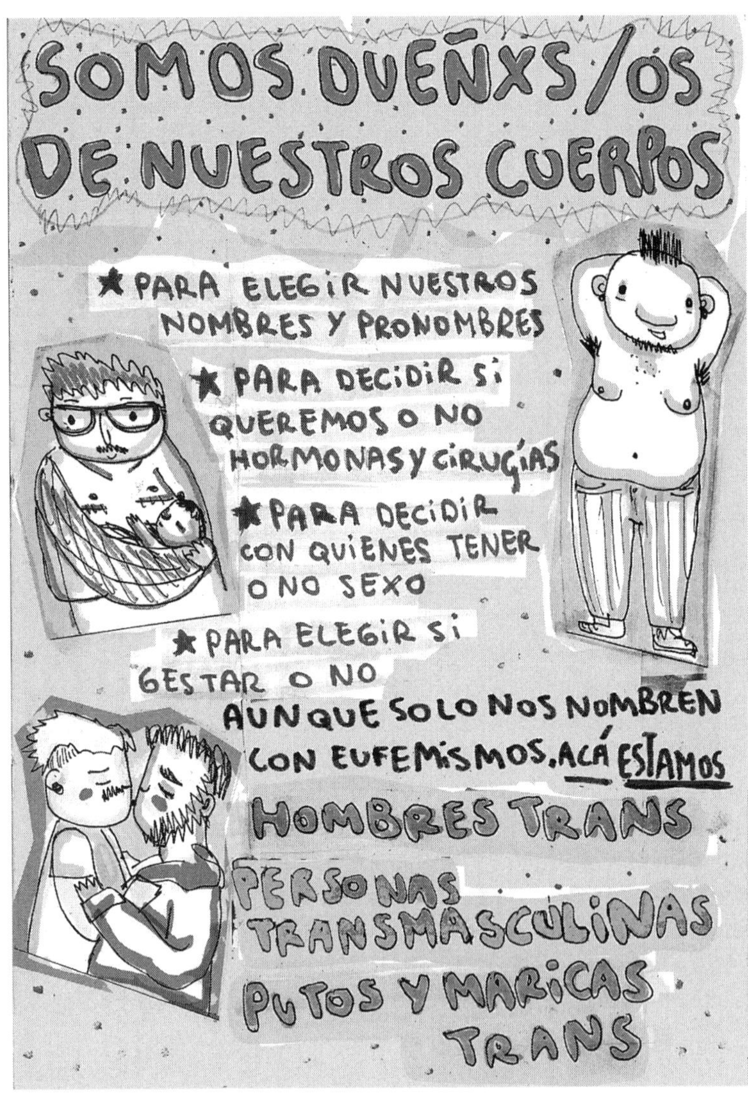
SOMOS DUEÑXS/OS
DE NUESTROS CUERPOS
★ PARA ELEGIR NUESTROS NOMBRES Y PRONOMBRES
★ PARA DECIDIR SI QUEREMOS O NO HORMONAS Y CIRUGÍAS
★ PARA DECIDIR CON QUIENES TENER O NO SEXO
★ PARA ELEGIR SI GESTAR O NO
AUNQUE SOLO NOS NOMBREN CON EUFEMISMOS, ACÁ ESTAMOS
HOMBRES TRANS
PERSONAS TRANSMASCULINAS
PUTOS Y MARICAS TRANS

Figure 10. Tirre Grillo, *Somos Dueñxs/os de Nuestros Cuerpos,* 2018. A line drawing by Argentine artist Tirre Grillo depicts several transmasculine figures accompanied by text in Spanish. In English, the text reads: "We are the owners of our bodies: to choose our names and pronouns; to decide whether or not we want hormones or surgeries; to decide with whom we do or don't have sex; to choose whether or not we want to carry a child. Regardless what we are euphemistically called, we are here. Trans men; Transmasculine people; Queer trans men/trans fags."

apply both to individuals and to groups. In practice, conflicts between claimants—generally in a landscape of inequitable power relations—perpetually shape these struggles.[33] The central problem for those working to determine the conditions of their own lives, particularly in a legal arena, is that these claims become contingent on demonstrating one's capacity for self-determination (Fisch 2015, 23). This requirement may reanimate and reproduce the very hierarchies of agency that lead to the necessity of sovereignty claims in the first place.[34] Yet in some instances, self-determination as a means of claims-making has become a lever for making materially redistributive claims against subjugating dynamics of power. This is particularly salient in anticolonial and Indigenous claims to territory and governance.[35]

For Stanley (2014), the "self" at stake in gender self-determination is that of the radical collectivity resisting various forms of capture, such as bureaucratic legitimacy or formally defined state-sanctioned protections.[36] "Antagonistic to such practices of constriction and universality," they write, "gender self-determination is affectively connected to the practices and theories of self-determination embodied by various and ongoing anticolonial, Black Power, and antiprison movements" (90). They ground the very act of "claiming of a self" in a Fanonian register as a gesture of collective refusal, contesting forms of knowledge that produce relations of subordinance and domination. Such refusals are continuous with Bierria's (2014) notion of transformative agency in confronting the supremacist convictions of hegemonic agency. Gender self-determination has, in recent years, become a means of joining together trans-, intersex, and other gender/sex outsiders who contest subjugating dynamics of power.

Emi Koyama (2003, 256) describes such collectivization and resistance as "transfeminism," which (among other things) endeavors to confront what she calls "society's taboo against the self-determination of our reproductive organs." These constraints are the forces that subject some of us to unwanted biomedical intervention while withholding it from others or that conditionally incorporate limited forms of trans- expression or embodiment into bureaucracies of state recognition (Gill-Peterson 2018; Koyama 2003; Spade 2015). In a broad sense, gender self-determination has become a collectivizing claim among (and beyond) trans- activists. Transfeminism considers its collectivities to be far-reaching. As I described in the Introduction, one group defined *transfeminism* as a "politics of resistance and alliance [that considers] domination to be a multilayered system that produces cross-oppressions, including transphobia" (OUTrans, n.d.).[37] As part of this collectivization, activists recognize various forms of gatekeeping (and pathologization) as expressions of medical paternalism and subjugation and thus target them as central barriers to self-determination.

Among trans- depathologization activists and advocates in the study, none defended stringent gatekeeping practices, and most actively worked to displace them. They frequently invoked gender self-determination or related concepts such as self-perceived need in the course of this work. As Amanda (interview, January 23, 2016) put it, confronting the relations of gatekeeping was key to "getting [trans-] people more power [and] getting people more access to resources." Activists, advocates, and some health-care providers sought to counter gatekeeping in a range of ways, many of which involved maneuvering within regulatory constraints and relations of domination. For the activist authors of the Gender Identity Law, for example, the notion of "self-perceived need" displaced biomedical or judicial authority.[38] For health-care providers in New York, clinic-based protocols and revised diagnoses enhanced patient autonomy and limited coercive requirements for mental-health treatment and diagnosis.

For some people advocating for poor trans- people in New York, gatekeeping went beyond medicine to describe coercive power dynamics of institutions such as prisons or shelters. Thus, it was not only the process of diagnosis that was an object of concern among activists and advocates but also judicial processes of legal and administrative legitimization and recognition. Most advocates were not invested in legal recognition per se. However, they saw these interventions as enhancing poor people's life chances. As Amanda (interview, January 23, 2016) said, "Diagnosis is a tool that helps people get things they need, and [in that sense] it's legitimizing . . . [but] I play with legitimization like fire, right? . . . I see that as a means to an end, but not an end to itself."

In this manner, the expressions of antigatekeeping at the heart of trans- depathologization were not confined to the realm of health and medicine. As Mark (interview, January 15, 2016), a New York–based advocate with whom I spoke, described, trans- health was not only about the "provision of what . . . might be called 'gender-affirming care.'" He said it also involves "the ability of trans people to survive and not be subjected because of systemic discrimination to an untimely death. . . . [Trans- health includes] the mechanisms that would enable trans- people to have control over their bodies, to have access to survival needs, and to be free from government surveillance and violence." These comments resonate with Anya's (interview, January 12, 2016) views on depathologized care in chapter 4, in which she expressed that freedom to access varying forms of trans- therapeutics—and, importantly, freedom from coercion—were key to enacting care without pathology. As Amanda and Anya emphasized, these claims to autonomy were not simply directed at claiming individual rights to access legitimized forms of care. Their interpretations of autonomy and self-determination instead also gestured at a collective refusal of state control reminiscent of paradigms of reproductive justice discussed in chapter 4.

For some of the respondents with whom I spoke in both sites of study, autonomy and self-determination were not only about individual claims for access to medical techniques and procedures but also linked to much broader objectives for transforming care relations. For example, during our interview, Talia (interview, August 3, 2013) said that she had been reflecting on the concept of health in general: "It's self-determined. . . . Maybe health is lack of oppression. Maybe health is agency, determining your own destiny."

Alondra Nelson's (2011) notion of "social health," as discussed in chapter 3, describes how the Black Panther Party's health activism "scaled up" from the individual body to the body politic. Likewise, collective trans- self-determination claims diagnosed biomedicine and its gatekeeping practices with the pathology of racialized transphobia.[39] In this landscape, activists focused on bioethical practices of informed consent to scale up to political refusals of pathologization and collective trans- self-determination.

For some respondents, such claims to self-determination extended well beyond the terrain of trans- health. As social worker Sylvia (interview, August 9, 2013) commented during our interview in her Brooklyn apartment:

> Although I'm very skeptical about individualism on a variety of levels, I think when it comes to decisions about one's own body, that's the only level that is ultimately morally defensible. . . . Trans- politics . . . [involve] transforming the medical system in a way that enables people to self-determine the basic conditions of their lives [as] a central part of its logic. [It] calls on trans- activists to make demands on the state and the health-care system, and [also] calls on trans- people and trans- advocates to transform the nature of those services in a way that prioritizes dignity and self-determination. Those are two great places to start for thinking about what a left health-care politics would look like.

The breadth of these objectives was echoed by other trans- advocates, such as New York–based advocate Amanda. During our interview, she commented that the goal of her organization's work was "to build power in low-income communities and communities of color. . . . A huge part of that is supporting someone's ability to self-determine" (interview, January 23, 2016).

For activists, self-determination and bodily autonomy were somewhat synonymous. These concepts both connoted broad collectivist claims to freedom from coercion or domination, in addition to the ability to determine the conditions of one's life. This understanding differs markedly from notions of personal autonomy centering rational, individually acting subjectivity that are mobilized in bioethics in the United States and increasingly in Argentina. Each distinct interpretation rests on differing theories of power. If activist interpretations implied collective reckonings with broader fields of medical and state power, bioethical interpretations focused more singularly on addressing the dyadic relation between provider and patient in the exercise of free will. Yet the shared use of these terms across social worlds enabled activists' claims to depathologization to be taken up and institutionalized by health-care providers, who found resonance and clinical precedence in the centrality of autonomy within bioethical frameworks.

Negotiating Transfeminist Care: Boundary Objects and Informed Consent

In chapter 1, I described how the gradual and incomplete institutionalization of depathologization has involved "cooperation without consensus" (Star 1993). Late feminist technoscience scholar Susan Leigh Star saw such coordinated work across social worlds as being enabled by what she and James R. Griesemer (1989) call "boundary objects." These are objects with "interpretive flexibility" that can move across different communities of knowledge while retaining enough shared meaning to accomplish coordinated work.[40] In Star and Griesemer's initial discussion of boundary objects, they describe them as being "plastic enough to adapt to local needs and the constraints of the several parties employing them, yet robust enough to maintain a common identity across sites" (393). In this sense, autonomy and its presumptive enactment through informed consent became boundary objects that could be interpreted in distinct ways by health-care providers and activists.[41] For providers, these signaled ethical and collaborative care (as well as protection from liability). For activists, in contrast, they heralded collective self-determination and freedom from racially stratified constraints to determining their conditions of life.[42]

To maintain their coordinated work, activists and providers were involved in "developing and maintaining coherence" of boundary objects across social worlds (Star and Griesemer 1989). Autonomy was an abstract concept on which both groups could agree, at least in its loosely constructed sense. For providers, informed-consent processes were ineluctably material and signified protocols, scripts, and contracts. For activists, they were abstract and politicized claims that could efficaciously supplant gatekeeping models of care and enact self-determination. A few activists and providers inhabited both social worlds and acted toward informed consent as both an emancipatory promise and a protocol-oriented process.[43] The boundary object of informed consent meant something different to actors in each social world, even as its plasticity enabled collaboration. However, these distinct interpretations and orientations of action were also accompanied by distinctly different political visions relevant to relations of care. These politics—specifically, those relevant to the governance of life and arrangements of power therein—ranged not only *between* social worlds but also within them.

As I mentioned at the outset of this chapter, informed-consent processes existed even within gatekeeping models, so for providers, consent-driven care meant figuring out how to substitute for psychiatrically or psychologically diagnostic care. This sometimes meant developing detailed conditions for care that they thought would guard against abuse, release them from malpractice liability, and establish patient agreement and authorization. In short, consent-driven care was about replacing an authoritative approach to care with a semistandardized, contractual, and collaborative approach. As Talia (interview, August 3, 2013) described:

> The problem was a lot of people might have been coming to us on hormones prescribed not by that nurse but some[one else]—who *knows* who they were!—and they weren't really given any information about what is going to happen, what's permanent, what's not. So we actually made it a requirement that everyone had to have that meeting with the hormone advocate. That hormone advocate is a licensed therapist, but it was not a therapy session. It was like a psycho-educational session where there was an assessment about ability to consent but the rest of it was more like an information-sharing time . . . to make sure they understood what the consequences may be versus benefits versus unknowns.

As she continued, she mentioned that the protocols she helped to develop in her former clinic were the result of patient resistance to gatekeeping. She explained the process as being a collaborative one, which began with what she described as somewhat of an "uprising" among patients:

> We looked at the Callen-Lorde protocol and we really tried to take the feedback from the people who were unhappy with

> how their process had gone, and then met as an interdisciplinary team for a good six months like every other week. And in that process [we] revamped our whole . . . step-by-step process, our actual written consents that people sign. We read the Tom Waddell protocol, and . . . took what we liked from Callen-Lorde and Tom Waddell and just . . . wrote our own thing.

This protracted work—the outcome of negotiations within the care team and among "unhappy" patients—resulted in a protocol and informed-consent contract that all actors could presumably and at least provisionally accept.

When put in this way, informed-consent contracts and protocols might seem to be awkward "tools for the job" (Clarke and Fujimura 1992) when it comes to activists' desires for radical transformations in dynamics of care provision, or what might be called transfeminist care. Thinking back to Callen-Lorde's sample informed-consent form with its technical lists and stark warnings, its simultaneous aims of education, collaborative decision-making, and contractual agreement are apparent. Moving from Boucher's image, for example, to the material contracts that accompany clinical practice induces some conceptual whiplash. It might indeed be difficult to recognize in such clinical forms the emancipatory self-determination that would lead to building collective power—particularly given the stipulation that providers are those charged with assessing people's supposed capacity to give consent in the first place.

Nevertheless, the struggle for trans- and travesti activists has been one of negotiation and collaboration in the midst of sustained (and sharply stratified) dispossession. As such, activists worked within the significant constraints of regulatory and biomedical infrastructures to intervene in the most sharply pathologizing and condescending forms of care provision by enacting consent-driven models. Even as they articulated "self-determination" in a register of transformative agency, the parameters within which they acted rendered elusive the desire to manifest transfeminist dynamics of care. Activists worked within the constraints of biomedical and regulatory infrastructure to enact insurgent agency (Bierria 2014).

As Argentine travesti activist Lohana Berkins asserted at a 2010 conference, "We are patronized, we are seen as inferior subjects, incapacitated, we cannot make decisions about our own lives. Others make decisions about us, about our bodies. They tell us what we can have and not have and how to be. Obviously, as good feminists, we disobey everything" (Redacción Marcha 2020).[44]

For Berkins, as for other transfeminists making claims about self-determination, the problem that is being addressed in displacing gatekeeping through consent-driven care is that of having decisions made for us about what happens to our bodies. Even in the form of a technical contract, activists identified consent-driven care as at least provisionally addressing some of the hierarchical dynamics between trans- and travesti people and care providers. Activists saw these as opening up a fissure through which to insert new claims—claims that were at least *inflected* by transfeminist claims to embodied autonomy, the rejection of medical paternalism, racial/sexological science, austerity and supposed deservingness, and the colonized imaginary. This was advanced through transfeminist care politics that addressed the uneven devaluation of life by exposing the asymmetrical structuring conditions that have restricted and coerced action. Disobedience and resistance to pathologization is what brought about the revolt. However, the constraints of clinical practice significantly tempered that revolt.

Activists nevertheless regarded informed-consent contracts as instruments through which some forms of depathologized care could be materialized. In the United States, these were only implemented in site-specific practices, which limited their reach. Even in Argentina, where consent-driven care formed federal law, activists noted that there was little enforcement or regulation—as Joaquín (interview, August 3, 2015) mentioned, recommendations and guidelines abounded, but providers were not compelled to implement changes. Still, in their mobility and flexibility, consent-driven care protocols could travel from site to site, instantiating a multitude of ways to confront gatekeeping practices. Continuous with Murphy's (2012) discussion of "protocol feminism," this required working within extant landscapes of health-care infrastructure. For Murphy, "protocol feminism" refers to the "standardizable and transmissible components of feminist practices" (29). Referring to 1970s feminist self-help as one mode of protocol feminism, she discusses how the instruments in question (menstrual extraction kits, vaginal self-exams, speculums, etc.) were a "reassemblage . . . crafted by appropriated and altering elements already available" at the time (30). Protocols—as how-to guides for taking specific kinds of actions and engaging in counterconduct within hegemonic arrangements of care—were thus intended to be flexible and mobile. Consent-driven care in trans- health activism also sought to reassemble dynamics of care in a transfeminist mode, and informed-consent guidelines and practices were one of the means by which they sought to accomplish this.

Social worlds, such as those of activists, advocates, and providers, comprise collectivities that share interests and coordinate action—but they are far from monolithic, and each social world ranged in its action toward consent-driven protocols. Like the self-help feminists at the center of Murphy's (2012) study, trans- health activists also acted toward these protocols in different ways and, in so doing, produced very different forms of knowledge about feminist biopolitics. This does not necessarily lead to a consistent or shared political position: "Biopolitics names life as the legible domain of politicization, yet still leaves open the question of how politics was itself mapped and given tactical shape" (37). In the open field of fashioning transfeminist biopolitics, activists, advocates, and care providers collaborated centrally around revising diagnoses (as discussed in chapter 2) and enacting practices of care, specifically through boundary-object work centered on informed-consent processes. Yet, the biopolitics they fashioned ranged significantly. If some trans- health activists found consent-driven care to meet their expectations for improved care relations and trans-self-determination, others recognized these transformations as the belated provision of a distinctly minimal form of agency.

Playing with Legitimization like Fire: Collaboration and Complicity

Even as activists, advocates, and some health-care providers ardently agreed on the centrality of self-determination as a means of contesting the hierarchical care relations of trans- gatekeeping, there was little consensus about just *how* to enact this in practice. The tactics and objectives that trans- depathologization proponents adopted ranged greatly depending on health infrastructure and primary foci of concern. As Amanda put it, trans- advocates often worried about the "flirtation with legitimacy" that accompanied the work to intervene in gatekeeping:

> You have to get just enough legitimacy to have the resources you need to self-determine and take power, but the more you get to the world of legitimacy, then the more regulated things become and the more they get prescribed, so the less self-determination you get. So, it's like walking this line. In some ways we're creating health protocols, in other ways we're trying to destroy health protocols. All in the name of just trying to help people have more control over what's going to benefit them, what's going to help them be healthier. (Interview, January 23, 2016)

In their work to demonstrate medical necessity to achieve publicly subsidized care, Amanda and other New York–based advocates were apprehensive about investing in tactics that upheld the privileged status of biomedicine. Embracing paradigms of consent-driven care—which were still squarely situated within the authorizing logics of biomedicine—enabled "walking this line" between legitimacy and self-determination.

In this sense, for Amanda and other advocates, it was not the case that legitimacy was desirable on its own. Rather, she and other advocates and activists wanted public governments to take responsibility for financing care. Without public subsidies for care, they recognized that conditions of self-determination would remain as stratified as ever. Yet, as Amanda asserted, state recognition and legitimacy were also accompanied by new forms of regulation that were at odds with principles of self-determination. These were the tensions inherent in the practice of care without pathology.

For activists and advocates in Buenos Aires, the legal codification of "self-perceived need" seemed to deflect new infrastructures of regulation and instead dismantled the arcane requirements stemming from dictatorial rule. In contradistinction to clinic-wide informed-consent policies in the United States, the provision of self-perceived need ultimately defined trans- people and travestis as having the last word in the care they sought. Yet the material possibility of actually accessing covered therapeutics was frequently thwarted by limited public-health funding, untrained surgeons, and hormone shortages.[45] Furthermore, the Argentine state's claims to being on the cutting edge of human rights meant that state actors—specifically those in the executive and the legislative branches of the government—still adjudicated the limits of "self-perceived need." As Antonio, the Argentine activist I discussed in chapter 1, commented, the Argentine framework of human rights remained insufficient to address the enabling conditions of subordination that shaped people's choices in the first place:

> Recognition is ground zero. [The Gender Identity Law involved] the right to identity, which is the most important. . . . Now, with or without recognition, people need to work, they need to study, and they need to go to the doctor. There are many other things where recognition is a necessary condition, but it's not enough. (Interview, July 25, 2015)

Antonio emphasized that even as medical gatekeeping practices among trans- people and travestis were formally eliminated, Argentine state actors still set conditions for governing life. As discussed in chapter 3, although the passage of the Gender Identity Law set into motion a series of claims for trans- and travesti reparations, for example, these have been far more difficult to enact as means of confronting state violence. Antonio continued:

> We can say that having a state that opposes human rights is terrible, but having a state that conceives of itself as the reincarnation of human rights is also terrible because at that moment if you are not the state, you are an enemy of the state. . . . The state is the maximum authority. Just like the church has the authority of interpreting the Bible, the Argentine government has the authority to interpret the human-rights framework.

As critics of human rights argue, such regimes of authority preserve rather than shift hierarchical relations of power (Hua 2011; Spivak 2005).

As boundary objects, autonomy and informed consent enabled materially effective challenges to gatekeeping models in trans- health. As incipient models of care, these worked to confront multiple barriers to care, whether in the form of classification, restrictive standards, economic stratification, or coercive care relations. In the past two decades, activists, advocates, and providers have collaborated and negotiated to implement consent-driven care as a new mobile and flexible standard. While it certainly has not displaced gatekeeping in all sites, it is no longer a marginal set of practices. Appearing in everything from transnational declarations of human rights to federal laws to clinical protocols, consent-driven care is becoming an unremarkable practice in the field of trans- health—and activists have announced this as a victory.

The material enactment of consent-driven care as a depathologized form of trans- health does not necessarily deliver on all of its promises, though, in large part because the notions of autonomy that all stakeholders can agree on are both distinct and stratified. Nevertheless, consent-driven care has become a primary site (in addition to diagnostic revision) through which activists, advocates, and providers have worked to depathologize publicly funded trans- health care in practice. The contracts, protocols, technical cautions, and clinical workflows of informed-consent practices were perhaps a far cry from the notions of freedom at the heart of self-determination or coalitional depathologization. Yet gender and its self-determination, as a "terrain to make space for living" (Snorton 2017, 175), became central and ambivalently successful tools of trans- depathologization in practice.

As activists, advocates, and providers worked out the quotidian practices that make up care without pathology, they confronted the tensions and impasses of medical paternalism, uneven resource distribution, and human rights. Yet, through the boundary objects of informed consent, self-determination, and autonomy, they fashioned modes of biomedical practice that at least provisionally intervened in hegemonic care politics. How, then, do these actions carry implications for enacting care without pathology beyond the domain of trans- therapeutics?

In a section of *Cumbia, copeteo, y lágrimas* (the epidemiological biography I discussed in chapter 3), activist and scholar Mauro Cabral Grinspan (2007, 147) contributes a passage about the limits of bioethical frameworks, especially among those who are "invisible to . . . a bioethics that is too satisfied with its own progressiveness—that which is limited, for the present, to those who are included within their restricted version of the world, and which ignores the existence of the rest."[46] Activists and advocates often interacted with bioethical frameworks with ambivalence or apprehension—in Amanda's terms, they approached these as if they were playing with fire. They frequently found such frameworks to be inadequate, particularly in their failure to comprehend the systemic racialized immiseration and stratified violence of transphobia. Yet they made interventions at clinic-wide, national, and transnational levels that in many cases formally shifted the locus of decision-making in trans- therapeutics and forced providers at minimum to respond to activists' demands for care without pathology.

Particularly among coalitional depathologization activists, contestations of gatekeeping were not simply about the ability to freely choose what would happen to one's body. They were also about rejecting the bureaucracies and ideologies of care that unevenly distributed access to the conditions required to live and thrive. Activists and advocates fought against gatekeeping practices to intervene not only in trans- pathologization but also in the logics of austerity in which these practices were embedded. Specifically, they expanded the possibility for depathologized care from wealthy people funding their own care to all travesti and trans- people, including those whose care was subsidized or covered by state funds.

Activist visions for collective self-determination had a profound effect on practices and dynamics of care. And yet, their codification into the formalized work of informed consent resulted in something that looked more like bioethics and less like revolution. Cooperation also remained starkly uneven—activist framings found their way into formal documents, but usually through a series of diffusions through scales of expertise and power. Gatekeeping thus functioned at the level of knowledge production as well as care. As Velocci (2021) points out, these interventions concede the domain of biomedicine as the proper site for decisions about bodies to be made. They write, "These [antigatekeeping] efforts continue to frame medicine as possessing a 'gate' that needs to be 'opened,' as though a slight tweak to clinical practice is the solution to the problems that clinical practice has caused" (476). Given these many concessions, there remains a simmering rage in this "cooperation without consensus" and its profound limits.

Yet the interventions into the politics of expertise and distribution that were made manifest through negotiations over consent-driven care undeniably shifted the terms and relations of care in trans- health. Activists' work to enact transfeminist care politics have thus raised critical questions about access to care, collective claims to life, racialized distribution of public goods, and depathologization, among others. These are relevant not only to the focused domain of trans- health but also to a much more capacious set of care practices that structure communication, diagnosis, financing, and notions about what "wellness" is. In this sense, transfeminist care politics—inclusive of the openings and limitations they have instantiated in health-care practice—offer substantial insights for the field of health-care politics more generally.

Next, I turn my focus to a group that has already, in a sense, been present throughout the book. While not all of the activists, advocates, and providers with whom I spoke could be described as coalitional depathologization activists, many could. And indeed, these were the study participants who most clearly worked to manifest care without pathology in its fullest sense. Chapter 6 will explore this group in more depth and detail.

6 Extending Depathologization

The Coalitional Approach

I spoke with Ana (interview, July 31, 2015), a travesti activist, at a downtown café in Buenos Aires. She had been part of the coalitional efforts to pass a comprehensive Gender Identity Law and was active in several other travesti struggles for access to health and employment. During our interview, she told me that she was fighting not just for depathologization but against criminalization and abbreviated life chances "and in favor of real economic, political, and social justice."[1] Ana said that during her work on the Gender Identity Law, she found herself at odds with the mainstream, mostly gay- and lesbian-led organizations that had proposed a more cautious and piecemeal approach to legislation.[2] During the struggle over what version of the law would ultimately be proposed, she said that the "gays with money" had condescended to travesti leaders, intimating that the latter group's approach was foolish and unrealistic. Now that the law had passed, she said with a laugh, *everyone* was claiming authorship.

The mainstream ex post facto supporters celebrated the law as a mark of the nation's steady political progress following the legalization of gay marriage in 2010. For Ana, it was instead a noteworthy victory within a protracted and ongoing "proletarian struggle." "It delivered a very strong message," she said, "to political and medical institutions and police . . . all of these institutions that systematically . . . mocked us, beat us, condemned us. . . . [It sent a message] because we made a decision to *do* things. And we can do many other things."[3] In short, it was evidence of the political power of a movement that centered their demands to address conditions of survival for poor travestis and trans- people.

Gesturing to our server as he walked away from our table, she explained that the travestis with whom she worked had more in common with him than with the well-off gay and lesbian leaders of mainstream organizations (and, she added, with me as a Global North–based researcher). While she was generally suspicious of bourgeois interests in travesti and trans- activism, she frequently forged cross-class coalitions with those whom she saw as "abandoning their personal interests" in political movements. She said these partners in activism distinguished themselves by their "actions, their lives, their other memberships and associations . . . how they show, on a daily basis, that they've learned from our respective positions." Ana explained that she was compelled to work with people who took an approach of "poner el cuerpo" when it came to activism and social change. As United States–based Argentine sociologist Barbara Sutton (2007, 130) explains, this phrase escapes direct translation, but might be partially described by the phrases "to put the body on the line" or "to give the body." Sutton argues that this concept has been especially central to feminist movements in Argentina and that the "embodied commitment" to which it gestures spans the public and spectacular forms of "participation in mass mobilization," as well as "the more hidden daily work of activism" (143). The phrase has also been readily applied to *piquetero* movements that mobilized as an informal labor movement (unrepresented by trade unions) to protest unemployment and austerity measures by physically blocking roads and major routes of travel.

In chapter 1, I discussed an orientation to depathologization activism that I termed "coalitional depathologization." What Ana was describing during our interview exemplifies this approach to trans- health activism. Unlike social-movement activists who focused their interventions or objectives on issues related solely (or seemingly solely) to transness, coalitional depathologization activists readily articulated cross-movement links and took part in political struggles on multiple fronts. This last chapter will return to some of the themes I discussed in chapter 1 related to cross-movement work when it comes to care without pathology. It will show how coalitional depathologization activists took trans- health activism's implicit fights against austerity and rendered them thoroughly explicit. In so doing, I show how coalitional depathologization activists pointed to different and more expansive desires when it came to trans- health.

In what follows, I begin by expanding my reflections in chapter 1 about coalitional depathologization, what it is, and what it looks like in practice. Next, I reflect on its orientations to *horizontal* modes of action, politics, and thought. I consider "the horizontal" in several senses: through horizontal relations of power, through an orientation to a political horizon, and through a horizontal commitment to collectivize beyond formations of travesti or trans- identity. Finally, I analyze how these coalitional and horizontal orientations led some activists to center political economy in their engagement with trans- and travesti politics. In this final section, I turn to their critiques of austerity and their engagement with debt—both sovereign debt and what activists called "debts of democracy." I conclude by discussing the stakes, possibilities, and limits of these approaches to depathologization.

Anticapitalism in the Clinic: Coalitional Depathologization in Practice

Ana considered it impossible to actualize horizontal care relations without simultaneously confronting the inequities of racial capitalism. As such, it made no sense to her to address biomedical pathologization without also mobilizing against economic marginalization and violence—nor did it make any sense to address these solely in the legal domain. Rather, the proletarian struggle she described needed to take place in many sites and through a multitude of tactics. In addition to her work on the Gender Identity Law, she had been involved in proposing a model for comprehensive care in public clinics for poor travestis and trans- people living in the *conurbanos* surrounding the city of Buenos Aires. These municipalities have significantly higher rates of poverty than the city proper, and public hospitals there—along with other municipal services—were comparatively poorly funded. Nevertheless, Ana and her comrades and supporters issued a charismatic proposal to develop *consultorios inclusivos*: "inclusive" or "trans-friendly" clinic days in hospitals. With the support of activist youth and enthusiastic municipal leaders, these models had taken root in at least four clinic sites, and each had a lively clientele on weekly scheduled clinic days.

Ana was proud of the Gender Identity Law's passage, but she had no illusion that it would put an end to pathologization and its persistent effects. Her work with consultorios inclusivos aimed to build spaces of practice that were somewhat more protected from pointedly pathologizing forms of care. She described how appointments during these clinic days were reserved not only for poor travestis and trans- people but also specifically for sex workers (whether travesti, trans-, or nontrans-) and for people seeking abortions (interview, July 31, 2015). While these were illegal until 2020, abortions were often performed prior to this time, but they remained most difficult to access for poor people (McReynolds-Pérez 2017). Consultorios inclusivos aimed to connect patients with supportive providers and to insulate people from the harassment that often occurred in standard waiting rooms. Rather than fundamentally shifting the stratified dynamics of medicine, Ana saw consultorios inclusivos as "another place for the resignification of politics," or as microcosms within which the practices and possibility of a broader vision of depathologization could be materialized.

The health, regulatory, and activist landscape in metropolitan Argentina is far from equivalent to that in the metropolitan United States. Nevertheless, I found remarkable continuities in critique, desire, and action among certain activists in both locales. For example, Mark (interview, January 15, 2016) was the New York–based advocate and attorney I mentioned in previous chapters. I interviewed him in his downtown Manhattan office, where he worked primarily as a litigator. On the wall behind him hung a series of radical political posters, including one depicting Black trans- liberation activist Marsha P. Johnson. Mark generally had a bleak view of biomedicine: "It wasn't until I started to really understand the legal system and . . . how health care worked in general . . . [that I] started to realize there was an entire . . . system that was essentially designed to make it impossible for some people to survive." Like Ana, he did not think that depathologization would immediately fix these systemically fatal hierarchies in medicine or the law, but he saw health care as a crucial site through which to amplify demands to address conditions of survival for marginalized trans- people.

> When I think of trans- health in a relatively broad way . . . I think about [it] as . . . the ability of trans- people to survive and not be subjected [to] systemic discrimination, to untimely death. . . . So I think of trans- health as the mechanisms that would enable trans- people to have control over their bodies, to have access to survival needs, and to be free from government surveillance and violence.

After outlining this broad notion of trans- health, which he later described as "self-determination," he lamented that his legal work on access to medical care was difficult to square with this "more robust idea of health." He said, "I don't think . . . we as lawyers [necessarily] conceptualize health care in a broader sense. . . . I think the law just doesn't really allow you to dream in that way, and I think people end up being really limited by what a legal case would allow you to accomplish."

Mark mentioned that people with whom he previously worked at a smaller-scale, direct-service focused legal project had mobilized a more expansive notion of health. "I think [health] meant not having to be subjected to a horrible shelter, or not being sent to prison . . . and as part of that, of course, . . . having access to hormones if that's what [clients] wanted." He explained that these more sweeping notions of health sometimes conflicted with the restrictions of legal work: "You're so constrained in terms of the advocacy stories you can tell to a court." He saw impact litigation as a prudent tactical approach through which to make immediate depathologizing and material demands on medicine and the state—but one that required provisionally narrowing a more sweeping political frame: "I mean, you have to tell a story and certainly I'm going to do that, [but it] doesn't mean I believe it. . . . But if it's effective, I don't really care."

I spoke with Sylvia (interview, August 9, 2013), the social worker and activist I mentioned in chapter 5, prior to the elimination of the state's Medicaid exclusion. For her, care without pathology was not a political end point but rather continuous with political and economic redistribution and revolution. She explained:

> Trans- health [has been] the starting point for beginning to think a lot about what it would take to turn back the tide on neoliberalism, to significantly increase taxation on the wealthy, to rebuild and expand the social wage, and to transform the provision of social services by the state into being more democratic, dignified, honoring the self-determination of particularly African American communities and immigrant communities, and queer and trans- people, and sort of rebuild [what a] democratic, egalitarian welfare state could look like.

She distinguished mainstream LGBQ freedom and rights projects from trans- health activism, explaining that the former were concerned primarily with issues of privacy or nondiscrimination. The latter, she asserted, might indeed foster the conditions to engage powerfully in class struggle. Specifically, she thought this had to do with how trans- health advocates and activists must enter into explicit engagements and make demands on institutional infrastructures in ways that LGBQ advocates and activists need not necessarily take up.

> Trans- health, on a very clear level, requires infrastructure of either the state or the market, [and] unlike LGB[Q] freedom, where you could say, "What we want is to be left alone in our bedrooms," trans- people require the actual acquisition of a material good that cannot be produced in one's own home. . . . So it forces advocates and trans- people into struggles around state provision and struggles around the shape of marketized and commoditized health care.

Sylvia's glib critique of mainstream LGBQ projects is perhaps too easy a dismissal, given the substantial materialist and feminist critiques emanating from queer of color theory. In Roderick Ferguson's (2004, 149) terms, this field "interrogates social formations as the intersections of race, gender, sexuality, and class, with particular interest in how those formations correspond with and diverge from nationalist ideals and practices." Given these interventions, reducing LGBQ politics to being "left alone in our bedrooms" is in fact more an indictment of a white supremacist "homonormative" queer politic, in Lisa Duggan's (2003) terms, or perhaps "homonationalism" in Jasbir Puar's (2007). In either regard, this is not representative of the fullness of queer/*cuir* politics writ large. Nevertheless, it is a useful contrast in thinking through the centrality of struggles over resources that characterize trans- health politics (as well as many strains of intersectional queer theory or activism).

Sylvia's Marxist commitments led her to conclusions that were similar to Ana's in terms of identifying collaborators in a broader politics of redistribution.

> I think care in Medicaid is an enormously important fight. . . . Trans- inclusion in the shelters, the defense of trans- prisoners, stopping police harassment and police violence for trans- people, providing more health-care access for trans- people. . . . Is there a way we can inflect our organizing that's informed by and rooted in a vision of a broader [working-class] left that our work contributes to rebuilding? (Interview, August 9, 2013)

In this sense, Sylvia frames trans- health activism as a distinctly working-class project—one that resonates for both trans- and nontrans- working-class people as a powerful means of making solidary and redistributive claims on the state in the absence of a robust working-class movement.

As I discussed in chapter 1, Ana, Mark, and Sylvia were enacting a form of trans- health activism I call "coalitional depathologization." Coalitional depathologization activists undertook what legal scholar and activist Dean Spade (2015) calls "critical trans politics" and what political scientist Cathy Cohen (1997, 444) calls "transformational politics." This is "a politics that does not search for opportunities to integrate into dominant institutions and normative social relationships, but instead pursues a political agenda that seeks to change values, definitions, and laws which make these institutions and relationships oppressive" (445). While all respondents in the study thought that trans- health should be a publicly available feature of health-care delivery systems, this subset of respondents specifically rooted these demands within a broader commitment to redistributive economics or labor struggles. Those who did drew strong connections between pathologization, economic marginalization, racialized surveillance, and abbreviated life chances—and thus saw depathologizing modes of redress to require a correspondingly expansive breadth of action.

Given this breadth in scope and commitment, what did biomedical care look like for coalitional depathologization activists—especially within institutions like public hospitals or benefits offices? Ana (interview, July 31, 2015) said that the effectiveness of consultorios inclusivos depended on the providers who staffed them sharing at least some understanding of the damage produced by pathologization of difference writ large and biomedicine's broader role in reproducing this. Adán, the primary-care physician I mentioned in chapter 5 who worked at a popular consultorio inclusivo, was one of the people she mentioned as someone who was good for the job. I interviewed Adán at his clinic and spent most of the day in the waiting room of the consultorio inclusivo prior to speaking with him. We were scheduled to speak midday during his lunch break, but he had to work through it. Every once in a while, he rushed out to let me know he would talk with me as soon as he was able. As I waited, I spoke with the patients there. Chairs were arranged in a circle, having been moved from their regular configuration in rows that faced toward the walls. We chatted and passed around snacks as people waited for their appointments. When we spoke on the phone to arrange the interview, Adán mentioned that it was common practice in the clinic to bring food to share and asked that I do so, too. In the afternoon, someone celebrated a birthday.

While I did not directly ask people in the consultorio inclusivo why they were there, some volunteered that they had come for hormone prescriptions or related care. Others were also there for a range of standard medical problems, even though they had to wait longer than on a regular clinic day. But they said they preferred to talk with Dr. Adán, and they liked the waiting room at the consultorio inclusivo anyway. I finally spoke with Adán—a Marxist and physician—about an hour and a half after the clinic was set to close. He shared some of the other reasons that patients had come, including one who was seeking misoprostol for a pharmaceutical abortion (interview, July 24, 2015).

In his ethnographic work on state bureaucracies and welfare programs in the Buenos Aires conurbanos, sociologist Javier Auyero (2012) reflects on extended forms of waiting. Arguing that poor people become "patients of the state," he posits waiting as a form of social control. The wait was certainly long, but it did not immediately seem to have the stultifying effect that Auyero describes. Rather, it carried the sense of "clinic as community" that often accompanies both feminist and queer health formations (Batza 2018; Murphy 2012). As Michelle Murphy (2012) shows, romanticizing this view involves an erasure of the ways hegemonic power still suffuses their operations. Nevertheless, it was difficult to ignore the fact that people seemed more or less content to be waiting there with each other. This—as well as the "structure of feeling" (R. Williams 1954) that more generally accompanies the trans-friendly clinic—emerges largely as a collective sense of relief at the possibility (however minimal) of being able to access previously unattainable forms of facilitating the conditions of life and well-being (Batza 2018).[4] For Ana, the availability of such spaces was certainly about fostering a communitarian sense of togetherness. More than this, though, she was interested in how consultorios inclusivos became one more site for the possibility of working-class coalitions to be forged and through which a movement for economic redistribution—led by Global South travesti and trans- people—could be imagined and mobilized.

This potential may also have been palpable for political actors who were wary of working-class and cross-class solidarities. In 2015, there were at least four robust consultorios inclusivos operating in different conurbanos. With the election of President Mauricio Macri later that year on a center-right neoliberal platform, the nation's robust social-welfare apparatuses became a primary target of a concerted economic austerity regime. Funding and state support for consultorios inclusivos dried up along with this systematic disinvestment in public-health programs in the nation (Gollan 2016). Diego Bocchio, one of the youth activists involved in starting a consultorio inclusivo in Morón, Argentina, says that officials initially framed dismantling the program as an economic necessity but soon undertook a systematic campaign of harassment (FM En Tránsito 2016). The program had resisted pressures to close through public protests and was able to continue operations for several more years. However, Bocchio reports that patients and staff became subject to a sustained campaign of blatant harassment, in which opponents of the program showed up for clinic days to intimidate patients and staff.

Ana's position on the potential for consultorios inclusivos to generate new popular critiques and solidarities was echoed in an editorial by leftist Argentine media collective Redacción La Tinta (2019). In an editorial article, they argue that clinic days involve the provision of "health as a basic right," which is "often almost impossible for those who do not conform to the heteronormative structures that seek to regulate [travesti and trans- people's] bodies."[5] Like Ana, Mark, and Sylvia, these authors see "thinking health as a right" as confronting a "patriarchal and pathologizing system" and as part of a broader project of ending institutional violence (Redacción La Tinta 2019). Similar to Sylvia, the collective thought that the *quality* of clinical care relations matter, but that hegemonic structuring conditions are what tend to shape care relations as hierarchical, pathologizing, and coercive. Sylvia (interview, August 9, 2013) saw this in terms of Marxist political economy, applying it to her understanding of racial capitalism in the United States:

> Class struggle is why we got neoliberalism, and class struggle is why we don't have universal health care. Class struggle is why we've got such pervasive . . . national oppression of African Americans. It's why we have mass incarceration and pervasive poverty and that we're not going to get very far in figuring all this out without figuring out the class war.

Indeed, this insistence on analyzing trans- health within political economy characterized coalitional depathologization activists like Sylvia, Mark, Ana, and others.

In their discussion of "trans political economy," Vek Lewis

and Dan Irving (2017, 4) describe "how contemporary 'architectures' of power differentially and unequally affect trans and sex/gender-diverse people across the globe." In various ways, coalitional depathologization activists made explicit claims for economic redistribution and transformations in state power against austerity politics. As such, their notion of care without pathology went well beyond the bounds of trans- health. Respondents who took this orientation to their work frequently compared differing modes of embodied autonomy, making commonsense connections between trans- therapeutics, access to safe and legal abortion, coverage for in vitro fertilization and other reproductive technologies, freedom from forced sterilization, and the prevention of surgeries on intersex infants and children. Some respondents also mentioned how disability connected to trans- health, paralleling the central clinical relevance of patients' life conditions over and above diagnosis- and prognosis-driven care. For example, Mark described some of the work he had done in his previous job:

> I was . . . building our disability justice lens and trying to think about confinement in different ways, about civil confinement not just criminal confinement . . . [and] provision of care in those settings . . . to sort of build more alliances with disability justice and [be] more mindful of . . . how our rhetoric and our advocacy at times was counter to a disability justice framework. (Interview, January 15, 2016)

From this perspective, trans- health is simply one among many forms of care that need not require a treatable illness. Even more important for this group, trans- health is only one among many forms of care that places the subject of care—not the provider—at the center of decision-making.[6] Coalitional depathologization activists insist that forces of marginalization shape the power relations between providers and patients to such an extent that autonomy requires far more than providers simply choosing to conduct their work differently. It is this position that distinguishes those who align themselves with coalitional depathologization from other depathologization activists and that connects their aims with those of reproductive justice and Green Tide feminists and disability justice activists. Here, self-determination (*autodeterminación*) becomes a mode of demand that seems to invoke distinctive power relations that exceed those that currently shape institutions such as biomedicine.

Coalitions and Horizons

For trans- depathologization activists in this study, *trans-* was never singular. By this, I certainly mean that they embraced the notion that there is no prototypical way to *be* trans- or travesti or perhaps to *inhabit* transness or travestismo. Yet even more so, I refer to the way they understood forces of marginalization to be kaleidoscopic, such that the subjugation of trans- people and travestis was inseparable from other forms of marginalization and subjugation. It was this variegated understanding of power relations that also shaped how coalitional depathologization activists understood the uneven contours of transphobia as well as the multisited modes of resistance to these (and other) subjugating forces.

In this sense, depathologization was never simply about revising a diagnostic classification, adjusting medical-financing schemas, or changing standards of care—though it often included all of these. Rather, fighting for high-quality accessible trans- health care for all was only one facet of envisioning and working to manifest (or in Kai M. Green and Treva Ellison's [2014] terms, "tranifest") a different world—one in which health care was not tied to profit, in which carceral institutions ceased to exist, and in which imperialism, racism, and ableism did not structure life and death. Coalitional depathologization activists thus drew on the long view of abolition frameworks of activism. These are most palpable today in paradigms of prison abolition, which strive to "eliminat[e] imprisonment, policing, and surveillance" (Critical Resistance, n.d.) and "require us to imagine a constellation of alternative strategies and institutions" (Davis 2003, 107).[7] Generally speaking, abolition-based movements focus on deep political transformations that seek to reassemble collective life and reject systemic forms of domination, coercion, and punishment.

The activists with whom I spoke engaged these visions in different ways, taking varying positions on actions and orientations that might bring about their desired objectives for social and political transformation. What they held in common, though, was their belief in the absolute inextricability of trans- and travesti- struggles from other forms of political struggle—and, indeed, their active participation in political coalitions. These included broad-based movements for prison abolition, economic justice, disability rights and justice, reproductive rights and justice, and universal health care.

In her classic article "Punks, Bulldaggers, and Welfare Queens," Cathy J. Cohen (1997, 457) muses on the possibilities for coalition work centered not on "straight or queer" identity but rather on a shared understanding of how to distinguish enemy from ally. In retrospect, her discussion of the "radical potential" of queer politics in the 1990s might appear unduly optimistic and limited in geographic and conceptual reach.[8] Yet, her political commitments resonate strongly with those of the coalitional depathologization activists I describe in this (and in the first) chapter. The radical potential to which she refers involves the formation of "strategically oriented political identities" that stem from a "nuanced understanding of power" (458).

In his preface to *Black on Both Sides,* C. Riley Snorton (2017, ix) calls Cohen's analysis "an echo from the future" that speaks to the imbrications of race and gender—specifically, the indistinguishability of Black and trans- lives mattering—in present political constellations of racialized gender. Likewise, coalitional depathologization activists in this study grounded their present-day coalitional work in the "then and there" of political desire for the future characterized by transformations in relations of care (to borrow from José Esteban Muñoz's felicitous description of queer futurities). Like Muñoz (2009, 35), coalitional depathologization activists also embraced a skeptical utopianism that, in his words, enabled them "to conceptualize new worlds and realities that are not irrevocably constrained" by institutionalized and other pathologizing forces—an orientation he calls "horizonal temporality" (25). For coalitional depathologization activists, the temporal horizon of care without pathology grounded its manifestation (or tranifestation) in present-day depathologization (and other) struggles—as part of both sustained mass movements and more ephemeral uprisings.

The notion of the "horizontal" was therefore important to coalitional depathologization activists in at least three regards. First, they organized their aspirations for power relations between care providers and patients into horizontal rather than vertical alignment. Second, and in the minor sense of the term *horizontal,* they looked toward a horizon to ground multiple forms of resistance to pathologization to imagine depathologized futures. Finally, they oriented their political affiliations expansively outward, and horizontally so, moving away from trans- subjectivity as the primary or singular center of gravity for trans- health and politics. These evoke Marina Sitrin's (2006) analyses of *horizontalidad* in Argentine working-class-driven coalition politics. Like abolitionist frameworks, horizontalidad centers "non-hierarchical and anti-authoritarian creation rather than reaction" and guided not only activists' goals but also their everyday practices (3). Such philosophies are also reflected in the organizing approaches of mutual-aid networks, which depart from hierarchical service-provision models to those of reciprocal and mutual support and decision-making (Spade 2020). When it came to coalitional depathologization, the *horizontal* was an organizing analytic for the ways depathologization and care without pathology were woven together—both ideologically and in the strategies and tactics of political action. These orientations directed the focus of their work on redistributing power and resources and on the reorganizing infrastructures and dynamics of care.

In so doing, coalitional depathologization activists were also casting their lot with a theory of change rooted in the transformative force of mass social movements rather than in the realm of legal, judicial, or executive power. In Bernice Johnson Reagon's (1983) classic reflection on feminist coalition politics, she describes coalition in terms of survival. Framing identity-based political formation (specifically, "'woman-only' spaces") in terms of "barred rooms" in which only people "like you" are admitted (358–60), she warns against the consequences of—among other things—maintaining universalizing insularity as a singular political project. "There is no chance that you can survive by staying inside the barred room," she writes. "The door of the room will just be painted red and then when those who call the shots get ready to clean house, they have easy access to you" (358). In Reagon's time, "having easy access to you" generally meant political targeting or abandonment by "those who call the shots." Through the late twentieth and early twenty-first centuries, this has also meant conditional inclusion and tokenism. As Lisa Duggan (2004) asserts in *The Twilight of Equality?*, the economic transformations of neoliberalism have been accompanied by ideological and political shifts. These include the emergence of a superficial and "stripped-down, nonredistributive form of 'equality'" that fits nondisruptively with the upward flow of wealth and resources and with the privileging of the individual over the collective (xii). Coalitional depathologization activists were as wary of these conciliatory dynamics as Reagon was of other forms of political targeting.

For example, Anya compared trans- health struggle with HIV/AIDS movements, asserting that the latter had become characterized by co-optation by state agencies and well-resourced NGOs and by the exclusion of supposedly disposable subjects, such as unhoused youth. For Anya, the formal incorporation of HIV/AIDS activism into state agencies and NGOs has been accompanied by a conservative shift. "That movement is one we can learn so much from," she commented, referring both to its bold political tactics and its eventual absorption into the hierarchizing structures of state agencies and NGOs (interview, January 12, 2016). Antonio expressed similar concerns about the Argentine government hiring more trans- and travesti workers in the public sector—a shift that was extended by provincial quota laws and in 2021 by the passage of a national law under President Fernández's administration. While Antonio was not hostile to the increased opportunities for those who have been systematically excluded from labor markets, he expressed concern about the anticipated depoliticizing and anti-coalitional effects of such inclusions:

> It is very difficult to build alliances when the main objective is accessing the state and participating in the structures of power, which are organized around state access. So if you have or belong to an organization where the boss of the organization has a

> public position in the state and ensures you a much lower public position in the state . . . Sorry, but there is no horizontal solidarity there! Everybody works within their own organization . . . [and] different trans- organizations that work with the [state] health system . . . control the access to waiting lists [for trans- therapeutic care], which ends up transforming [it] into a political good. (Interview, July 25, 2015)

For both Anya and Antonio, participation in formal or NGO sectors curbed trans- activists' ability to effectively critique their mystifications and simultaneously limited possibilities for building effective alliances demanding horizontal redistribution of goods, wealth, and resources (including, but resolutely not limited to, trans- therapeutics).

Lisette, an Argentine trans- activist who worked in trans- advocacy, shared these positions but was somewhat circumspect about whether mass movements could indeed be effectively mobilized. "You have to get your . . . feet on the street and nobody wants to do that," she commented during our interview in a Buenos Aires café (interview, July 16, 2015). "Everybody wants to sit . . . somewhere and change the world with a dry martini in hand," she continued. Her skepticism contrasted with Ana's assertion that the organizing that led to the Gender Identity Law's passage sent a political message that travesti and trans- activists "can do many other things" (interview, July 15, 2015). Ana saw ample evidence in the mass political power that travestis and trans- people had mobilized—often alongside gay/lesbian/bisexual, working-class, and student movements—to resist criminalization, pathologization, exclusion, and marginalization. In short, she was optimistic about the willingness of a working-class travesti-led coalition of people who were willing to take to the streets and poner el cuerpo—put their bodies on the line for political change.[9]

"Putting one's body on the line" and coalitional approaches to mass movement-building have a long history in trans- politics in the United States, as well as Argentina. In this sense, Spade's "critical trans politics" have indeed been manifested—often in broad coalition—for nearly as long as discernible trans- movements have been active. As I describe with Elliott Fukui elsewhere (Fukui and Hanssmann, 2022), New York's Street Transvestite Action Revolutionaries (STAR) House was eminently involved in a broad effort to synthesize working-class movements and movements for Black and Puerto Rican liberation, anti-imperialism, housing, and health-care struggles with the politics of racialized gender and sexuality. STAR's work involved not only housing young, unhoused street transvestites (to use the language they used to describe themselves at the time) but also participating in street protests for gay as well as third-world liberation. "Putting one's body on the line" also evokes Robert McRuer's (2018) discussion of crip times. This notion critiques the fetishization of compulsory able-bodied/mindedness that austerity regimes brandish. It also describes the commitment of antiausterity activists—including many who were queer and disabled—to take creative and embodied action in public to protest austerity and to model different orientations to collective life. As I discussed in chapter 3, and as María Soledad Cutuli (2012), Lohana Berkins (2007b), and Josefina Fernández (2004) describe, travesti and trans-led struggles against capitalism and criminalization in Argentina were also foundational to the formation of trans- and travesti politics in the nation, even as more recent expressions of these politics have submerged or disavowed these histories.

These disavowals are expressed in varying forms, from the ableism of trans- activists who double-down on the "*We're* not mentally ill, but *they* are!" narrative to the co-optation of "creditworthy" trans- people for Citibank's "True Names" advertising campaign. In these and other examples, trans- health and trans- politics have turned inward, overlooking the mutable effects of pathologization beyond "transphobia" or viewing assimilation into dominant culture as a political triumph. Each is symptomatic of the chilling triumphs of racial neoliberalism. Yet, coalitional depathologization activists continually insist on the importance of working beyond Reagon's "barred rooms." As Antonio emphasized, "At the end of the day . . . the right to transition-based health is part of the right to health" (interview, July 25, 2015). For coalitional depathologization activists, care without pathology became a lens through which to view and act politically with others who were produced as pathological and criminalized subjects through racialized, classed, and (dis)abled norms of sex/gender/sexuality.

Vultures, Sovereign Debts, and Debts to Democracy

In Buenos Aires in 2014, I was walking in the Congreso neighborhood to my apartment when I saw a series of posters and graffiti on the side of a building. The posters read, "Fuera Buitres de Argentina," or "Vultures Out of Argentina"—and the graffiti read simply, "Fuera Yanquis," or "Yankees Get Out." They were each engaging a cross-hemispheric controversy that pitted Argentina against United States–based hedge-fund managers. The origins and intricacies of Argentina's significant sovereign debt are many. For the sake of this book, it suffices to say that neoliberal economic reforms and the institutions adjudicating financial globalization played an outsized role in its formation and accumulation, as well as in the international and domestic power struggles that emerged in its wake.[10] Argentina's default on its sovereign debt in 2001 led to an unprecedented economic crisis that resulted in half the population falling below the poverty line and sparked mass public protests. One unanticipated effect of this was the rise of "reclaimed" or "recuperated" businesses—including hotels (such as the Bauen), factories, and hospitals, which workers took over, usually adopting a horizontal work structure. For some travestis, these became sources of work and housing (as with the Nadia Echazú Textile Cooperative and the Hotel Gondolín).

A more nefarious effect was the entry of hedge funds, like Elliott Management and its subsidiary NML Capital Ltd., buying up defaulted debt titles. Also called "vulture funds" by critics, these particular companies are run by Republican Manhattan billionaire Paul Singer. Other hedge-fund managers who had also purchased Argentina's debt at pennies on the dollar agreed to restructured debt payments. Singer, however, pushed relentlessly for the full payout. During my 2014 stay, the nation was being sued by Singer's company in a U.S. district court in New York to pay its debts in full. Judge Thomas P. Griesa ruled in favor of the company.[11] In 2015, the hedge fund received $2.4 billion from Argentina's government.[12]

What, though, did vulture funds have to do with trans- politics? Perhaps more than initially meets the eye. Paul Singer was not only a vulture-fund manager, he was also one of the major funders that in 2013 compelled the Human Rights Campaign (HRC)—one of the major proponents of same-sex marriage campaigning in the United States—to expand its global reach. In the HRC's press release about the new program, Singer commented, "Some of the worst offenders [of LGBT persecution] also happen to be the same regimes that have dedicated themselves to harming the United States and its democratic allies across the globe." During a conversation at a Buenos Aires café in August 2014, Antonio expressed frustration with his activist counterparts in the United States for failing to make the connection between Singer's debt vulturism in the Global South and the imperialist saviorism of his global LGBT philanthropy. As feminist scholars of "NGOization" point out, the lopsided dynamics of global wealth have in recent years been translated into well-funded NGOs (Bernal and Grewal 2014; Dutta and Roy 2014; Álvarez 1999). These are often located in the Global North and exert a heavy influence on what local forms of activist work are fiscally supported (or denied support) in regions experiencing global disinvestment.[13]

Given this, it would stand to reason that coalition-based projects related to trans- labor rights and economic redistribution would be unlikely candidates for global HRC funding. As Antonio explained, it was the mainstream and elite gay- and lesbian-led organizations—some of whom had coalesced around Argentina's 2010 same-sex marriage campaign—that had initially struggled hard against trans- and travesti-led organizing efforts for a more comprehensive Gender Identity Law (as discussed in chapter 3). Concerns about figures like Singer indirectly influencing global LGBT politics were therefore all the more chilling to Antonio and others, particularly since it was likely to generate political fissures that might be exploited and because it would amplify conservative agendas to larger audiences. Antonio said that he had seen scores of United States–based activists complain on social media about Singer's entry into global LGBT politics and about the similarly trans- exclusionary history and conservative political approach of the HRC more generally.[14] He commented, "And then they laugh about Argentina being irresponsible with its money. The same people had no idea about the politics behind Argentina's debt and the vulture funds that have taken advantage of it." Speaking of Singer, he continued, "It's the same guy!" (field notes, August 27, 2014).

The following year, in a formal interview with Antonio, he remained angry at what he saw as the ignorance on the part of activists outside of Argentina of the imperialist and neoliberal politics shaping the nation's sovereign debt. Unlike some of the other activists with whom I spoke, Antonio did not identify as a *Peronist* and distanced himself from the state government.[15] Yet, he was vocal in his support for then President Kirchner's refusal to pay off vulture funds and bristled at the implication that the nation's debt reflected fiscal or political irresponsibility. "The disdain is . . . very strong from [the Global North]. . . . [They claim that] 'Argentina doesn't pay its debts.' Well, no!" Within these dynamics, which he saw as a manifestation of imperialist condescension, refusal was a means of anti-imperialist resistance—and indeed an anti-imperial resistance that was eminently intertwined with the forces that were likely to significantly shape local trans- politics for years to come. Through this transnational transfeminist analysis, Antonio attuned to these dynamics, as Amanda Lock Swarr and Richa Nagar (2010, 5) put it, as indicative of the "multiple ways in which they (re)structure colonial and neocolonial relations of domination and subordination."

Austerity politics—in both the large scale of the nation-state or the more moderate scale of state, provincial, or municipal economies—depend on the figure of the "irresponsible spender" and the "free rider" that it supposedly enables.[16] Through this lens, economists and media analysts represent Argentina as running under an imprudent government that spends excessively on social and economic programs and fails to privatize in accordance with the modern economic paradigm of economic neoliberalism. On a different scale, policymakers and popular media portray New York

City's municipal budget as similarly reckless, particularly when it comes to public-benefits programs such as Medicaid. At each level, lawmakers, economists, and policymakers advocating for austerity have urged belt-tightening regimes, generally focused on public programs for poor people, to implement economic prudence, limit spending, and reduce debts. Jenna Loyd (2017, 57) describes these attempts to pin debt on so-called entitlement programs as "deploying the purse as a weapon" (riffing on James Madison).

If state actors advocating austerity wielded notions of public benefit and good governance as weapons, some trans- and travesti activists—in conversation with others, including piqueteros and other confrontational working-class movements—wrested these out of their hands and fought back. For example, trans- and travesti activists and advocates mobilizing for the Gender Identity Law took to the streets to demand access to identity, health care, decriminalization, and depathologization as "debts of democracy" (*deudas de la democracia*). Trans- and travesti depathologization activists were far from alone in this framing; as legal scholar Kelsey M. Jost-Creegan (2017) points out, a variety of social movements in Argentina have mobilized it, from feminist movements to migrants to health-care-access movements. She describes this framing as an "innovation of Argentine social movements" in the wake of military dictatorship and sustained state violence and repression (168). Coalitional depathologization activists like Antonio and Ana took this as a debt to be repaid not only by the public provision of trans- therapeutics but also by the broader redistribution of economic resources, political power, and life chances against forces of racialized imperial power, medical power, and state power.

In New York, Sylvia took a similar view (interview, August 9, 2013). When I asked her about the ultimate political objectives of movements for trans- health, she responded, "Maybe it ends when we have a respectful, self-determined provision of medical services to trans- people provided in a system of universal single-payer health care with a democratically controlled worker state. Maybe." Her aspirational yearning is emblematic not only of the capaciousness of coalitional depathologization but also of the self-determined orientation that drives care without pathology.

Alongside Antonio, Mark, Ana, and others, Sylvia recognized something like New York's Medicaid fight for the public provision of trans- therapeutics as a narrow victory. On one hand, it certainly enabled a means of grappling with austerity politics and racialized and classed health disparities. On the other, it did so in a constrained manner, with significant exclusions, and in the broader landscape of a largely exclusionary and highly profit-based health-care system. In other words, it was a small concession, given the sweeping transformations she thought were necessary.

If depathologization activists in general sought to shift relations of care, coalitional depathologization activists understood this to require far more than regulatory, financial, or diagnostic tinkering. Rather, it required constructing a political analysis and a mass movement that went beyond the immediate needs of trans- people and travestis to broader desires for political transformation. As Antonio commented, "It's not about building a community, it's about building a movement" (field notes, August 27, 2014). Furthermore, if depathologization activists implicitly contested austerity by making claims for the legitimacy of trans- therapeutics as a social good, coalitional depathologization activists brought fights against austerity explicitly to the fore. Austerity regimes, among other forces, became a primary shared antagonist for them and for their coalitional partners, and debt—in addition to care—became a principal set of relations to transform.

Specifically, coalitional depathologization activists refused debt as a justificatory means to restrict ostensibly scarce collective resources. Rather, they reversed common notions of what was owed and to whom. In a related analysis, Lucí Cavallero and Verónica Gago (2021) describe how the development of international feminist strikes illuminates coalitional links between movements against gendered violence and in favor of transnational economic justice:

> Femicides and travesticides are inseparable from this geography of capital that imposes increasingly violent forms of dispossession and exploitation around the world. Saying "the debt is owed to us" in the international feminist strike *inverts*

> the burden of the debt: it recognizes us as the creditors and it forces investigations about debt to start in households and on the streets. (47)

In this regard, if coalitional depathologization activists were creditors, the debt of trans- and travesti dispossession was far from settled through the provision of public coverage for trans- therapeutics. Rather, there were far greater debts to settle, and they did not plan to stop at the concessions they had collected on to date.

Significant research remains be done on coalitional depathologization activism among trans- and travesti and other movements. Not only would this illuminate more of the interconnections between movements—perhaps more akin to social-movement permeability than "spillover" in David S. Meyer and Nancy Whittier's (1994) terms—it would also help us begin to grasp the emergent politics of care without pathology. As I mentioned in the last section, these movements oriented toward horizons of redistribution and, broadly speaking, justice.[17] As part of stretching toward those horizons, they worked to fashion notions of health and health care that were dignified, equitable, and nonhierarchical—in short, that were futures of a different world to come.

Argentine feminist historian Emmanuel Theumer (2018) describes how Lohana Berkins made clear her understanding of the relatedness of travesti and anticapitalist struggles. He quotes a quip for which she is famous in Argentine social movements: "In a world of capitalist worms, it takes courage to be a butterfly."[18] In Berkins's assertion, Theumer reads multiple meanings:

> She stressed a double displacement. First, the traditional Marxist capital/labor polarization and second, the feminist male/female polarization. . . . The antagonism between capital/gender suggested by Berkins is not confined to sexual difference . . . but instead opposes the allegorical multitude of butterflies to parasitic capital. The courage to become butterflies warns about the impossibility of recognition without redistribution and restitution. It pushes issues of representation

> into those of coalition, the harmony of consensus to the successive interference, the dialogue to the political conflict.[19]

Indeed, it is precisely the "impossibility of recognition without redistribution and restitution" that might be considered a paradigmatic position for coalitional depathologization activists.

Likewise, coalitional depathologization activists developed notions of health for trans- people and travestis that shaped clinical practice, especially in sites such as the consultorios inclusivos. These clinics served to insulate people from the thorniest elements of pathologizing care (not to mention waiting-room harassment). Catering largely to poor travestis living in the conurbanos, they also served people seeking abortions, nontrans- sex workers, and many others. Some community-based clinics in New York evoked a similar sense. Collectively, these endeavors were some of the ways activists made manifest theories of coalitional depathologization. They prioritized the needs of those who have been sharply marginalized in health and biomedicine and in racial capitalism and neoliberalism and worked to aspire to horizontal relations of care for all (even as they were certainly unable to manifest these fully).

Coalitional depathologization activists were under no illusion, though, that "parasitic capital" had been vanquished through the introduction of a few scattered sites of practice where care relations were being enacted differently (and against significant constraints). These were few and far between, plagued by funding and staffing shortages in the best of times and subject to closure with the intensification of austerity measures. Nevertheless, Ana had high aspirations for spaces like these sites for the "resignification of politics" and class solidarity formation. Whether or not her hopes were realized in these spaces, they did carry a certain promise for horizons of practice. And indeed, many coalitional depathologization activists marshaled a prefigurative or aspirational politics that they hoped to manifest through experimentation with the insufficient present.

It was not only through experiments with care relations that coalitional depathologization activists worked. They also strove to redefine the notion of debt and responsibility. New York– and

Buenos Aires–based trans- and travesti activists engaged in such resignifications in the statistical collectivization work about which I wrote in chapters 3 and 4. For many of these activists—specifically, those who made explicit links between trans- and travesti employment marginalization and labor-movement struggles or between travesticide and broader antiviolence movements—coalitional depathologization guided the ways they rethought the sources of harm and risk. Further, they insisted on the necessity for less hierarchical notions of care. Such expansive desires anchor the ongoing potentials—perhaps, as Cohen (1997) wished for, even radical ones—of trans- and travesti politics that center coalition and redistribution over isolation and concession. Cohen's "echo from the future" has also portended the difficulties and fissures in coalitional approaches—and the tensions from within trans-/travesti and Green Tide movements illustrate only one example of this. Nevertheless, these approaches might chart a path not only for depathologization but for the eventual enactment of broader health-care infrastructures that are accessible to and that care well for everyone—and perhaps that change the terms of medicine to fit the visions of care without pathology.

Conclusion

During the 1990s and 2000s, trans- depathologization activists in the United States, Argentina, and beyond were dreaming up a future. Plans were crafted in street protests, in popular assemblies, at the margins of interdisciplinary scholarly discourse, and in clinic waiting rooms, chatrooms, and conference rooms. These movements took notes from similarly pathologized subjects who rebuffed psychiatric authority and rejected patienthood, such as gay and lesbian depathologization activists. Yet many among them were uninterested in rending ties to biomedicine altogether. In this regard, they tuned into the guiding claims of disability activists, reproductive-health activists, and antiausterity and transnational feminisms to develop visions for depathologization that enacted care without pathology.

Care without pathology envisions a transformed landscape of care politics, practices, and objectives. It facilitates, asks, and collaborates where hegemonic frameworks of care have directed, diagnosed, and pathologized. These relations—distilled into practice by care without pathology—have begun to take a very partial hold in biomedicine, limited as they are by infrastructures of care and economy. This book explores how trans- and travesti knowledge has intervened in biomedical authority by interrupting and reformulating its relations of care, forging practices based largely in horizontalism.

While these models often fit awkwardly (if at all) within infinitely variable and unevenly supportive extant infrastructures of care, the demands of care without pathology nevertheless prompted considerable changes. For example, its proponents forced debates in domains of nosology, clinical dynamics, financial infrastructures, conceptualization of risk, care guidelines, and standardization of care. Trans- people and travestis have not been alone in enacting such changes—AIDS activists, reproductive-justice and disability-justice activists, feminist strikers, illness communities, and many others have also transformed landscapes of care provision. And still, the specific story of trans- health raises into relief what happens when care without pathology—at least partially and at least in theory—exerts force on an institutionalizing field of care in the twenty-first century.

In her study of feminist self-help health practice in the twentieth century in the United States, Michelle Murphy (2012, 32) describes how feminist health "critically diagnosed and redirected the exercise of power" within biomedicine. In *Care without Pathology,* I argue that trans- health activists undertook a similar project of developing a politicized diagnosis to contest enduring and shifting forms of pathologization. By contesting pathologization and redefining racialized transphobia as the true pathology shaping regimes of care for trans- people and travestis, activists formulated a powerful political diagnostic that could be applied in both narrow and expansive ways to rethink health politics. However, as Murphy also points out, the dynamics of feminist self-help were never external to the infrastructures and conditions within which they operated. In this sense, feminist self-help was not only a diagnosis but also a symptom of its entanglements with nation, geopolitics, racial capitalism, and other stratifying conditions of care and life chances within which its practices were embedded (32). She characterizes this as the collective condition of "living the contradiction" amid the uneven landscapes of care and biopolitics (Murphy 2012, 177–81). Likewise, similar contradictions in trans- health reveal the tensions that render "self-determination" a concept that is as compatible with regimes of bioethics and neoliberal economies of self-entrepreneurship as it is with collective assertions for universal access to care.

Revising Paradigms of Care

As I followed these phenomena over time, I witnessed what some have identified as a paradigm shift that claims to mark a partial catharsis of the pathologizing impulses of "transsexual medicine" and to make way for the depathologizing arrival of "trans- health" (Singer 2006; Pyne 2014; Saldivia Menajovsky 2018). In this book, I have traced the multiple revisions inaugurating the genesis of trans- health: from psychopathology to difference, from etiology to disparity, and from economic burden to social benefit. Running through these is a mode of thinking about trans- people that is also under (contested and conditional) revision: the apparent shift from object to subject. This is indeed the claim that animates trans- studies and trans- activisms: specifically, that trans- people know things about ourselves and know what conditions support our thriving (even in situations of considerable constraint). Importantly, this is as much about the broader conditions of life—housing, economic means, education, and freedom from violence among them—as it is about health care. Following activists who centered the public provision of care meant that these broader conditions were consistently part of conversations about trans- health, rather than *only* being about the entrepreneurial capacity to become "self-made" through trans- therapeutics (Irving 2009; Aizura 2018).

Indeed, if depathologization has been an anchoring concept for trans- activism, revision has been the means through which it has been concretized in health-care practice. In its dictionary form, *revision* connotes an act of review or reexamination for the purpose of correction, amendment, or improvement. In its rarer use, though, the term emphasizes the optical thrust of its Latin root ("to see"). *Revision*—sometimes hyphenated as *re-vision*—also means "the fact of seeing a person or thing again; an instance of this; a fresh or new vision of something" (*OED Online*).[1] This is indeed the doubled sense of the term that Adele E. Clarke and Virginia L. Olesen (1999) adopt in developing a diffractive optics to account for the varied practices of women's health and healing. In this book, I show how the revisions that have characterized trans- health's emergence have also unfolded in both senses of the term.

In the past decade, classificatory changes to both the *Diagnostic and Statistical Manual* and the *International Classification of*

Diseases have changed not only the criteria for diagnosing transness but also its ostensible status as an illness in the first instance. Legal and regulatory changes have accompanied these modifications to diagnostic knowledge and practice, including the passage of Argentina's 2012 Gender Identity Law and the elimination of New York State's Medicaid exclusion for trans- therapeutic care in 2015. Clinics, hospitals, health systems, and state laws have also adopted various models of consent-driven care, shifting the locus of medical decision-making in trans- therapeutics (at least at some level). Finally, coalitional depathologization activists have made concrete connections between trans- health and broader movements for redistribution, decolonization, racial justice, and collective self-determination. Depathologization—whether in its narrow or expansive form—has been at the heart of these transformations.

It might seem as if activists' and advocates' focus on trans- therapeutics risked displacing a broader set of desires or demands for broader forms of trans- health, or even for a more generalized set of redistributive politics, mutual care, decolonization, or emancipation. Indeed, as I began my project, I initially resisted the gravitational pull to concentrate on trans- therapeutic practice. I wanted to veer away from the tendency for trans- therapeutic care to become a synecdoche for the varying needs of trans- people and travestis, particularly since many people have little or no desire to pursue trans- therapeutic technologies of care, at least under the auspices of biomedicine.

However, the more I learned about how activists, advocates, and some providers were approaching depathologization, the more I realized that sweeping claims were frequently *embedded* within certain demands for care without pathology—albeit to varying degrees. This was perhaps most evident in the explicitly synthetic and expansive demands emanating from coalitional depathologization, but it also animated more contained or modest depathologizing claims. Furthermore, the shift away from illness and toward wellness was only one dimension of depathologizing projects. In contrast to this one-dimensional take on depathologization, proponents of care without pathology issued deeper demands.[2]

For example, struggles for the public provision of trans-therapeutics have been a central stage on which activists have made the broader claim that trans- health, and by extension, the flourishing of trans- life, is a social good. Implicit in this demand is that publics reorient to forms of collectivization that are not (strictly) pinned to productive citizenship, racialized respectability politics, calculations of modernity, and the varying forms of inclusion and rights that are predicated on whiteness. Of course, it is not the case that public coverage is the only or singular means of accessing these technologies. In addition, poor trans- people, travestis, and trans- people of color (among others) have long found alternative and nonbiomedically sanctioned means of meaningful enactment and embodiment of sexual/gender nonnormativity. However, the public demand for noncriminalized health-care access signals broader demands for wealth and resource redistribution and the eradication of austerity measures. These, in turn, scale up to poor-led, *piquetero*-inspired, and grassroots politics in trans- and travesti activism.

These were the movements I studied that also posited trans-health and trans- life in its radical multiplicity as modes of existence that profoundly enrich the worlds they inhabit. In this sense, trans- health and trans- life were asserted as a social good in a broad sense. In this regard, the flourishing of trans- multiplicity was figured as a desirable horizon not only for trans- people and travestis but for all. This was indeed one of the key contributions of care without pathology. Especially as care without pathology accompanies *furia travesti,* welfare warriors, coalitional depathologization, antiausterity activism, and transnational transfeminisms, this orientation to care suggests that divesting from subordinating structures bodes well for broader collective thriving.

Of course, there is a sense in which the transformation of trans- health into a social good was also a commodified and commodifying process. This becomes apparent in both a political and an economic sense, as trans- people become pawns for governments and private capital to diffuse dissent or leverage capital accumulation—whether this is about nation-states' smug superiority about their modern embrace of trans- and travesti subjects or about global finance or for-profit health systems recognizing a market in transness. This is where "living the contradiction" also becomes a project of discernment.

Changing "Medicine" into "Health"

As part of these broader confrontations with subordination, trans- health has become one of the testing grounds for rethinking biomedical authority. These dynamics evoke what Steven Epstein and Stefan Timmermans (2021) trace as recent changes to the "cultural authority of medicine."[3] Among these changes is an increased emphasis on concerns related to "health" and "wellness," which often transcend biomedical domains per se (243). To be sure, trans- health activism is implicated in these dynamics. Transsexual medicine has in large part ceded ground to trans- health, including its widening reach well beyond the bounds of biomedical practice.

Yet the turn from "medicine" to "health" is not an inherently radical one. Indeed, "health" is a concept with an abundance of baggage, as even a brief excursion into the texts related to eugenics, racial science, and sexology would demonstrate. The seemingly limitless diffusion of both "health" and "biomedicine" into all realms of life has instantiated as much weaponization as deliverance. These have circulated moralizing, racializing, and marginalizing definitions of what counts as a "healthy life," often in individualizing ways that obscure structuring dynamics that differentially compromise life chances (Clarke, Mamo et al. 2010; Metzl and Kirkland 2010). As such, the centrality of "health" in trans- health activism might raise eyebrows among those who are understandably eager to elaborate on forms of trans- and travesti life *beyond* health and biomedicine.

Indeed, both trans- of color theory and anticolonial or decolonial trans- studies have issued powerful rebukes to the breathlessness that often accompanies white trans- studies' enthusiasm for the molecular alterability and embodied plasticity facilitating trans- embodiment.[4] Affective investments in biomedical technologies were certainly present among the people with whom I spoke, but the particularities of these investments ranged widely. In my observations, a few providers (and others) were attached to the technicities of hormones and surgeries to perform a sort of emancipatory magic, and certainly a few were less troubled than others that capital-generating infrastructures and state apparatuses had begun to (conditionally) incorporate transness.[5] Most, though, were keen to the racialized, classed, and abled exclusions that made these conditional inclusions possible. Certainly, Mark, Amanda, Sylvia, and Anya argued as much when they pointed out contradictions of care and criminalization in New York. Ana also underlined this point when she claimed working-class affinities as central to her trans- politics, which were as focused on exclusions from labor as on those in health care. Similarly, Antonio and Joaquín asserted that their work on the Gender Identity Law involved a herculean effort to render trans- and travesti subjectivities as medicalized or as nonmedicalized as people wanted them to be. As such, I contend that these debates about public coverage for trans- therapeutics, ironically enough, opened the door for grappling with the materiality of trans- and travesti life in its stratified forms, in its different and often constrained relations with medicalization, and in its radical subjective indefinability. In this vein, the requirement for trans- health to adapt to varying needs—by place, by individual, across time, and across infrastructure—has been key to depathologization and the elaboration of care without pathology.

Care without Pathology follows an emergent set of currents in health-care practice, and the shifts I trace are far from comprehensive. As stef shuster (2021) shows, many care providers remain apprehensive about surrendering to uncertainty, leading them to reassert their hold on expertise not only concerning biomedicine but regarding sex/gender. Conflicts still abound, and stark divisions remain between the beneficiaries of depathologizing forms of trans- health and those who still struggle to access it. Even more disconcertingly, as Mark described, depathologization has in some regards further forsaken or intensified pathologization for people whose access to care has relied tenuously on pathologizing standards, such as those who are locked up in prisons or detention centers. Depending on how it is advanced, by whom, and for what ends, depathologization can—oddly enough—become an instrument of pathologization or repathologization. This is precisely why it remains crucial to attend to the diffuse webs of pathologization, both historical and current, within which trans- people and travestis are differentially interpellated.

Nevertheless, it matters a great deal that care without pathology is being elaborated within public domains in Argentina, the United States, and transnationally. *Care without Pathology* has interrogated the multitude of ways in which these changes matter and has focused on some of the more generative means through which these approaches were made manifest. Still, it would be a mistake to recognize the stories I tell here as reflective of a leveling in the distribution of depathologized care. Even within the growing but limited diffusion of depathologization, infrastructures of care remain sharply stratified. In Argentina as well as in the United States, health-care infrastructures define the very concept of health in terms that reproduce racialized, classed, and abled subordination (see Bridges 2011; Auyero 2012). Still, these emergences offer up a set of possibilities for thinking and rethinking the relations between social movements and the politics of health and biomedicine.

To date, examinations of depathologization have been generative but have focused primarily on trans- health's ostensible exceptionality. I contend that examining trans- depathologization as one expression of a broader set of struggles rather than as a singular or unique phenomenon will enable a more lucid interpretation of the stakes and effects of how biomedicine and social movements grapple with care. Trans- health is not an *exception* to biomedical practice but rather emblematic of its contemporary transformations, including biomedicine's reckoning with resource distribution and the politics of care.

Do You Have Any Regrets?

In addition to the paradigm shift that ushered in the field of trans- health, the last decade has been replete with reactionary assaults against even the incipient appearance of depathologization and care without pathology. Legislative efforts to limit, bar, and even criminalize trans- therapeutics are only one example of how these struggles are playing out. As I mentioned at the outset of the book, in the United States and the United Kingdom in particular, TERFs are seizing the airwaves (despite their concerns that they are being silenced). They stand shoulder-to-shoulder with Christian fundamentalists who would erstwhile send them hell-bound to disparage what they call "gender ideology," proliferating forms of pathologization and villainization in the midst of the turn to depathologization. Among these TERFs, children's book authors, concerned parents, and radical feminist separatists all offer up armchair perspectives on the potential harms of trans- therapeutics, often defining trans- therapeutics as offering young people a masculinizing and misogynistic escape from the constraints of womanhood or (perhaps even more curiously) the chance to supposedly colonize womanhood through means of feminization. Stories about regret and the specter of detransitioning form the primary justifications for hitting the panic button and calling for an end to trans- therapeutics. In England in 2020, Keira Bell's case against a National Health Service–commissioned clinic challenged its informed-consent model for providing trans- therapeutics, especially for adolescents.[6] Bell, who previously identified as trans- and has since detransitioned, maintains that she made a "brash decision as a teenager" and "couldn't sit by while so many others made the same mistake" (Turner 2020). The High Court's initial ruling was for the plaintiff, establishing that people under the age of sixteen should not be legally permitted to consent to trans- therapeutic care. This decision was overturned on appeal less than a year later, but it has already had a chilling effect in the provision of trans- therapeutic care in the nation.[7]

Research into medical regret is perhaps best elaborated on the topic of cancer treatment and prevention. Making significant decisions in the face of uncertainty is the standard when it comes to navigating existent as well as anticipatory forms of cancer (Nye 2012; Jain 2013; Fernandes-Taylor and Bloom 2011). Within this domain, experiences of regret are common—not only for actions taken but also for those *not* taken (Fernandes-Taylor and Bloom 2011). Concerns about regret among trans- people are not new—as Beans Velocci (2021) points out, mid-twentieth-century transsexual-medicine providers standardized care and developed professional treatment guidelines in large part to guard against legal repercussions related to anticipated regret. Currently, there is a pointed resurgence in these claims. However, this is emanating less from those who provide these forms of care and much more from the odd coalition comprising Christian fundamentalist lawfare and reckless TERF saviorism—each of which claims to "protect the vulnerable." "Regret," in these regards, becomes weaponized as a basis for claims to ban or limit trans- therapeutics or intensify gatekeeping given the reality of regret, even in its rare appearance (Narayan et al. 2021). In stark contrast with a field such as oncology—which accepts regret as an inherent part of medicine, uncertainty, and the vicissitudes of recovery—reactionaries are targeting trans- health with remarkable vitriol. Painting its proponents as dupes or villains, they have leveled their most vigorous critiques at depathologizing regimes in trans- health.

It was Bell's case that prompted Ky Schevers, a United States–based "ex-detransitioner," to go public about the rhetoric of regret and prohibition. As she asserts in a media interview, "Trans people deserve access to support, and it makes no sense to shut down people's access to medical transition just because some people end up detransitioning" (Urquhart 2021). Schevers had previously been a vocal member of detransitioned people working with women who identified themselves as "gender critical" to target and demonize trans- activism—and particularly trans- health care—as harmful. She, along with this group, promulgated the notion that misogyny and trauma are in fact the primary motivators for pursuing medical transition (when it comes to people pursuing masculinization). Later, Schevers published a blog post entitled "Feeling Regret about My Detransition and Past Activism" (2021). In it, she writes, "I regret my role in creating that community and how I worked to spread its theories and 'alternative treatments' for gender dysphoria. I regret the time and energy I invested in transphobic detrans activism." Schevers goes on to discuss wishing she had embraced herself in her full gendered complexity rather than pathologizing her transness. She attributes these past errors to transphobia, which in its internalized and externalized forms "can take so much from trans people, so much of our time and energy. We have so much to give the rest of the world, our loss is everyone's loss."

Her grappling with regret (not to mention social good) is instructive. Schevers is no longer concerned with medical regret and the fact of trans- therapeutics, even as she is no longer pursuing precisely the same therapeutic path as she had previously. Rather, she is expressing regret for the fact of transphobia and her earlier participation in its diffracted forms of weaponization. Now Schevers has joined forces with her partner, Lee Leveille—who describes himself/herself as a "former (de)trans organizer"—to run a website and research project named Health Liberation Now! Described as a "free, trans-run resource analyzing the social and political forces acting in opposition to health liberation for transgender, detransitioned, retransitioned, and gender diverse people, as well as those questioning their gender," they draw on the techniques of epidemiological biographies to offer "proactive resistance strategies . . . in pursuit of trans health liberation" (Health Liberation Now!, n.d.). In addition to providing biographical grounding in their shared history as former detransitioners, Schevers and Leveille also provide an interactive databased "map of influence" that accompanies a report charting the origins and associations of antitrans- conversion therapies. The map is intended to aid trans- (and detransitioning, retransitioning, and otherwise gender-nonnormative) people in avoiding the dangers of coercive therapy and enmeshment in expanding global webs of antitrans- recruitment. For Schevers and Leveille, uncertainty and dissatisfaction are simply experiences that are to be expected in anyone's search for meaningful life, including within the sometimes-meandering pursuit of trans- therapeutics. In this regard, they place people who have transitioned, detransitioned, or retransitioned in a close and generative kinship with each other. However, they emphasize that this kinship can only thrive after an absolute break from TERFs, right-wing pundits, and conversion therapists.

Taking a lead from coalitional depathologization, Schevers's efforts to grapple with regret might be turned outward even further. In this sense, perhaps regret *does* deserve a prominent place in discussions about trans- health. Not as a means through which to demean or undermine individual therapeutic paths that trans- people may take, but instead to express the dissatisfaction of living in a world that, in its racialized transphobia and classed vitriol, is insufficient to our collective flourishing. Such structural regret is the structure of feeling that names the conditions of a world that might otherwise have been and, indeed, that may still be to come. In this sense, the mobilization against these structural forms of regret is one of the animating forces of care without pathology.

Trans- Health Circles Back

In 2014, the Tierra Violeta Cultural Center in Buenos Aires (the site that hosted Agustina Guimaraes García's *Furia Travesti* show and performance) hosted a community seminar on depathologization. Led by Mauro Cabral Grinspan, the seminar explored "the process of reform and revision of the ICD-10 as an historic opportunity for trans activism" (Centro Cultural Tierra Violeta 2014). Unlike the celebratory tone of much discourse on depathologization, the seminar's description was strikingly ambivalent. It named depathologization as an "emancipatory struggle" but conceded that "the very terms of that emancipation are also in dispute."[8] For some activists, the description explained, depathologization has been about facilitating access to rights and care without the need for diagnostic requirements. For others, it has meant eliminating diagnoses and "subvert[ting] . . . the medicalized ordering of bodies."[9] In either regard, its conceptual approach has carried a risk in its relation to biomedicine: specifically, the perils of the illness–care conundrum. To put too much distance between transness and biomedicine could mean losing access to its modes of care. However, failing to separate trans- subjectivities from therapeutic domains may perpetuate the very biomedical currents that racialize, subordinate, and marginalize in the first place. The seminar's description thus likened depathologization's objectives to a Möbius strip and situated the illness–care conundrum as a framing question for the seminar.

The circularity of the Möbius strip is also an apt metaphor for trans- health's broader revisions to twentieth-century transsexual medicine. The infrastructures that matter to trans- health also mattered to transsexual medicine. As politics, practices, implications, nominal diagnoses, and objectives of contemporary trans- health formations have shifted, the infrastructures on which they run remain limited in their flexibility. Scholars of trans- health and politics have aptly elucidated the colonial, medicolegal, and racial histories of trans- pathologization—and even depathologization's turn to environments of structural violence have not taken full stock of these. Such insights point to how these ghostly pathologizing legacies live on in diagnostic criteria, care guidelines, and clinic protocols. These ghosts still haunt the landscapes of trans- health practice and field formation, depathologization efforts notwithstanding. This has to do with the malleability and persistence of subordination, to be sure, but it also dwells within the durability of infrastructures. As Susan Leigh Star reflected in 1999, "Infrastructure does not grow de novo; it wrestles with the inertia of the installed base and inherits strengths and limitations from that base" (382). Such inertia relates not only to the protracted pace of bureaucratic change. It also correlates with the ways that multiple and imbricated infrastructures hold each other in place. For example, insurance regimes pin diagnostic codes to the possibility of care coverage. Fears of malpractice litigation are only alleviated by the existence of care guidelines. State identification documents are difficult to change not only because of the classifications systems on which they rest but also because they circulate within legal infrastructures of immigration surveillance and fraud prevention. In this regard, depathologization is in a perpetual confrontation with these varied and interwoven systems of care, surveillance, financing, governance, distribution, and punishment. Practices associated with the field of trans- health are qualitatively different from those of transsexual medicine. And yet, infrastructural inertia keeps trans- health's novel interventions from veering too far from the familiar constraints of transsexual medicine.

The contributions that care without pathology has provided to the institutionalizing field of trans- health are certainly legion. In this manner, activist revisions have in large part influenced formation of a field whose practices are distinctly different from frameworks of transsexual medicine. As I have discussed in chapters 2 and 5, this was accomplished in part through changes to diagnoses and protocols. Perhaps even more significantly, though, activists provided new ways to view trans- health and care politics. For example, the community-based studies I discussed in chapters 3 and 4 reworked notions of "risk" and "population" to produce different accounts of what is at stake in trans- health. In stark contrast with paradigms of transsexual medicine, they asserted that what mattered most profoundly for trans- people was not pathology of the psyche but rather the varying and differentially violent social hierarchies within which gender-nonnormative people dwell. These paradigmatic differences matter, and they are indeed what opened up the possibilities for coalitional depathologization that I discussed in chapter 6.

However, these partial transformations cannot entirely separate from the elastic scaffolding and techniques of power organizing trans- therapeutic care (not to mention biomedical practice more generally). Indeed, the transformations of biomedicalization (Clarke, Mamo et al. 2010) scarcely leave an "outside" from which to contest medical power. Instead, as I mentioned in chapter 6, activists engage in "counter-conduct" to shift the politics, hierarchies, and terms of biomedicine without fully divesting from its commitments (Murphy 2012, 29). Trans- health thus takes on the properties of the tail-eating serpent (Mehen or Ouroboros): recreation through return or transformation through absorption. Transsexual medicine is hardly a site for redemption, and trans- health has thus been shaky ground on which to forge the worlds that the activists I studied most desired.

Nevertheless, despite the infrastructural limits of depathologizing revisions, coalitional depathologization activists took seriously the refractive potential of revisioning in its most sweeping forms. They envisioned transformations in care, politics, and distribution that would shift dynamics of power. They sought to enact this not only in the space of the clinic but in the varied realms of economic distribution, political power, and collective self-determination. For them, revision was anything but revisionist. Instead, it was an opening through which a broader political coalition could be formed. The infrastructural inertia they encountered became less of a limit to action and more of a prismatic account of political wrongs that shape the present world. Through this refractive view, coalitional depathologization activists identified the true *pathology* as dwelling not only in the racialized pathologization of transness but also in the broader pathologies of wealth consolidation, racial capitalism and neoliberalism, eugenic desire, and imperialism. Alongside these refractive diagnostics, they worked to develop expansive blueprints of how to counter these interrelated forces. For these activists, the shift to trans- health was only one front in a much deeper and more enduring struggle.

In this sense, activists, advocates, and providers alike saw health as a site through which politics and care practices could be refigured and refashioned. They worked on these through a variety of techniques: coding creatively, developing regulatory interventions to redistribute resources, fashioning methodological innovations, and forging coalitions well beyond the realm of health and medicine. Some respondents were more insistent than others on the relevance of concerns beyond medicine that make up "health." Coalitional depathologizationists, for example, viewed health politics as wholly inseparable from a broader set of politics concerning subjugation, racial capitalism, colonization, labor politics, disability, migration, and so on. Biomedicine, in this sense, was a site of significant constraint when it came to political possibility and horizon, but it was still a site for collective struggle.

This story does not begin and end with the audacity and subsequent abdication of biomedical authority, nor with the extraordinary triumph of a social movement. It does not presume that changes in trans- health have emerged solely through legal or organizational changes, or through structural dialectics. Rather, it engages a complex set of forces, currents, and emergences—representational, methodological, political, economic, infrastructural, and geopolitical—that both reproduce and reconfigure stratified practices of care. Tracing the emergence of trans- health provides an important instance of how health-care formations grapple with politics of difference. As the "transgender tipping point" begins to recede into recent history, these analyses are relevant not only to the futures of trans- health (as well as those implicated within them) but also to shifting commitments in health care and other biomedical practices more broadly.

What Comes Now?

In August 2020, I attended a seminar with legal and trans- studies scholar Paisley Currah entitled "Can We Stop Talking about Transphobia Already?" He opened the discussion by conceding that we probably *cannot* yet stop talking about transphobia but that it remains a deeply insufficient way to engage difference and differential exposure to violence, immiseration, and other harms. By way of illustration, he joked that a hypothetical white trans- student at a liberal-arts college in the Global North who proclaims to be at increased risk of arrest because they are trans- is instead far more likely to be in greater danger of getting a job at an investment firm (Currah 2020). During the question-and-answer period, Currah was asked to reflect on what steps could be taken to best address the health and well-being of trans- and gender-nonnormative people. He replied, "The moves that would help the *most* transgender people *the most? None* of them are transgender-specific" (Currah 2020). He argued that fights for universal health care and against income inequity and imprisonment would improve life conditions for most trans- people far more than focusing on antidiscrimination provisions. While it was indeed a bad thing that the Trump administration was trying to change rules like Section 1557 in the Affordable Care Act to explicitly exclude trans- people, for example, he thought that focusing unduly on such exclusions missed the forest for the trees.

Argentine activists have used legislative tactics to address some of the material conditions to which Currah was referring, as in the health provision of the Gender Identity Law, the trans- and travesti employment quota requirement, and reparations laws. However, these have had a limited effect amid regulatory constraints and the persistent structuring effects of austerity regimes. As I mentioned in chapter 3, a twenty-two-year-old trans- man named Tehuel de la Torre disappeared from his home in San Vicente, a small town about thirty miles south of Buenos Aires, in 2021. He went missing after going to what he thought was a restaurant job interview. A campaign called "¿Donde Está Tehuel?" ("Where Is Tehuel?") has followed online and in the streets. To date, two suspects have been detained, but the particulars of his disappearance remain a mystery. On social media, an illustration of Tehuel in a blue shirt against a pink background has circulated with the text "May Tehuel Be Found: Please Share as if He Were Cis."[10] Returning to Currah's point, though, it is not only transness versus cisness that contributed to his disappearance and the legal impunity for presumptive violence that has followed but also the web of conditions that led him to pursue low-income work in a partially informalized economy.

These are the conditions to consider as we think collectively about the present and future of trans- health. As I have shown, trans- health far transcends processes of confirmation, affirmation, or therapeusis when it comes to enacting and embodying sex/gender. In contrast, it consists in the broad assertion that people generally know a great deal about their conditions of life and what kinds of care they require. They also recognize the historically sedimented constraints they are up against in pursuing this—even if only implicitly. Such knowledge leads to the claims for care without pathology that I have traced throughout this book. As I have striven to make clear, this is not *only* a feature of trans- health. It is also a means of rethinking biomedical care and power, redistributing wealth and resources, and addressing the differential conditions of life that enduring regimes of pathologization have materialized. Indeed, we might be guided by the tenets of care without pathology as we rethink care and power in matters of health and thriving. Its experiments may provide a blueprint through which we might organize the deeper forms of justice and collective self-determination that activists have been imagining all along.

Acknowledgments

Nobody writes alone. This was the unofficial motto of the writing group that led to this book seeing the light of day. Nobody thinks alone, either. Here, I thank some of the primary supporters, mentors, collaborators, friends, and respondents who made this book possible.

First and foremost, I thank the feminist scholars and activists who trained me, mentored me, and showed me that scholarship can imagine new worlds into being. UC San Francisco's Sociology Department was a wonderful intellectual home, and I was especially fortunate to work with Adele Clarke and Janet Shim as dissertation committee cochairs. Adele's tenacious support and ebullience kept me afloat, and her intellectual dexterity and rigor sharpened my analysis immeasurably. Janet's considered and insightful readings and collaborative approach deepened and broadened my thinking and set the bar for the kind of mentor I strive to be. Across the bay at UC Berkeley, committee members Mel Chen in Gender and Women's Studies and Lawrence Cohen in Anthropology encouraged me to experiment in thinking well beyond the bounds of my discipline. Their creative and lively approaches to inquiry inspired me to follow my intuition, even when it took me in unexpected directions.

I can still scarcely believe the privilege I had to join the Women and Gender Studies Department at San Francisco State after graduating from UCSF. Kasturi Ray, Julie Hua, Leslie Quintanilla, Martha Kenney, Deb Cohler, Nan Alamilla Boyd, and Jillian Sandell are colleagues beyond compare, even as we no longer share the same department. The STS Hub and the Health Equity Institute were also cherished intellectual homes at SF State—Laura Mamo, Martha Kenney, Dawn-Elissa Fischer, Martha Lincoln, Supriya

Misra, Ikaika Gleisberg, Clare Sears, Blanca Missé, Jesus Ramirez-Valles, and many others were among those who workshopped early chapter drafts or talked out ideas with me. Recently, I've had the extraordinary opportunity to join the faculty in Gender, Sexuality, and Women's Studies at UC Davis. I am already grateful for support from my new colleagues—Wendy Ho, Beenash Jafri, Rana Jaleel, Ava Kim, Amina Mama, and Joanna Regulska—as well as colleagues in the Feminist Research Institute. I'm looking forward to our shared work together.

UCSF provided enviable intellectual community in my graduate training. In addition to my committee members, other faculty at UCSF in Sociology, Nursing, and Medical Anthropology were instrumental in my scholarly development. Howard Pinderhughes, Catherine Bliss, Leslie Dubbin, Shari Dworkin, Vincanne Adams, and Kelly Knight at UCSF provided key support and insights. In addition to Mel and Lawrence, UC Berkeley faculty also provided warm mentorship and support. Charis Thompson was a grounding force and informal mentor, as were Juana María Rodríguez and Leslie Salzinger. My classmates and writing partners also played critical roles in developing the project. Lawrence's UC Berkeley Care seminar was my introduction to graduate school. As part of this, conversations with Raphaëlle Rabanes, Victoria Massie, Pierre Minn, and Jason Alley, among others, planted the seeds for this project. Later, our UCSF (plus) writing group helped these seeds to grow. Membership shifted over time but included Kate Darling, Sonia Rab Alam, Dilara Yarbrough, Krista Sigurdson, Jen James, Natalie Ingraham, Jarmin Yeh, Heather Dron, Rima Praspaliauskiene, Jamie Chang, Mike Levesque, and Taylor Cruz. Oliver Rollins and Martine Lappé graduated too soon to officially write with us, but they were also keen and incisive readers. Kate, Sonia, and Dilara were especially generous in reading the roughest, earliest, and messiest of chapter drafts.

Scholars and mentors beyond these institutions have also been key in bringing this project to fruition. Emily Thuma, Alisa Bierria, Aren Aizura, Dean Spade, Chandan Reddy, Janelle Taylor, Gillian Harkins, Lamble, Sharyne Shiu-Thornton, Finn Enke, and Paisley Currah initially encouraged me to pursue what felt like a belated entry into graduate training, and I am glad I listened.

Early on, Nayan Shah and Priya Kandaswamy helped me to develop analyses that proved central to my analyses. Conversations with Cindy Bello were intellectually formative, and her wisdom about navigating graduate school was indispensable. In particular, Emily, Alisa, Priya, and Dean have helped me to bridge intellectual thought and political action as decades-long interlocutors and co-conspirators. Chandra Lekha Sriram—whom we lost in 2018—and Amy Ross showed interest in my project in its formative stages, and their dedicated support proved critical to its development. Mauro Cabral Grinspan, Emmanuel Theumer, Nick D'Avella, Soledad Cutuli, Josefina Fernández, Francisco Fernández Romero, and Mabel Bellucci helped me to develop a better understanding of Argentine activism and social movements. Steven Epstein, Héctor Carrillo, Natalie Boero, Julia McReynolds-Pérez, Katie Hasson, Lezlie Frye, Emily Thuma, Kate Darling, Natali Valdez, Sonia Rab Alam, Emily Vasquez, Aren Aizura, Dean Spade, Melissa Creary, Lauren Berliner, Kalindi Vora, Eda Pepi, Ben Hegarty, and Brooke Lober (among others) organized panels and events in which I had the opportunity to take part. These helped me to sharpen my arguments, consider new questions, and draw new connections.

More people than I can possibly name provided support, guidance, and feedback at critical times over the course of my graduate training. Among them are Kalindi Vora, Joe Hankins, Ben Singer, Dan Travers, Aihwa Ong, Alondra Nelson, Zakiyyah Iman Jackson, Susan Stryker, James Pfeiffer, Zakiya Luna, Eric Plemons, Quinn Grundy, Florencia Rojo, Katie Hasson, Anna Jabloner, Gowri Vijayakumar, Melissa Creary, Rosanna Dent, Paisley Currah, Hale Thompson, Michael Polson, Natali Valdez, Sara Matthiesen, Mark Fleming, Sid Jordan, Anna Torres, James Battle, Hil Malatino, Francisco Fernández Romero, Jacob Lau, Cole Rizki, Emiliano Litardo, and Mauro Cabral Grinspan. I also remain indebted many years later to my undergraduate mentors and instructors, particularly Jill Morawski, Jennifer Tucker, Joe Rouse, Jessica Shubow, and Kate Rushin. Christina Crosby, who passed away in 2021, was also an early mentor, and I am still guided by her careful, critical, and generous approach to intellectual inquiry.

As this project has moved from dissertation to book, many readers and interlocutors have aided me in the long process of clarification. Among those who read full chapters, I want to offer special thanks to Emily Thuma, Aren Aizura, Julie Hua, Martha Kenney, Toby Beauchamp, Jennifer Singh, Ben Hegarty, Dean Spade, Soledad Cutuli, Lamble, Mimi Kim, Josefina Fernández, Martha Lincoln, Lilly Nguyen, Rima Praspaliauskiene, Dilara Yarbrough, Finn Enke, Lilly Irani, Kalindi Vora, Sal Zárate, Leslie Quintanilla, Saiba Varma, Belkys Garcia, Francisco Fernández Romero, and Mark Fleming. I owe particular debts of gratitude to Finn, Lamble, and Josefina for reading and responding to multiple chapters and to Toby and Jennifer for their immeasurably helpful feedback and engagement with the project as a whole. The book is much improved after their careful readings and suggestions.

I'm delighted to have been able to publish with the University of Minnesota Press. I'm especially grateful to my editor, Jason Weidemann, for his vision and steadfast support throughout the process. I was also very lucky to work with Ziggy Snow as my copyeditor. Working with the entire production team has been a dream, and I thank all who have been involved.

There were many people who supported me when the work was in a fledgling stage. My SSRC DPDF program cohort in Critical Approaches to Human Rights nurtured the earliest inklings of my project, and their feedback and support were instrumental in assuaging my doubts about it. Special thanks to cohort members Jaime Morse, Alexa Hagerty, J Sebastian, Laura Matson, Greg Hervouet-Zeiber, Justin Pérez, and Samar Al-Bulushi and to field leaders Amy and Chandra. Taking part in the São Paulo Advanced School on Biotechnologies, Biosocialities, and the Governance of the Life Sciences, the California STS Retreats, UC Berkeley's Reproductive Justice Working Group, and the UC Berkeley Speculative Visions of Race, Technology, Science, and Survival Conference also provided wonderful spaces for thought.

Erica D'Andrea offered critical research support and intellectual engagement related to chapter 5. Along with Erica, many students have also helped me to think through key elements of the book. There are too many to name, but Tara Gonsalves, Sarah Lewis, Carolina Osoria, Laura Kent, Kate Amunrud, Sabrina Enomoto, Evelyn Soria, Syreeta Young, Cavar, and Bex MacFife are among them.

As a weird sociologist, I feel lucky to be able to reflect on artistic production as part of my work. I want to thank all of those who shared their art as part of this project, especially Tirre Grillo, Roan Boucher, and Florencia Guimaraes García. In addition, I am wildly grateful to have worked with Marcus Rogers (https://thisgoldenhour.com) on the cover art for this book. His care, collaborative vision, and enthusiasm are beautifully reflected in the painting he so generously provided to represent the project.

I was privileged to have many people support my fieldwork in both New York and Buenos Aires. People put me up, helped me connect with respondents, and met my work with care, curiosity, and enthusiasm. During my fieldwork in New York, I made many fortuitous connections and reconnections. Particular thanks to Ronica Mukerjee, Nathan Levitt, Lara Comstock, Bran Fenner, Soniya Munshi, Gabriel Foster, Tara Mateik, Belkys Garcia, Pooja Gehi, Elana Redfield, Martine Lappé, Dani Heffernan, Luce Lincoln, Leeroy Kang, Nadir Souirgi, Pooja Rangan, and Josh Guildford. Prior to my first fieldwork trip to Buenos Aires, Nick D'Avella supplied me with books, maps, housing advice, friendly contacts, and crucial knowledge about life and research there. Julia McReynolds-Pérez graciously met me on my first day of fieldwork. My three seasons in Buenos Aires were enriched by many new friends and interlocutors. Special thanks to Mauro Cabral Grinspan, Sergio García, Francisco Fernández Romero, Emmanuel Theumer, Elián Katz, Karen Bennett, Lucas Morgan Disalvo, Maria Luisa Peralta, Mabel Bellucci, Peter Pank, Soledad Cutuli, Pabli Balcazar, Pao Lin Raffetta, Charlotte Jenkins, Leo Silvestri, Blas Radi, Emiliano Litardo, Iñaki Regueiro De Giacomi, Julia Amore, and the late Diana Sacayán and Lohana Berkins (may they rest in power). A very special thank you to all the respondents who took the time and energy to speak with me during my ethnographic research. Without them, this book would not exist.

I was fortunate to receive fellowship funding for the fieldwork and completion of this project. This was made possible with the generous support of the Social Science Research Council's Dissertation Proposal Development Fund, the National Science Foundation's Doctoral Dissertation Improvement Grant in Sociology (Grant #1519292), UCSF's Social and Behavioral Science Program's

Estes Research Fellowship, and the Graduate Division's Dean's Health Science Scholarship. Support from SF State's Presidential Award for Professional Development of Probationary Faculty enabled me to develop the missing chapters.

Generosity also arrived in the form of administrative support. UCSF staff members, particularly Brandee Woleslagle and Cynthia Mercado-Scott, helped me more times that I could count. Thank you also to my transcriptionists, Javier Moreno-Pollarolo, Murtado Bustillo, and Sabina DelRosso. Many more have devoted invisible labor to bringing this book into the world, and I gratefully appreciate all of it.

A version of chapter 3 was initially published in *Social Science & Medicine* 247, as "Epidemiological Rage: Population, Biography, and State Responsibility in Trans- Health Activism," copyright Elsevier, 2020. It is reprinted with permission, and it benefited greatly from the feedback of an anonymous reviewer.

Perhaps most crucially, the love and support of friends, comrades, and family (chosen and otherwise) have sustained me. The friends I made during my twelve years in Seattle have remained close to my heart, despite having been in California for just as long. From the beginning, my dear friend Elizabeth Payne nurtured my dreams and encouraged my slightly irrational decision to move and start a new career. I am grateful to have maintained connections with many others, as well. Among them: Sarah Brown, Emily Thuma, Sid Jordan, Dean Spade, Calvin Burnap, E. T. Russian, Darius Morrison, Kaden Mack, Angélica Cházaro, Devon Knowles, Chandan Reddy, Bridge Joyce, Gabriel Foster, Gillian Harkins, Amy Vanderwarker, Luke Newton, gita mehrotra, and Alix Kolar. While our friendship precedes our time in the Northwest, Sara Jaffe has also provided consistent love and encouragement.

In the Bay Area, I have encountered a rich community of friends, many of whom have supported me in a myriad of ways over a decade of research and writing. I will not attempt to name them all (though I hope you know who you are). I will mention several who have provided an especially anchoring force or direct support in my endeavors to bring this project into being. Sabrina Wu, Paolo Chico, and the rest of our little pod provided insulation from Covid-imposed loneliness. The tiny house in our temporarily shared home provided just the room-of-one's-own that I needed. The world got small during this time. Among those of us who kept each other going, even amid the contraction: Holly Maeder Sheehan, Molly McClure, Dunya 'Alwan, Puck Lo, Ismalia Gutierrez, Adrienne Skye Roberts, Mark Fleming, Adele Carpenter, Florencia Rojo, Leeroy Kang, Elliott Fukui, Ikaika Gleisberg, Kalindi Vora, Emily Thuma, Sid Jordan, Chaya Mangel Pflugeisen, and many others. My parents, Joan and Dennett, and my sister, Nicole, have also provided concrete support and respite through visits and adventures with my wonderful nephews Jono, Drew, and Adam.

Finally, after many years of running in the same circles, Esteban Rodriguez came into my life right around the time when revising a dissertation into a book seemed an impossible task. As usual, his thoughtfulness, care, and unwavering encouragement have been instrumental in making the impossible possible, and I couldn't be more thankful.

I dedicate this book to the lovers and fighters—both living and no longer here—who are imagining and enacting less treacherous worlds into being. Thank you for the levity and forcefulness that keeps us striving, working, thinking, and struggling. Onward!

Notes

Introduction

1. *Trap* is a slang and generally derogatory term for trans- people, usually trans- women, that implies an intention of tricking straight men into sexual relations. The group's use of the term is, like *queer* and many other terms, an instance of affirmative reclamation.

2. For reasons that I will address later in the Introduction, I generally use the word *trans-* with a hyphen instead of *transgender* or variations like *trans.*

3. Within a few days, event leadership did an about-face and invited the group to present at the conference.

4. Gender Identity Law, Law No. 26.743, May 24, 2012 (Arg.).

5. For more, see Cabral 2012; Cabral and Viturro 2006; De Mauro Rucovsky 2019.

6. There are many debates within trans- activism and trans- studies about legal gender markers. Some people take the position that not only should trans- people be able to change these but there should also be more options available in addition to "male" and "female." In fact, in 2021, Argentina passed a national law enabling people to select a nonbinary gender marked "X" (Decreto 476/2021). Similar changes have passed at a state regulatory level in the United States, including for California and New York driver's licenses and IDs. Other scholars and activists take the position that state governments do not need to track anyone's gender and that adding options simply creates more problems for people who could be targeted. See, for example, Currah 2022.

7. A notable difference is that community clinics generally have not provided specialized care, such as surgeries, and thus have referred people to surgeons—who have not always accepted insurance. Integrated hospital-based care networks have usually included in-house surgeons.

8. Specifically, the Human Rights Campaign added the presence of "at least one transgender wellness benefit" as a data point for their Corporate Equality Index in 2006 (Human Rights Campaign 2006, 3).

9. As I write this book, gender-affirming care for minors in particular

has become a national controversy. As of April 2023, eleven states have passed bans or restrictions on care for people under the age of eighteen, and twenty additional states are considering bans. Some of these criminalize care for transgender minors, including Alabama, which has designated it a crime punishable by up to ten years in prison. Oklahoma passed a law that blocks minors from gender-affirming care altogether and bars any state or private insurers from covering gender-affirming care for youth or adults. A pending bill in Florida would ban companies from covering gender-affirming care for trans- people, would prohibit trans- minors from accessing it, and—chillingly—would empower state courts to take temporary custody of minors in the case of their parents or guardians supporting them in accessing trans- therapeutics. By the time this book goes to print, it is likely that more bans will be in place.

10. This is not to say that classed and racialized stratification do not also structure these conversations. As Vanessa Grubbs (2017) points out, profound racialized disparities are reflected in rates of kidney transplantation: Black patients received only one in five of donated kidneys despite making up a third of candidates. Structural racism also conditions the ways that people are held responsible for conditions that require care, so it is not the case that debates about cost are not primary concerns elsewhere (see Fleming et al. 2019). Nevertheless, the question of cost and public subsidies has become a somewhat singular and primary pressure point in debates about trans- therapeutics.

11. I will discuss the term *travestis* in more detail shortly. For now, this can be understood as a term used in the Spanish- and Portuguese-speaking Americas to describe some groups of transfeminine people. In Argentina, this is a politically reclaimed term that is most often used by poor people who are marginalized and criminalized based on race, class, and employment. While they collaborate with people who describe themselves as "transgender," they do not generally use this term to describe themselves.

12. For discussions of the Gender Identity Law, its emergence, its effects, and its limits, see Cabral 2012; Hollar 2018; De Mauro Rucovsky 2019.

13. Jules Gill-Peterson (2018) emphasizes that the field was not altogether new, but was in fact built on a half-century of medicalization and experimentation on children's sex starting in the early twentieth century.

14. See chapter 6 of Kyla Schuller's (2021) *The Trouble with White Women* and Ruth Pearce, Sonja Erikainen, and Ben Vincent's (2020) introduction to a special issue of the *Sociological Review.*

15. As Kyla Schuller (2021) points out, though, these views are wholly consistent with the possessive forms of politics she describes as "white feminism."

16. In this book, I generally use the term *nontrans-* instead of *cis.* In so doing, I follow Finn Enke and Jules Gill-Peterson in troubling *cis* as an identificatory subject position. For Enke (2012), *cisgender* does the troubling work of solidifying the notions of "woman" and "man" as stable and self-evident. For Gill-Peterson (2021), *cis* is a more useful tool to describe changes to sex/gender systems in the midcentury. As she writes, "Cis isn't an identity. It's a diagnostic, a description of a system organized to subject people to the authority of institutions: the state, medicine, law . . . and the university."

17. Sociologist stef shuster (2021) discusses the structuring force of anxiety around expertise in their book on transgender medicine.

18. There are those—trans- people included—who welcome evidence that transness is real (which many equate with being biologically identifiable), especially when multipronged antitrans- campaigns hinge on the idea that trans- people are simply delusional. However, these studies frequently underestimate the complexities of social relations and culture, and they reduce authenticity to tissues, organs, and neurons. For more on sexed brain research, see Jordan-Young 2010; Llaveria Caselles 2021. For more on the notion of the social construction of reality, see Thomas and Thomas 1970; Berger and Luckmann 2011. For more on biological determinism, see Subramaniam 2014.

19. On opacity and desubjectifying resistance to biomedical capture and trans- of color critique, see Gill-Peterson 2018. In invoking this here, I am not suggesting that trans- health has suddenly become accommodating to heterogeneity. As in the twentieth-century cases about which Gill-Peterson (2018, 615) writes, racialized objectification, anti-Blackness, and dehumanization continue to structure biomedicine—including trans- health.

20. For example, nontrans- women who undergo mastectomy regularly opt for gender-affirming breast implants, while nontrans- men with breast growth (gynecomastia) may choose surgery to remove this tissue. These are generally covered by insurance. In addition, the parents of intersex infants, children, and teens are often coerced into consenting to so-called gender-affirming care in the form of genital/gonadal surgeries or hormone treatments on behalf of their children (usually without children's assent or knowledge). These procedures and treatments are also generally covered by insurance. When it comes to trans- people, however, even accessing gender-affirming care has been difficult, let alone having these forms of care covered by insurance. In its very origins, institutionalized medicine's approach to gender-affirming care for trans- people has been defined by maximizing exclusions to access or coverage (Velocci 2021). In sum, coverage for gender-affirming care generally only becomes controversial when trans- people pursue it.

21. I use *decolonial* here as a term that is part of a set of conversations about Latin American decolonial studies that center on the rejection of colonial hierarchies of knowledge and social organization. Aníbal Quijano's (2000) work on the coloniality of power and knowledge has centrally engaged these critiques, as has María Lugones's (2007, 2010) work on the coloniality of gender and decolonial feminism. Scholars such as Eve Tuck and K. Wayne Yang (2012) issue the critical reminder that "decolonization is not a metaphor" and that practices—including anticolonial practices—are not in fact "decolonizing" in the absence of land return. Max Liboiron (2021) attends to distinct histories and trajectories in specific place-based orientations to "decolonial" thought and practice. I use *decolonial* here to signal debates related to Latin American subaltern studies because this is the terminology these scholars use to describe their work.

Provincializing is a term that postcolonial scholar Dipesh Chakrabarty (2001) uses as a means of decentering the epistemological hegemony of the Global North (or West, depending on the analytical division of the world) and displacing the metropole as the center of knowledge and action. In these analyses, Chakrabarty and other subaltern studies scholars, such as Gayatri Chakravorty Spivak (1999), work to center marginal knowledge as a center of theory of analysis. More recently, trans- studies scholars have also urged the provincialization of *transgender.* Through this lens, for example, Aren Z. Aizura (2018) critiques the transgender origin stories that emanate from Europe and the Global North, which conceptualize transness through regimes of truth, classed entitlement, and whiteness. Aniruddha Dutta (2012, 2013) takes a similar position, as do other scholars who strive to displace *transgender* as a universalizing umbrella term of gender, sex, and sexual variance or nonnormativity.

22. While I have been drawn to this quotation previously, Toby Beauchamp reminded me of its profound relevance to trans- politics.

23. When I discuss *transness,* I exclude the hyphen for the sake of simplicity. However, I urge readers also to regard this term in its most capacious and variable form.

24. Thanks to Aren Aizura for thinking with me on this point, building on his work and our previous exchanges on "provincializing" *transgender.*

25. Aizura (2018), Nael Bhanji (2011), and others adopt this approach to discussing transness. Drawing on Jacques Derrida's (1978) extension of Martin Heidegger's notion of *sous rature,* terms "under erasure" are stricken out in text while remaining visible. I have not adopted this typographical practice here, but the reader is free to imagine this visual cue. To claim a term as being under erasure in the Derridean sense is to concede to both the inescapability and insufficiency of language's constraints.

26. For more, see Berkins 2007b; Wayar 2018; Cutuli 2012, 2017; DiPietro 2016; Rizki 2019; Simonetto and Butierrez 2022. Some of these works emphasize the importance of *sudaca* theorizing (a reappropriated derogatory term originating in Spain to describe South Americans, and which currently speaks to Global South knowledge production, often through implicit or explicit critiques of the epistemological imperialism of the Global North). Anthropologist Don Kulick (1998) published a book-length study on travestis in Brazil, emphasizing at once the interlaced subjectivities of travesti and sex worker, as well as the cultural politics of public scandal. While there are marked differences in Brazilian and Argentine identifications with the term, some of the aforementioned scholars critique Kulick's work as ahistorical in its burial of the political histories and present conditions of travesti life.

27. In a somewhat confusing but pitched debate on Anglophone social media platforms like Tumblr, *trans** was first celebrated as an expansive intervention and then disparaged as exclusionary. Its institutional life was brief. The youth-led advocacy and training project Trans Student Educational Resources (TSER 2016) published a statement entitled "Why We Used Trans* and Why We Don't Anymore." In it, they proclaim, "In the end, we decided to stop our use of the asterisk because of how unnecessary and inaccessible it is and its common application as a tool of binarism and silencing trans women. We encourage you to do the same. We are in the process of removing all asterisks from our web site, publications, and infographics."

28. Thanks to Francisco Fernández Romero for drawing my attention to this as a specific intervention (which we discuss in more detail in a forthcoming coauthored article).

29. Chiang (2021, 4) refers to this term to signify the "different scales of gender transgression that are not always recognizable through the Western notion of transgender."

30. For example, see the special issue on "*Cuir*/Queer Américas" in *GLQ* (Pierce et al. 2021); Viteri 2017. In a different geopolitical topography, Dutta and Roy (2014) reflect on the partial resignification of *transgender* in India, and Evren Savcı (2021) reflects on the mobility and translation of LGBT terminology in Turkey.

31. For example, some trans- people bristle in particular at the connotation of external and authoritative sanction implied by the description "gender-confirming." Yet this was the preferred language among United States–based legal advocates to address diagnosis discrimination against trans- people, since gender-confirming procedures for nontrans- people were generally covered. For example, hair removal for nontrans- women and breast removal for nontrans- men were covered as gender-confirming procedures, but they were not for trans- people.

32. Eric Plemons (2017) mobilizes this term in *The Look of a Woman*

to emphasize the shifting therapeutic logics within which primarily surgical interventions for trans- people are mobilized. Specifically, he describes how trans- therapeutics work within broader logics of treatment to link treatment rationales with outcomes (7). I draw on Plemons's emphasis on therapeutic processes and on patient-initiated claims in trans- medicine, but I depart from his surgical focus. As such I consider *trans- therapeutics* to include a wide variety of processes and procedures related to trans- embodiment and enactment.

33. I also attended a trans- health conference in Philadelphia with several providers from New York City. My early pilot work also included the Bay Area. In addition, while not part of the city of Buenos Aires proper, I visited some of the outlying areas (*conurbanos*) of Buenos Aires. These are among thirteen districts that are a short distance from the Autonomous City of Buenos Aires but are administered by their own municipal governments. Nevertheless, there is extensive daily travel and exchange between the city and these areas.

34. It is difficult, particularly in sociological symbolic interactionism, to parse methodology from epistemology. This field has historically refused a stark separation between these (Blumer 1986; Strauss and Corbin 1998). Through "theory-methods packages," Star refers to the coconstitutiveness of ontology, epistemology, and practice. Star (1989) and Adele Clarke (2005) extend the perspectives of Straussian grounded theory and its methodological rooting in symbolic interactionist and philosophical pragmatist epistemologies (e.g., Strauss and Corbin 1998).

35. Science and technology studies scholars examine the politics, history, culture, and philosophy associated with science and technology (sometimes also called "science, technology, and medicine studies," or STMS). This field emphasizes that technology, culture, and scientific practice are value-laden and inseparable, and they shape how people know and act toward the world. As Maria Puig de la Bellacasa (2011, 86) puts it, "Ways of studying and representing things can have world-making effects." For a concise discussion of the field, see C. Thompson 2005, ch. 1.

36. Both *technoscience* and *biomedicine* are portmanteaus that are conceptually taken up in STS to define how the linked realms of technology, science, the biological and life sciences, and medical practice are increasingly permeable. For more, see Latour 1987; Haraway 1990; Löwy 2011; Clarke, Mamo et al. 2010; Murphy 2012.

37. Other authors who generatively engage trans- and queer rural life include Mary L. Gray (2009), Jules Gill-Peterson (2018), Ryan Lee Cartwright (2021), C. Riley Snorton (2017), and Eli Clare (1999).

38. I had plans to return to Buenos Aires in 2020 to follow up on interviews and some open questions related to my preliminary conclusions. The global pandemic made this impossible.

39. This differs somewhat from the group that stef shuster (2021) interviewed for *Trans Medicine,* who became involved in trans- medical care in large part through interactions with specific patients. In contrast, my study skews in the direction of supportive providers. As such, their positions are not necessarily generalizable to a broader cross-section of care providers.

40. Situational analysis involves what Clarke (2005) calls "positional analysis" to understand "the discursive positions taken and not taken" in the data (Clarke, Friese, and Washburn 2016). In this regard, any particular individual may assert multiple and even conflicting positions—and this positional mobility and heterogeneity arose frequently as activists and providers negotiated trans- health.

41. I garnered this information from surveys that people completed prior to interviews. I missed the opportunity to ask participants about immigration status and disability, which also would have been important information.

42. Josefina Fernández (2004), Lohana Berkins (2007b), María Soledad Cutuli (2012, 2013, 2015), and others have each written extensively on these dynamics.

43. "Que susciten equívocos respecto del sexo de la persona a quien se impone." These were legislated specifically by the Law of the Practice of Medicine, Dentistry, and Collaborated Activities (Law No. 17132, Jan. 31, 1967 [Arg.]) and the Law of Names (Law No. 18248, June 24, 1969 [Arg.]). For a more detailed analysis, see Cabral 2012.

44. Medicare—the government program that subsidizes care for people who are over sixty-five or have disabilities—operates federally. Medicaid, in contrast, is jointly financed by states and federal funding. This safety-net program covers some low-income individuals, families, and children, and eligibility requirements, including income requirements, are set state by state.

45. During my fieldwork, I spoke with a trans- activist who expressed only tempered excitement about the Medicare program lifting its ban. When I asked her why she seemed hesitant to define this as a victory, she laughed sardonically and said, "Because we'll be dead by the time we qualify."

46. Specifically, Section 1557 of the law implemented Title IX antidiscrimination provisions. Patient Protection and Affordable Care Act, Pub. L. No. 111-148, 124 Stat. 119–1024 (2010).

47. As legal scholars point out, antidiscrimination rules often have little bearing in action, particularly given the burden of proof in establishing discrimination claims (particularly given the founding assumptions about animus rather than structural inequity related to discrimination in the first instance). See Spade 2015; Siegel 1997.

48. For example, the annual Trans March in the city—called the Trans Day of Action for Social and Economic Justice—has historically been organized by TransJustice, a political group led primary by low-income trans- and gender nonconforming people of color. Racialized police violence and harassment and housing access are among the issues that have been centered in this event. Annual Trans March events in other major cities have often included, but maintained less of a focus on, these issues.

49. For more on reproductive justice, see Ross and Solinger 2017; Luna 2020; Silliman et al. 2004. For more on Green Tide activism, see Palmeiro 2018; Sosa 2021. For more on disability justice, see Piepzna-Samarasinha 2018; Sins Invalid 2019.

50. David Valentine (2007) and Joanne Meyerowitz (2002) assert that "sex," "gender," and "sexuality" as discrete domains emerge from sexology.

51. For example, see Amin 2018; Aizura 2018; Gill-Peterson 2018; Meyerowitz 2002; Skidmore 2011; Snorton 2017; Valentine 2007. For historiographies engaging relevant themes related to sexuality, sex, race, embodiment, and coloniality more generally, see Arondekar 2009; Sengoopta 2000; Stoler 1995.

52. For detailed reflections on varying paradigms of eugenics (including Larmarckian versus Mendelian notions of heritability), see Gill-Peterson 2018; Miranda 2018; Schuller 2018; Stepan 1991; Turda and Gillette 2014. Of these, Marisa A. Miranda, Nancy Stepan, and Marius Turda and Aaron Gillette focus especially on eugenics in the Americas, particularly in Argentina and Mexico.

53. Eugenics were only one part of the assemblage of positions that made up the Argentina Nacionalismo ideology that formed in the early twentieth century. Whitening regimes in Argentina were situated as eugenic projects, which enabled their framing as matters of health and "hygiene" (Salessi 1995; Aguiló 2018). As Jorge Salessi (1995, 116–17) emphasizes, these campaigns defined *social illnesses* as encompassing sexual/gender pathologies, class solidarities, racialized class, and antiauthoritarianism (among others). Ignacio Aguiló (2018) details how each of these were intertwined with race, despite this being disavowed by Argentina's supposed racelessness. For more, also see E. D. Edwards 2020; Hooker 2017; Campos and Novella 2017; Miranda 2018; Stepan 1991; Briggs 2002; Schuller 2018; Stern 2005.

54. During my fieldwork, respondents in Buenos Aires across class strata spoke openly about their experiences in therapy. In fact, Argentina has the highest concentration of mental health providers in the world—about seven times the concentration of therapists in the United States (WHO 2018).

55. The *DSM* is published by the U.S.-based American Psychiatric Association, but its circulation and consequences are much broader. In fact, its diagnoses make up most of the mental health chapter of the World Health Organization's *International Classification of Diseases,* the diagnostic system used in most of the world.

56. Collusion between psychiatry and state violence has a longer history. As Marco A. Ramos (2013, 250) discusses, during the period of successive military dictatorships from 1966 to 1983, psychiatry became an "ideological tool used for both leftist resistance and military oppression." At some level these political splits remain, as do legacies of psychiatry's politicization.

57. See, for example, Edelman 2011. Until recently in New York, the possession of multiple condoms could be grounds to arrest a person for sex work solicitation. "Walking while trans-" riffs on the phrase "driving while Black," which gained prominence in the United States in the early 1990s to name the phenomenon of racialized police profiling that led to disproportionate traffic stops among Black drivers. "Walking while trans-" is also relevant to the policing of public space in Argentina, where geographer Francisco Fernández Romero refers to regimes of "walking while travesti" (pers. comm., October 24, 2020).

58. There are rich literatures engaging these and related topics emanating from thinkers across the Global North and South. See, for example, Aizura 2018; Berkins 2007b; Cabral Grinspan 2017; Di Pietro 2016; Fernández 2004; Gill-Peterson 2018; Pérez and Radi 2020; Rizki 2020; Schuller 2018; Spade 2015; Skidmore 2011; Snorton 2017; Wayar 2018.

59. Medicine, psychology, and psychiatry are not the only sites through which such classificatory exuberance has been routed. Anthropologists, among others, have also taken part in efforts to map the particularities of sex/gender nonnormativity. These efforts have often taken place through the colonizing and racializing dynamics of ascribing primitivity to those whose actions, expressions, or desires do not align with sex/gender differentiation. See Towle and Morgan 2002; Boellstorff et al. 2014.

60. For example, Todd Sekuler (2013, 15) maintains that in the early 2000s, France represented itself as a "forward-thinking and rights-protecting nation" by legally depathologizing trans- health. However, he argues that state actors used this ostensibly trans- supportive move to shore up a xenophobic national agenda by vilifying ostensibly transphobic immigrants. In this process, depathologization activists were unwittingly enrolled into the "racial policing of the French nation-state" (27). In addition, disability activists criticize the ways trans- depathologization has disavowed mental illness by relying on ableist narratives of respectability and claims to mental wellness (Cavar and Baril 2021).

61. For example, at the U.S. Professional Association for Transgender Health (USPATH) symposium in Los Angeles in 2017, Kenneth Zucker's talk caused much controversy. Zucker is a prominent psychiatrist whose position on gender nonnormativity as pathological has raised ire among both activists and providers, though he remains very engaged in revision projects. At the symposium, activists interrupted Zucker's talk to question his presence and reject his stances on trans- health. This was followed by a highly politicized debate among providers and activists about the place of pathologizing providers in trans- health, and it resulted in an apology being published online by USPATH. The apology was removed soon thereafter (Sand Chang, pers. comm., 2017). At a health professional summit in Buenos Aires in 2019, Argentine activist Mauro Cabral Grinspan chastised largely Global North–based providers for coming to Argentina to enjoy its tourist attractions but not to learn from activists' experiences of depathologizing care through the Gender Identity Law (Sand Chang, pers. comm., 2017).

62. "Discriminalizar, desestigmatizar, desjudicializar y despatologizar las identidades trans."

63. Spade (2015) takes a similar position about legal study in his discussion of administrative violence.

64. Indeed, transness also colludes with whiteness to sharpen biopolitical divides and preserve forms of conditional admittance for certain subjects. See Aizura 2018; Gill-Peterson 2018; Reddy 2011; Snorton and Haritaworn 2013; Spade 2015.

65. The Gondolín garnered local fame after the travestis who were staying there (including Argentine travesti activist Mónica León) filed a complaint about the dismal and dangerous conditions in the hotel. The owner charged travestis exorbitant rates, recognizing that he could take advantage of their precarity and largely cash-based income. The hotel was summarily shut down after the complaint, but travestis who were living there remained and collectively organized to improve living conditions.

66. Hotel Bauen was owned collectively by its workers until 2020, when the Covid-19 pandemic severely affected business.

67. Although it was published too recently to deeply engage Beatrice Adler-Bolton and Artie Vierkant's (2022) excellent *Health Communism*, theirs is an excellent companion book to this one. Particularly relevant here is their insight about the enduring pairing of "eugenic and debt burdens" with respect to surplus populations. They argue that this framework simultaneously shapes both modern health-care systems and capitalist economic relations more generally and that patient activist groups have pushed back against such logics to resist both entrenched medical hierarchies and broader capitalist economic relations.

68. I arrived a bit late to *Crip Times,* Robert McRuer's (2018) excellent book on the centrality of disability to struggles against the related phenomena of neoliberalism and austerity regimes. In it, he stages (queer) crip politics as a present and potential (though by no means preordained) intervention to politics of austerity. He traces how crip activism against austerity has taken shape in large part through proposed social transformations that privilege interdependence across radical difference, contrary to austerity's fixation on "deservingness" for the few (tied to both manufactured economic scarcity and compulsory able-bodiedness/mindedness). His book is also a generative companion to this one and delves even more deeply into austerity regimes and antiausterity movements.

69. According to Lewis and Irving (2017), trans- political economy builds on feminist political economy to attend simultaneously to free market and neoliberalizing economies and gendered and sexualized dynamics of labor and capital accumulation.

70. Here, Goldberg (2009) builds on Cedric Robinson's (1983) notion of racial capitalism, which contests Marxist theories about capitalism's emergence and argues that structures of capital accumulation hinge on racialized devaluation and dispossession. Goldberg extends this to engage neoliberalism's intensification of capitalist relations. In racial neoliberalism, he asserts, disinvestment from social welfare and focused investment in private capital accumulation and securitizing regimes produce profoundly divergent conditions of racialized life—the effects of which are chalked up to individualized failing rather than structured and systemic deprivation.

There are other dimensions of trans- health that extend beyond racial and economic stratification, such as questions of disability, citizenship, and age. My focus on the former issues reflects the primary foci of the activists with whom I spoke at the time I conducted my research. Many activists included broader concerns in this work, but the relevance of racialized class was a site of the most intensified discussion and action.

71. In the United States, racialization has largely proceeded through the interrelated regimes of settler colonialism, enslavement, eugenics, anti-immigrant legislation, and imperialist nationalism. Argentina's nation-building legacies are not wholly dissimilar, but its genocide against Indigenous people and its expulsion (or denial of the existence) of Afro-descended people were arguably more entangled with whitening regimes that aimed to secure the distinction of Europeanization and supposed progress in the Global South. This rendered whiteness significantly more permeable in Argentina in comparison with the United States (in which the one-drop rule prevailed), but wealth and education

were among the requirements for admission. These dynamics were later enfolded into an anticommunist fascism that conflated poverty, Indigeneity, Blackness, non-Catholicism, gender nonnormativity, and provincial life (among others) as dangers to the nation. For more on racialization and its differing trajectories in each region, see E. D. Edwards 2020; Finchelstein 2014; Hooker 2017; HoSang, LaBennett, and Pulido 2012; Goldberg 2009; Ward 2009.

72. See Spade (2015) for a legal critique of trans- antidiscrimination legal tactics, which he engages through critical race theory.

73. Cole Rizki (2020) writes about how the dictatorship and fascist state violence are active and present forces within contemporary Argentine social movements, including in trans- and travesti politics.

74. On neoliberalism's elaboration in Chile under Pinochet and its subsequent uptake in the U.S. Reagan administration, see Barder 2013.

75. For an excellent analysis of biomedical entrepreneurialism in trans- health, see Aizura 2018. He mobilizes Clarke, Mamo, and colleagues' (2010) notion of "biomedicalization" and Janet K. Shim's (2010) "stratified biomedicalization" to discuss the Foucauldian concept of "entrepreneurialism of the self" as it relates to trans- health and medicine. Aizura argues that this is not so much about freedom from medical subjection as it is reflective of the submission to economic subjection (167–69).

76. Fifty-five senators voted in favor, zero opposed, and eleven abstained.

77. The Gender Identity Law was preceded in 2010 by the Right to Protect Mental Health Law, which legally excluded the psychiatric use of diagnoses to pathologize people on the basis of political affiliation, cultural group, sexuality, religion, morals, or beliefs (among others). Right to Protect Mental Health, Law No. 26.657, Dec. 3, 2010 (Arg.).

78. For example, Malta, Sweden, France, Ireland, Belgium, Denmark, India, Chile, Bolivia, Colombia, Ecuador, and Uruguay all passed gender identity laws in the years following Argentina's, although Malta's (followed closely by Argentina's) was arguably the most expansive. Many of the other bills lacked key provisions around gatekeeping, self-determination, and care coverage.

79. There were also contestations among activists that the law remained too binary in availing people the option of gender reclassification only as "woman" or "man"—which, for many travestis, are not the primary positions they claim (De Mauro Rucovsky 2019; Wayar 2012). Activists such as Mauro Cabral Grinspan counter that it is the state's binary infrastructure rather than the law that produces this problem. These debates have extended into disagreements over Argentina's recent law to adopt a third gender option ("other" or "*otra*") on national IDs.

80. While significantly expanded, advocates report consistent denials

for procedures such as facial feminization surgery (Sylvia Rivera Law Project 2017b). Eric Plemons (2017) asserts that changing notions of sexed embodiment center facial structures as one of the preeminent sites of relational gender.

81. This draws on perspectives from various legal studies fields, including critical race theory (e.g., Harris 1993; Delgado and Stefancic 2001), which examines how racialized subordination is legally encoded by interrogating its conditions of emergence and operation. This field (along with law and society, Latino critical race theory, and others) presumes that laws are not necessarily operationalized in such a way that they perform the work they claim to perform.

82. In Robin D. G. Kelley's (2008, xii–xviii) revised edition of *Yo' Mama's Disfunktional!*—which urged grassroots community groups to make more, better, and stronger demands on the state—he answers to Grace Lee Boggs's critiques that such imperatives amount to a failure of imagination beyond state forms. He concedes this point but maintains that mounting state-focused demands is indeed part—though certainly not the whole—of a broader "politics of liberation" (xviii).

83. The original text appears in French. I have used the translation offered by Espineira and Bourcier (2016).

84. Foucauldian biopolitics analyzes the workings of power that administer aggregate life through the figure of population (Foucault 1990). The characterizing shift in governing power was the move from "make die and let live" to "make live and let die." In Michel Foucault's account, biopower involved individualizing disciplinary power combined with population-level interventions shaped by state racism to mark certain groups as advancing society and others as its drains. In biopower, embodied life became particularly central to politics and governance. Achille Mbembe (2003) argues that Foucault failed to account for regimes within which entire populations are exposed to death, developing the concept of necropolitics to account for populations under the siege of war, enslavement, and colonialism. C. Riley Snorton and Jin Haritaworn (2013) productively extend this as "trans necropolitics" to describe the stratifying dynamics among white trans- subjects claiming rights by mobilizing trans- of color death.

85. Clarke (2010) refers to the varied assemblages of health politics as "healthscapes," drawing on Arjun Appadurai (1996). Clarke, Mamo, and colleagues (2010) also describe the dynamics of life's administration and biomedicine's expansion as "biomedicalization." More recently, Steven Epstein and Stefan Timmermans (2021) describe broad cultural shifts from "medicine" to "health," which incorporate increasingly expansive sites of practice, expertise, and intervention that far exceed spaces of clinical practice and medical research.

1. Care without Pathology

1. Activist engagements range when it comes to this assessment. While groups like STP center transphobia as a structuring phenomenon for health-care regimes worldwide, transnational groups like GATE and regional groups within and beyond my sites of study call for a differentiation of the racialized, sexed/gendered, economic, and regional conditions within which transphobia takes shape in health care.

2. Medical sociologist Laura Mamo (2010, 173) engages a related concept in her exploration of biomedicalization without pathologization relevant to the neoliberal subjectification of lesbian consumers of technoscientific reproductive technologies. Adele Clarke, Janet K. Shim, and colleagues (2010, 47–48) describe biomedicalization as the increasingly complex and technoscientifically enmeshed ways that biomedicine saturates life "not only from the top down or the bottom up but *from the inside out.*" Mamo's discussion of biomedicalization as no longer requiring pathologization or medical classification relates to the subjectifying suffusion of biomedical (and markedly stratified) choice in reproductive technology markets. In this important critique, Mamo shows how social imperatives of normativity and inclusion converge with logics of neoliberal choice in biomedical fertility markets. She argues that such shifts have, at least in part, entrenched persistent forms of economic stratification that enable the pursuit of "perfectible" humanity for some against the unavailability of even basic forms of care for others. "Care without pathology" is therefore a concept that must be analyzed as inseparable from the political economic forces that enable its operation and in relation to shifting bounds of normativity and marginality.

3. The Medicaid exclusion was in fact lifted in March 2015, following a class-action lawsuit that was filed against the State of New York by a group of attorney advocates (Department of Health, New York State 2015). Prior to this, any procedure code with the *DSM*'s Gender Identity Disorder diagnosis (now Gender Dysphoria) would be rejected for reimbursement. Endocrine Disorder became a standard work-around during this time, since it raised fewer flags for hormone treatment reimbursement.

4. Nearly from the beginning of Trump's presidential term, his administration worked to reinterpret this regulation to *exclude* gender identity. In June 2020, the Trump administration announced that it planned to roll back these protections by amending the Health Care Rights Law (Section 1557) of the Patient Protection and Affordable Care Act (H.R. 3590, Pub. L. No. 111-148, 124 Stat. 119 [2010])—the provision that prohibits discrimination in health care, insurance, and other programs receiving funding from federal sources. While this does not amount to congressional authorization of the reinterpretation, and while the U.S. Supreme Court decided

in favor of interpreting Title VII federal employment discrimination prohibition to include gender identity and sexual orientation as part of sex discrimination, the administration's actions have produced significant confusion.

5. In this sense, Argentina's Gender Identity Law is distinct (at least in theory) from Brazil's legal provisions guaranteeing "sex-reassignment surgery" as a basic health right. As Carmen Alvaro Jarrín (2016) discusses in their ethnographic account of publicly funded hospitals in Rio de Janeiro and Belo Horizonte, pathologization of transsexuality in these clinics became a means of denying both pathologized medicalization and desired care to travestis whose narratives did not align with diagnostic criteria, even as people identified as nontravesti transsexuals were considered to be legitimate subjects of care.

6. Notably, many activists are quick to point out that nearly all of these are also provided—and frequently covered—for nontrans- people as part of treatments and procedures to enhance gender normativity. Surgeries on intersex infants are some of the most contested among these, given what many argue is the impossibility for infants and children to provide informed consent. Adults often elect to pursue other kinds of gender-confirming procedures that have long been legitimated as being medically necessary. For example, among nontrans- women with hirsutism (unusually prolific hair growth) or nontrans- men with gynecomastia (breast tissue development), treatments and surgeries are frequently justified as both necessary and reimbursable (see Latham 2017). Indeed, the available language about "gender-confirming" procedures was part of what drove advocates to describe trans- therapeutics in these terms, since this supported their legal position that public and private medical payors were engaging in diagnosis discrimination. This detail became somewhat lost in subsequent debates among trans- activists about whether "gender-confirming" was a demeaning way to describe such processes and procedures, since trans- people do not need our gender expressions to be "confirmed" by anyone—particularly the medical establishment. This is only one example of the ways such terminological debates, even those that are extraordinarily valid in their positions, become somewhat unanchored to the conditions of their historical emergence.

7. Further, as Jarrín (2016) points out through her ethnographic work in Brazil, even in public health-care systems that generally cover plastic surgeries and that consider trans- therapeutic surgery to be a public right, as in Brazil, exclusions remain in the ways that providers assess people's eligibility as a proper subject of care. Specifically, she shows how such exclusions are enacted within clinics to separate "transsexuals" from "travestis" and to define only the former as qualified subjects of care.

8. As I mentioned in the Introduction, the providers with whom I spoke were generally unrepresentative of providers more generally, as they regarded themselves as particularly supportive of trans- health. For an account of providers who were somewhat more hesitant or cautious in their approach to trans- health and gatekeeping, see shuster (2021). It remains worth noting, however, that even outside of a pathologizing frame, the structures of trans- health in the United States place medical providers—even supportive ones—squarely in a position of authority when it comes to knowledge and care regarding trans- people.

9. Although *depsychopathologization* and *depathologization* are often used synonymously, the former explicitly signals projects that focus on psychiatric or psychological regimes of pathologization (which trans- depathologization often also implies).

10. As Eve Kosofsky Sedgwick (1991) and others point out, it was not long after this removal that Gender Identity Disorder was entered into the *DSM*. She saw this as a new route through which psychiatry could perform early intervention into childhood effeminacy in boys in its continued efforts to prevent homosexuality.

11. Even before the formal legalization of abortion in 2020, clandestine abortions were readily available for those with the means to pay for them. As sociologist Julia McReynolds-Pérez (2017) shows, feminists waged sustained battles for access to abortion as struggles not only against sexism but also against racialized class inequity.

12. Some Argentine activists and scholars have drawn directly on RJ paradigms to advance claims about trans- health. For example, Argentine philosopher Blas Radi (2020) draws on RJ to analyze surgical requirements for legal gender classification and lack of explicit reproductive protections for trans- people as a means of passive eugenics. In fact, he critiques the limits of the Gender Identity Law in the realm of reproductive health, asserting that, despite eliminating sterilizing surgery as a legal requirement for gender reclassification, it fails to address other reproductive rights.

13. Guardianship is the legal status that formally places adults with disabilities under the care of a legal guardian (whether a parent or another adult). Andrew Dilts (2012) discusses racism and guardianship laws, Theresia Degener (2017) analyzes guardianship in the context of human rights models of disability, and Luisina Castelli Rodríguez (2020) explores the concept at the nexus of disability and feminist activism.

14. "La rebeldía no se tutela. Las discas y locas no vamos a parar hasta ver arder la sociedad hasta sus cimientos para construirla sin escaleras, ni psiquiátricos, ni CIES, ni cárceles, ni barreras." Thank you to Francisco Fernández Romero for directing me to these Buenos Aires–based disability activist groups.

15. For the visual map that Mingus, along with Cara Page, Patty Berne, and others produced to represent the medical-industrial complex, see Mingus 2015.

16. *Sex reassignment* is sometimes used by trans- people to describe surgeries or other trans- therapeutics. More often, it is a clinical term used to describe trans- therapeutic surgeries.

17. Health-care reform in Argentina (and elsewhere in Latin America) has not tended as much as the United States toward gatekeeping per se as a major strategy in health-care reforms. Nevertheless, Argentina's health system has in the last few decades undertaken (or been coerced into adopting) closely related economic reforms. Argentina was among many nations that adopted the terms of the so-called Washington Consensus that the International Monetary Fund (IMF) and World Bank required in exchange for significant loans in the late 1980s and early 1990s. Former president Carlos Menem enthusiastically adopted these neoliberal reforms, including in the domain of health care (Machado 2018). While implementation of these reforms has ranged by nation and administration, they share logics of cost containment, privatization, free-market orientation, and decentralized decision-making in marked contradistinction to the public, collectivist tenets of Latin American social medicine (Hartmann 2016). Argentina's recent history with neoliberal reforms is a tortuous one: from its role as the IMF's star pupil in the 1990s to its 2005 departure from the organization under President Néstor Kirchner, from subsequent President Cristina Fernández de Kirchner's refusal to pay debts to former President Macri's renewed IMF membership, requested bailout, and ultimate failure to reinvigorate the national economy. This book cannot do justice to the fullness of these intricacies, but for the purpose of this chapter, it suffices to say that the logics of medical gatekeeping gesture toward the broader austerity measures of free-market privatization and profit through cost containment. In this sense, the broader milieu within which trans- health gatekeeping unfolds remains shaped by these economic dynamics in both geographic locales.

18. This statement should not imply that such dynamics have ceased—in fact, despite significant transformations, suspicion and distrust on the part of care providers remains persistent to this day. However, contestations to this conduct and approach have gradually entered mainstream discourse, which stands in contradistinction to twentieth-century transsexual medicine.

19. Before changing its name to WPATH, the professional organization was named after sexologist Harry Benjamin: the Harry Benjamin International Gender Dysphoria Association (HBIGDA).

20. Scholars such as Sander L. Gilman (1985), Ellen Samuels (2014),

and Jules Gill-Peterson (2018) offer rich and varied accounts of some of these imbrications.

21. Joey L. Mogul, Andrea J. Ritchie, and Kay Whitlock (2011), as well as others analyzing queer criminalization, are quick to point out that racialization matters greatly to the intensity of surveillance or violence among criminalized groups. Whiteness, wealth, ability, and masculinity generally insulate subjects from the effects of criminalization, even though the protection afforded by these subject positions is in some situations tenuous or transitory.

22. Other scholars understand these forms of criminalization as historical extensions of "colonial queerness," or the introduction of "institutional actions against sexual difference" that accompanied the European invasion of the Americas (Domínguez Ruvalcaba 2016, 31).

23. "Los llamados edictos policiales–que no son exactamente leyes sino reglamentaciones internas de la policía–permiten detener a cualquier persona sospechosa de prostitución, homosexualidad, vagancia, ebriedad, etc., y recluirla sin intervención de la Justicia, en la cárcel ¡por plazos que oscilan entre los 30 días en Buenos Aires y los 90 en Córdoba!" Perlongher's missive was published posthumously.

24. The American Medical Association (AMA) and American Public Health Association responded to major ethical breaches in prison-based health care by establishing standards of care in the 1970s. In the 1980s, the AMA established the National Commission on Correctional Health Care.

25. Philosopher Andrea J. Pitts (2018, 15) identifies some of the problems related to the deficiencies of prison-, jail-, and immigration-detention-based health care as being related to the "conflicting goals of health care and those of punitive institutions."

26. *Adams v. Federal Bureau of Prisons,* 716 F. Supp. 2d 107 (D. Mass. 2010). On September 30, 2011, a settlement was announced in *Adams v. Bureau of Prisons* that reversed the federal freeze-frame policy that had prevented trans- prisoners from beginning transition-related care unless they could prove that they already started it prior to incarceration. Currently, regulations do not enact a blanket policy that requires a current medical hormone prescription or other forms of sanctioned medical care in order to be eligible for its continuation in federal United States prisons. Nevertheless, current claims are evaluated on a case-by-case basis, which provides little protection from denials and relies heavily on a stringent gatekeeping logic.

27. I use the term *activist providers* to describe people working as care providers who were explicitly activist in their framing and who took part in street-based or other direct-action organizing in addition to their caregiving work. This is distinct from, albeit related to, the concept of "insider-providers" that I have developed elsewhere (Hanssmann 2016).

28. Of course, there are many other kin relations when it comes to depathologization—harm reduction, intersex activism, HIV/AIDS treatment and prevention, Health at Every Size, and many more. While I do not explore these here, each merits exploration, as they exemplify various forms of care without pathology.

2. Unruly Terms

1. Trans- people have circulated anecdotes on social media using the hashtag #TransHealthFail. These include videos and other posts describing uncomfortable, degrading, and sometimes dangerous interactions with health-care providers.

2. The problem list was developed in the late 1960s as an area in the medical chart that "helps [physicians] to define and follow clinical problems one by one and then systematically to relate and resolve them" (Weed 1970, 3). Intended as a less-standardized space for clinical reflection and synthesis, its uses are multiple, and it does not always work as intended.

3. The notion of fraudulence haunts trans- health and medicine at every turn, the "truth" of patients' sex/gender was a central point of contention and anxiety for several generations of trans- medical providers (Gill-Peterson 2018; shuster 2021). Transness continues to be popularly represented as fraudulent gender expression (see Spade 2015).

4. Among the notable exceptions are Aren Z. Aizura (2018), Jules Gill-Peterson (2018), C. Riley Snorton (2017), and Dean Spade (2015).

5. Here, I use *intersectionality* in Crenshaw's original sense—as an explicitly institutional critique of the failures of law to account for multiplicities of marginalization across race and gender—rather than in its more diffuse popular sense.

6. While these publications both precede and come after the formal period of study, I found it important to analyze the full spectrum of historical and contemporary classifications to ground the broader situation within which these debates were (and continue to be) unfolding.

7. María Lugones (2007, 190) proposes "colonial gender" not as a preexisting colonial gender system that was *imposed* on colonial subjects but rather as a new gender system through which colonized life was then organized and known. This included emphases on "biological dimorphism [and] the patriarchal and heterosexual organizations of relations" as concepts underpinning "differential gender arrangement along 'racial' lines."

8. For more on these histories across the Global North and South, see Aizura 2018; Berkins 2007a; Cabral Grinspan 2017; DiPietro 2016; Fernández 2004; Gill-Peterson 2018; Rizki 2020; Schuller 2018; Skidmore 2011; Snorton 2017; Spade 2015; Wayar 2018.

9. As Evan B. Towle and Lynn M. Morgan (2002, 472) assert, "third gender" entered anthropological literature in the 1970s. Even prior to this, though, anthropologists studied sex/gender variance through a reductive and colonizing lens. See also Boellstorff et al. 2014.

10. In the 1990s, trans- people in the Global North also began claiming a kindred siblinghood with these anthropologically mediated representations—a dynamic that Towle and Morgan (2002) call "romancing the transgender native."

11. This was written as "Trans-sexualism" in the *ICD.*

12. Scholars and advocates engage each of these domains and more in detailed accounts. I cannot do justice to each of these analyses, but I direct readers to these thoughtful engagements. On crises of authority and politics of expertise, see shuster 2021; Epstein 2021. On epistemological shifts, see Drescher 2013. On access and equity, see Gorton 2013. On depathologization, see Suess, Espineira, and Walters 2014; Stop Trans Pathologization 2012; Cabral Grinspan 2017; Burke 2011; ICATH, n.d.; Epstein 2021. On transnational legibility, see Aizura 2018; Lynne 2021.

13. See Bowker and Star 1999. With respect to the importance of practice relevant to classification in trans- studies, see Aizura 2018; Plemons 2017; Gonsalves 2020.

14. While this is a new diagnostic classification for the *DSM, gender dysphoria* is an older term that was coined by sexologist Harry Benjamin in the 1970s.

15. In this book, I emphasize the breadth, instability, and mobility of these classifications. It is beyond the scope of this project to provide a detailed account of each of the debates and histories involved in classificatory development over time. For detailed accounts of these processes across the twentieth century (including their basis in eugenic and racial science), see Gill-Peterson 2018; Snorton 2017; Skidmore 2011. For debates about psychiatric and medical classification—especially as it unfolded in the *DSM* in the late twentieth century—see shuster 2021; Burke 2011; Drescher, Cohen-Kettenis, and Winter 2012; Drescher 2010; Gorton 2013. For detailed discussions about recent revisions to the *ICD,* see Epstein 2021; Gonsalves 2020; shuster 2021.

16. While *DSM*-5 contributors framed *dysphoria*—which originates from the Greek term for *distress*—as a novel intervention, it is in fact far from a new concept. In 1973, following the growth of university-based gender biomedical centers offering surgeries, Stanford psychiatrist Norman Fisk suggested "gender dysphoria syndrome" as an improved means to assess patients' *degree* of nonnormativity. "As originally intended," he wrote, "the term *transsexual* was to specifically identify a person who was not to be confused with a homosexual or a transvestite" (Fisk 1974, 387). In this manner, *gender dysphoria* was revived and rebranded to

meet a contemporary moment. Its appearance in the *DSM* bridged Fisk's spectrum model with activists' notions of nonpathological plurality. The former served to index intensities of pathology, and the latter defined the environments within which trans- people live as sources of stress of social subjugation.

17. Cohen-Kettenis is a Dutch psychiatrist and researcher who has been a longtime member of WPATH. Drescher is a U.S. psychiatrist and psychoanalyst who has long advocated against the pathologization of gay identities in psychiatry and who has worked as a provider-advocate in favor of trans- depathologization. Meyer-Bahlburg is a professor of clinical psychology in the United States and studies conditions related to intersex and gender dysphoria, often focusing on hypotheses pertaining to brain chemistry. Pfäfflin is a German psychoanalyst and retired university chair of forensic psychopathology.

18. For a detailed discussion, see Kamens 2011.

19. Damien W. Riggs and Clare Bartholomaeus (2018) describe how some of these tensions played out at the WPATH Conference in Buenos Aires in 2018.

20. In stating this, I wish to characterize a general tendency, though the field of psychiatry in Argentina is no more monolithic than anywhere else. In addition, the psychodynamic approach has also been pathologizing vis-à-vis sex/gender nonnormativity (Farji Neer 2018). Indeed, Argentine psychiatrists colluded with law enforcement in the nation to produce criminalizing frameworks restricting travestis from public space (Fernández 2004, 34).

21. The presumption that transness is indeed a condition of the psyche is increasingly contested, following in large part the turn to the soma that theorized sexual orientation in genes and brains (see, for example, see O'Riordan 2012). While there is not space to explore this in detail within this book, Eric Llaveria Caselles (2021) addresses the "epistemic injustice" of neuroscientific brain mapping studies of transness.

22. For a detailed account of the *ICD* revision process and its central debates, see Epstein 2021.

23. As an ethnographer, I signed up as a contributor and was prompted to disclose any potential conflicts of interest. One of the questions included asked if I or members of my family have been diagnosed with any of the conditions on which I might comment. I checked the box.

24. The trans- diagnosis was only one of many proposed revisions in the *ICD-11*, and it was not the only classificatory diagnosis that was met with controversy. For a discussion of some of these debates, see Stein et al. 2020.

25. In fact, some argue that this process of declassification was legalized in 2010, with the passage of the Derecho a la Protección de la Salud

Mental, or the Right to Protect Mental Health. Among other provisions, the national law excludes medical diagnoses that apply to collective identity or membership vis-à-vis politics, sexual identity, or alignment with prevailing beliefs or social standards. However, some study participants mentioned that certain psychiatrists continued to issue socially pathologizing diagnoses despite the existence of this law.

26. The Medicaid exclusion for gender-confirming care was lifted in March 2015, following a class-action lawsuit that was filed against the State of New York by a group of attorney advocates (Department of Health, New York State 2015). Prior to this, codes with the *DSM*'s Gender Identity Disorder diagnosis (now Gender Dysphoria) would be rejected for reimbursement.

27. Karin Knorr Cetina (1999) and Geoffrey C. Bowker and Susan Leigh Star (1999), among others, theorize about work-arounds, largely in the milieu of technological work. For these STS scholars, work-arounds are a critical part of infrastructures that enable interactions between humans and technologies that do not always proceed at face value or as intended.

28. Some of these debates assert that there is less distinction between this than previously assumed. This converges with recent turns in mental-health professions to "biologize" certain "conditions." This is presumed to "reduce stigma," in addition to "scientizing" psychiatry (see Pitts-Taylor 2016). For more on the biologization of transness in neuroscience, see Llaveria Caselles 2021.

29. Work-arounds are part of navigating the "administrative violence" that Dean Spade (2015) describes as characterizing the encounter between trans- people and institutions, with its most antagonizing operations affecting those who are most exposed to state bureaucracies—namely, poor people, people with disabilities, and people of color.

30. Sociologist stef shuster (2019, 2021) also discusses these dynamics at length in their discussions of gatekeeping and informed consent.

31. In 2015, the Health Information Technology Certification Criteria published rules about the requisite inclusion of sexual orientation and gender identity in electronic health records (Office of the National Coordinator for Health Information and Technology 2015). Hale M. Thompson (2016), Taylor M. Cruz (2020), and Cruz and Emily Allen Paine (2021) show that these transformations strove to integrate more "social factors" into care practice. However, they also assert the limitations of such changes in terms of disparate and stratified exposure to harm via disclosure (H. Thompson 2016) and a lack of focus on the conditions that produce inequities in the first place (Cruz 2020; Cruz and Paine 2021).

32. Here, I want to speak briefly to an important point that Gill-Peterson (2018) makes regarding "unruliness." Gill-Peterson discusses

embodied unruliness, but this may also extend to the classificatory and linguistic realm. Specifically, she links unruliness to sexed plasticity as a capacity for transformation and, in a eugenic mode, as the purported phenotypic embodiment of whiteness. In this regard, "unruliness" does not automatically possess a political position, though it is often celebrated within trans- studies and activism as if it necessarily contests rather than underwrites power.

33. For a discussion of biomedical stratification, see Shim 2010.

34. For a historical analysis of this phenomenon, see Gill-Peterson 2018.

3. Epidemiological Rage

1. The monologue was delivered in Spanish, and the translation is mine. *Travesticides,* or *travesticidios* in Spanish, is a reconstruction of *femicides* (*femicidios*), formally criminalized and informally protested in Argentina and in various regions of South America, Central America, México, and beyond. Jill Radford and Diana E. H. Russell (1992) advance the concept of "femicide" to describe gendered violence and murder, describing it as "the killing of women by men simply *because* they are women" (xiv), and other feminist scholars extend the concept. Argentina has federal legislation specifically addressing gendered violence, but activists complain that it has not been budgeted for or implemented substantively. A movement organized under the banner Ni Una Menos (#niunamenos, meaning "Not One (Woman/Travesti) Less") undertook coordinated protests in the summer of 2015. Lohana Berkins (2015) published an opinion piece in the leftist paper *Página 12* at the height of the coordinated Ni Una Menos protests in June of that year, asserting that "travesticide is also femicide" ("el travesticidio también es femicidio"). Feminist organizers of the nationwide protests were mixed in their reception to the presence and claims of travestis who asserted their inclusion in this coordinated movement, with some expressing that travesti concerns were distinct. The political implications of femicides in Argentina is important to consider not only for the feminist and coalitional claim that travestis are making under the Ni Una Menos banner but also because these classed and racialized femicides are frequently linked in media reporting to sexualized and reproductive struggles around abortion, pregnancy, and sex work. Media frequently mention gendered intimate partner violence that occurs in response to women who are pregnant or intending to get an abortion, as well as violence against sex workers by their johns.

2. After being excluded by some Ni Una Menos activists, travestis specified "no more travesticides" ("Basta de travesticidios"). This became

a rejoinder to both the exclusionary definition of feminized violence adopted by some Ni Una Menos activists and the perpetrators of violence against travestis (Radi and Sardá-Chandiramani 2016).

3. The question of racialization remains somewhat submerged, however. Argentina's particular racial formations have taken shape in programs of expulsion, disavowal, and a broad institutionalized erasure of Blackness and Indigeneity through regimes of "whitening" in the late nineteenth and early twentieth centuries (Aguiló 2018). Erika Denise Edwards (2020) traces these histories of racialization into the eighteenth century in her discussion of Afro-descended women in Córdoba and the institutionalized erasure of Blackness. I discuss some of these dynamics in the book's Introduction, as they shape some of the conflation of race and economic class in travesti and trans- politics.

4. Disability was not explicitly taken up by epidemiological biographies, although scholars assert the inextricability of disability from geographically specific processes of racialization, sexualization, and gendering (e.g., Samuels 2014; Erevelles 2011).

5. The critiques of state securitization that were advanced by epidemiological biographies did not necessarily extend beyond the direct and specific realm of policing, criminalization, harassment, and violence against travestis and trans- people (as is the premise of Toby Beauchamp's [2019] crucial work on transgender politics and stratified surveillance in the United States). However, as travesti and trans- political coalitions and activist histories demonstrate, activists' positions against state violence and securitization were legible against a larger backdrop of postdictatorship suspicion about institutionalized state force. Thus, these conceptual shifts that I trace might be read as an inchoate critique of state surveillance writ large.

6. Sociological analyses of risk are key to a broader analysis of the behavioral focus of most population-health risk assessments. While relevant here, I will take up this discussion in more detail in chapter 4. For the sake of this chapter, I treat *risk* as the set of conditions that researchers identify as strongly affecting health outcomes.

7. An exception involves select Argentine health research publications that define state violence as a public-health issue (e.g., Spinelli 2004). These nevertheless mostly focus on the historical phenomenon of health during the nation's dictatorship rather than ongoing modes of state violence.

8. Other studies that bear mention include the following: Capicüa 2014; Cabral 2009; Frieder and Romero 2014.

9. All translations from Spanish made by the author.

10. As María Soledad Cutuli (2015, 301) points out, founders were able to access funding from the National Ministry of Labor in the wake of the

economic crisis to start the cooperative, though at this time the Argentine state was certainly not working to address employment exclusion for travestis.

11. Before her death, Berkins requested that Fernández (2020) publish her biography, *La Berkins.*

12. "Las travestis, las transexuales y las transgéneros participemos activamente de la producción de conocimiento acerca de nuestras vidas, necesidades y deseos."

13. Without knowing the specifics of how this research unfolded, it is difficult to comment on the power dynamics that might have taken shape between institutionally affiliated academics, independent researchers, and travesti researchers. However, it is notable that few academic researchers at the time (or currently) authored collaboratively with travesti activists.

14. Intersex and transmasculine activist Mauro Cabral Grinspan was also involved in these studies, but it was not until several years later that transmasculine activism gained a more robust public presence in Argentina.

15. "Los que se exhibieren en la vía pública con ropas del sexo contrario."

16. "¿Qué es la policía? Por un parte, que los organismos estatales sigan siendo violadores sistemáticos de los derechos humanos nos habla de prácticas y mentalidades autoritarias aún hoy presentes en el Estado, que no han sido removidas durante la democracia. Así, el llamado 'Estado terrorista' (que refiere a esa extraña combinación en la que quien debería custodiar las leyes es su principal violador), el Estado vuelto contra la sociedad, sigue siendo una realidad cotidiana para un conjunto de sectores subordinados."

17. "Pibas y pibes chorros, travestis, transexuales, transgéneros, villeros y villeras, prostitutas, morochas y morochos y migrantes somos sometidos a una doble violación de nuestra ciudadanía y nuestra integridad: la primera, al ser sometidos/as a situaciones de violencia; la segunda, al no poder apelar a una instancia superior para denunciarlas, porque es desde esas instancias mismas que partió la agresión." These are rough translations of slang terms that defy translation, especially "morocho/a"—a term that is generally coded in feminine terms, and while vague enough to describe hair as well as skin color, is often mobilized as a mode of expressing phenotypic colorism within Argentina's racial regime.

18. "La información recogida en esta encuesta (tanto como el trabajo de otras organizaciones que defienden los derechos humanos) hacen imposible pensar los abusos policiales como problemas individuales de los miembros de la fuerza que los lleva adelante. Por el contrario, se trata de una violencia institucional. Esto no debe llevarnos a pensar que entonces

el o la policía que nos pega, nos maltrata o nos agrede sea inocente; sino que es el o la responsable individual de un hecho de responsabilidad mayor que recae, en última instancia, en una decisión política."

19. In a similar vein, Cole Rizki (2020) discusses a 2016 protest campaign by the political group La Brecha. The title of Rizki's article borrows from his 2018 interview with the group: "No state apparatus goes to bed genocidal then wakes up democratic."

20. "No van al hospital porque saben que interviene la policía. En ese caso se van a la calle ven cómo se pueden curar."

21. "La salud no es considerada un bien social sino una mercanda que se adquiere a traves de mecanismos de mercado."

22. "La economía hospitalaria no soporta despilfarrar en nosotras suministros, medicación genérica, cama, comida y cuidados de enfermera/os sobreexigidos/as y mal pagos/as. Nos toca morir en la calle mientras otras/os soportan el VIH con un mínimo de calidad de vida."

23. "Tal como hemos señalado, la declamación formal del derecho a la atención adecuada de la salud no nos alcanza, es preciso elaborar politicas públicas que traduzcan este derecho en posibilidades concretas para nosotras aquí y ahora."

24. It is beyond the scope of this article to detail transnational dynamics, histories, and politics that produce varied categories of gendered/sexualized difference. See Lewis 2010; Namaste 2000, 2011; DiPietro 2016; Simonetto and Butierrez 2022; Cutuli 2013b. PJ DiPietro (2016) emphasizes the irreducibility of travestismo and Indigeneity in Argentina, linking its persistent criminalization to "whitening" regimes constitutive of the nation's founding. Fernández (2004) routes travesti subjectivity not though Anglophone "gender identity" but in political opposition to modes of sexualized criminalization that Paul Amar (2013, 3) calls "moral security."

25. "Los integrantes de la comunidad trans son en general personas con las más bajas expectativas de vida y con mayor dificultad para la escolarización, y son expulsados, en general, de los sectores laborales. Sufren una enorme discriminación y violencia social." Sesión Ordinaria (Especial), "Derecho a la Identidad de Género," Period 129, Meeting 10 (November 30, 2011), Argentina Congress, https://www.diputados.gov.ar/diputados/fsola/discursos/debate.jsp?p=129,10,13.

26. For a discussion of Abuelas de la Plaza de Mayo's role in DNA identification to locate children who were stolen during the dictatorship, see Smith 2016. For a discussion of the contested quantification of the disappeared during the Dirty War, see Brysk 1994.

27. "La salud es algo colectivo, que no es un proceso de enfermedad individual de una persona, sino que es una construcción social colectiva."

28. As Martínez and Vidal-Ortiz (2021) explain, *travar* has a complex translation. It is a verb that plays on the term *trava,* which is a somewhat reclaimed but still derogatory term referring to travestis. In addition to this, though, *travar* is pronounced like *trabar,* a term that means "to jam." This double meaning, the authors argue, is of critical importance for the travesti theorists who mobilize it (668–69).

29. Examples include CORREPI, n.d.; "The Counted," n.d.; Mapping Police Violence, n.d. Between 2015 and 2018, former Argentine president Mauricio Macri's austerity policies sparked protests to which police responded with violence. Relatedly, Macri and other officials have also downplayed estimates of people who were disappeared during the right-wing dictatorship from 1976 to 1983.

30. Claiming state responsibility is a critical reframing that epidemiological biographies had a part in instantiating (building on previous anti-authoritarian movements in Argentina). However, this move also requires a flattening of the multifaceted, multiple, and often contradictory faces of the state—which is indeed resolutely not a singular or coherent entity. I am grateful to Evren Savcı for a generative conversation about this point.

31. I am indebted to Alisa Bierria and Emily Thuma for drawing attention to this aspect of activists' efforts as reflecting another inflection of statistical collectivization.

32. Drawing on Max Weber's (1978, 302) notion of life chances, Spade (2015) describes how "reduced life chances" for trans- people are shaped not straightforwardly by errors of transphobia but rather by interrelated conditions of administrative violence, economic stratification, racialized/sexualized criminalization, and medicolegal power.

33. "La declamación formal del derecho a la atención adecuada de la salud."

34. The Madres and the Abuelas de la Plaza de Mayo (the Mothers and the Grandmothers of the Plaza de Mayo) used the phrase "debts of democracy" ("deudas de democracia") in their activism following the disappearances of young leftists during the military dictatorship. Kelsey M. Jost-Creegan (2017) describes how this phrase and framing has been reanimated in recent social movements in Argentina. Julia McReynolds-Pérez (2017) describes its uptake in activism for legal access to abortion. Cole Rizki (2020) also elaborates alliances between travestis and the Madres de la Plaza de Mayo.

35. The phrase "militant mixed methods" borrows from Colectivo Situaciones (2005), a radical former research collective in Buenos Aires, that employed what they called "militant research."

36. Ezra Berkley Nepon (2016) uses the term *dazzle camouflage* to describe the specificity of queer performance.

4. Saving Lives, Saving Money

1. As an organization that was involved in direct service as well as legal support and organizing, they were some of the first to learn from their clients and members about a crackdown on reimbursement for hormone prescriptions for trans- Medicaid recipients in the state.

2. The question of public coverage for trans- therapeutics in other realms, such as in prisons and jails, remains a critical site of development for similar themes—though the intensification of criminalization introduces an even more pointed public critique around supposed deservingness. *It's War in Here: A Report on the Treatment of Transgender and Intersex People in New York State Men's Prisons* (Sylvia Rivera Law Project 2008) by the Sylvia Rivera Law Project is one epidemiological biography on this topic that I do not analyze here but that is nonetheless important to these broader themes.

One distinction between most resources I identified as "epidemiological biographies" in New York versus Buenos Aires was that the majority were produced by nonprofit nongovernmental organizations. Many of these organizations ran broad, grassroots organizing programs, some of which included directed research efforts (Sylvia Rivera Law Project [2017a], for example, held a "Participatory Research Night" to collect data and build methodologically on a republication of *It's War in Here*). It bears noting that the professionalization and institutionalization of community-based research in the United States (and beyond), as well as the professionalization of social movements through what many refer to as the nonprofit-industrial complex, likely had some effect on the conditions of development and circulation of epidemiological biographies in New York.

3. For a sustained discussion on how solidarity and the social contract were instantiated through the political technology of insurance, see Ewald 2020.

4. There has been some resistance, particularly among trans- people, to the term *gender-confirming* to describe trans- therapeutic surgeries. However, advocates tended to use this language because it was already being used to describe the surgeries or procedures that nontrans- people sought (and often had covered) to "confirm" their gender expressions.

5. Raymond's (1979) text targeted trans- women specifically as either antifeminist dupes or as enacting a violent "colonization" of womanhood. She writes, "All transsexuals rape women's bodies by reducing the real female form to an artifact, appropriating this body for themselves" (104). Specifically, she views trans- women as "literally possess[ing] women's bodies," asserting that "transsexuals merely cut off the most obvious means of invading women, so that they seem non-invasive" (104). Raymond reserves most of her ire for trans- women rather than trans- men,

but her repetition of false arguments about fraudulence and danger have unevenly affected trans- lives in cultural, political, material, and legal domains.

6. While states exercised more control over Medicaid regulations with respect to trans- therapeutics, few offered explicit policies for coverage until about 2014. New York and other states held blanket exclusions. Other states had no specific regulatory guidelines and covered these on a case-by-case basis. While states supposedly exercised their own prerogative in Medicaid policy, state programs did not escape federal scrutiny. For example, after Washington State Medicaid covered two surgeries for trans- people between the years of 2000 and 2006 (which cost the state a total of $113,000), Iowa senator Chuck Grassley told then governor Christine Gregoire that he planned to have federal inspectors audit such use of funding (Thomas 2006).

7. Welfare Reform Act, New York State, Office of Temporary and Disability Assistance, Chapter 436 Welfare Reform/Restructuring of the Department of Social Services, S. 5788/A.8678 (November 20, 1997). https://otda.ny.gov/policy/directives/1997/ADM/97_ADM-20.pdf.

8. For a sustained reflection on the collusion between neoliberal and neoconservative welfare retrenchment in the 1970s and 1980s, see Cooper 2017. Melinda Cooper extends the feminist argument that welfare reform marked disproportionate racialized policing of gender and sexuality. Specifically, she asserts that neoliberals and neoconservatives understood macroeconomic problems as being *directly* linked to what they saw as "an ominous shift in the sexual and racial formations of the Fordist family" (Cooper 2017, 24). In other words, they defined economic crises as moral ones.

9. As informants were quick to note, the amendment limited a long list of procedures and interventions that were not eligible for coverage, including presurgical fertility preservation, breast augmentation, facial feminization or masculinization, electrolysis unrelated to vaginoplasty, tracheal shaves, and voice therapy. It explicitly excluded what it described as "cosmetic surgery" or procedures "solely directed at improving an individual's appearance." N.Y. Comp. Codes R. & Regs. tit. 18 § 505.2(l) (2016).

10. *Cruz v. Zucker,* 195 F. Supp. 3d 554 (S.D.N.Y. 2016).

11. *Casillas v. Daines,* 580 F. Supp. 2d 235 (S.D.N.Y. 2008).

12. A federal regulation (42 C.F.R. § 440.230) prohibits the arbitrary denial or reduction of coverage for patients based only on diagnosis, illness, or condition.

13. 42 C.F.R. 440.230(d). The same provision was cited in *Moore v. Medows* (563 F. Supp. 2d 1354 [2008]), a court case that took place in Georgia. Plaintiffs argued that Medicaid could not contravene an assess-

ment of "medical necessity" issued by a physician about supportive nursing care for a girl with severe disabilities. A federal district judge decided in favor of the plaintiffs, asserting that physicians rather than the state Medicaid program should have the last word on medical necessity. The Eleventh Circuit Court reversed this decision, arguing that a "private physician's word on medical necessity is not dispositive."

14. *Ravenwood v. Daines* was not filed by the advocates with whom I spoke, and there was some concern among them at the time that a second case would set a dangerous legal precedent. While the activist attorneys with whom I spoke were considering an appeal after the *Casillas v. Daines* case, they were soon urged by poverty lawyers not to do so as to avoid setting a negative legal precedent that would affect broader action for poor people attempting to bring action against Medicaid under section 1983, which in essence gives Medicaid and other public beneficiaries the ability to take individual action against government programs. As study respondents explained, appellate poverty attorneys were concerned that a negative ruling would compromise the already-narrowing capacity to bring 1983 claims to court. As such, they decided not to do so. For more on 1983 claims, see Rao 2009. *Ravenwood v. Daines,* No. 06-CV-6355-CJS, 2009 WL 2163105, at 13 (W.D.N.Y. 2009).

15. Section 1557 prohibits discrimination in health care for a number of protected characteristics. While the rule mentions sex as one of these, it was initially somewhat unclear whether gender identity was understood to be included within this. After significant pressure from activists and advocates, the Department of Health and Human Services under Obama eventually clarified that, from a regulatory standpoint, discrimination on the basis of gender identity would be recognized as sex discrimination. This rule was later the target of the Trump administration's 2020 effort to eliminate language about gender identity, remove sex-discrimination protections, and redefine *sex* as "the biological binary of male and female that human beings share with other mammals" (Affordable Care Act, 42 U.S.C. § 18116, 85 Fed. Reg. at 37178). Alongside mass public mobilization, several lawsuits blocked these provisions from taking effect.

16. TransJustice is "a political group formed by and for trans and gender-nonconforming [TGNC] people of color" (TransJustice 2006, 227) and is part of the Audre Lorde Project, an organization in New York City that organizes LGBTQ people around issues related to community wellness and social and economic justice (Audre Lorde Project, n.d.). They held the first Trans Day of Action for Social and Economic Justice in 2005. The statement associated with this event asserted that "the specific issues that TGNC people of color face mirror those faced by

broader communities of color in NYC: police brutality and harassment; racist and xenophobic immigration policies; lack of access to living wage employment, adequate affordable housing, quality education, and basic healthcare; and the impacts of US imperialism and the so-called US 'war on terrorism' being waged against people at home and abroad. These issues are compounded for TGNC people of color by the fact that homophobia and transphobia is so pervasive in society. As a result, our community is disproportionately represented in homeless shelters, in foster care agencies, in jails and prisons" (228).

17. SRLP had partnered with poverty law organizations since its inception, but during this era, poverty law and health law organizations began prioritizing trans- health as a concern and working in direct and sustained collaboration with SRLP and other trans- health-focused attorneys. This marked a turning point in their willingness to devote significant time and resources to this issue.

18. GLAAD is a media advocacy organization that was formed in the mid-1980s to address homophobia in reporting. Initially called the Gay & Lesbian Alliance Against Defamation, the organization is now known only by its acronym. Currently, it works with media and entertainment industries to reshape narratives concerning LGBTQ communities.

19. One of the study's authors was a primary organizer in the Health Care for All! coalition. Most study respondents (70 percent) used "health-related public benefits," including Medicaid. The multiracial team of nineteen researchers were majority trans- women or gender nonconforming people, with the majority being low-income and BIPOC.

20. The research collective's name is in fact borrowed from the title of Premilla Nadasen's (2004) book on the Black women activists at the fore of welfare-rights organizing in the 1960s and 1970s.

21. These were not the first documents to circulate that made the case for trans- health-care coverage through the lens of economic rationality (for example, San Francisco conducted citywide research and Oregon conducted statewide research about the anticipated versus actual costs of insurance). However, the "Eliminating the Medicaid Exclusion for Transition-Related Care in NYS" fact sheet and campaign infographics were distinct among these in their narrative of a speculative story about cost savings in the realm of mental health and suicidality, in addition to self-medication.

22. Justin Tanis (2016) makes a compelling argument to recognize the interpretive limitations of this figure, emerging as it does through a nonrandomized sample in the National Transgender Discrimination Survey, as reported in Grant et al. (2011). This is an oft-cited resource that surveyed over six thousand trans- people on a variety of items relevant to discrimination. While Tanis encourages taking this figure with

a grain of salt, he nevertheless also argues that such statistics still reflect profound inequities and uneven access to resources, support, and care. As in the case of life span figures, however, these statistics also conceal profound racialized, classed, and other differences (though the survey disaggregates these somewhat).

23. Murphy's (2017, 5–6) discussion of the "economization of life" signals a late twentieth-century "regime of valuation" that has come to delimit present landscapes of political thought and action. Specifically, they describe how quantification has produced intertwined notions of "population" and "economy" to ascribe differential value to different forms of racialized and classed life in terms of quantified contributions to macroeconomy. (The link to disability vis-à-vis Murphy's broader argument is a somewhat curious elision in their otherwise outstanding analysis of differential valuation and distribution of life and life chances.) In rendering aggregate life calculable, the economization of life works to define some lives as worth living or saving and others as expendable for the sake of robust and sustainable national economies. These calculative modes of thinking have ossified over time, Murphy argues, culminating in a collective inability to think beyond the "container" of macroeconomies and beyond life as anything but "human capital." Arianna Planey (2021) has deftly engaged Murphy's work to critique the deficiency of the Triple Aim in its failures to take up inequity and uneven cost burdens in health care, focusing on racialized disability and care practices.

24. In this context, *deference* refers to a concept in administrative law where courts yield to the ways that agencies interpret laws or regulations. Generally, courts have tended to defer to agencies' regulatory interpretations unless they are demonstrably wrong. Recently, the Supreme Court has taken a somewhat different turn by requiring more congressional oversight for agency decisions that are interpreted to be of major national significance.

25. Here, she builds on scholars who interrogate neoliberalism in its diffuse manifestations beyond economic reforms to culture, subjectivity, and sexuality. See, for example, Berlant 2011; Cheng 2010; Ong 2006; Duggan 2003; Bernstein 2018.

26. Various social-movement activists and scholars aligned with the politics of prison abolition describe the imaginative politics that transcend present limits as moving toward a "vision of a restructured society in a world where we have everything we need" in Mariame Kaba's words (2021, 2). Many scholars extend Gorz's (1964) notion of a "non-reformist reform," often developing criteria that can shift conditions of power or distribution in the meantime as social movements continue to call and work for deeper political transformations. For more on politics of prison abolition and nonreformist reforms, see Spade 2015; Gilmore 2007; Kaba 2021.

27. This True Name feature was launched in 2019 through Citibank's

joint venture with Mastercard. This specifically gave trans- and nonbinary customers the option to use a "self-identified" chosen first name on credit cards. Citibank released an ad campaign for the card option during Trans Awareness Week.

5. Crashing the Gate

1. "Derecho al libre desarrollo personal. Todas las personas mayores de dieciocho (18) años de edad podrán, conforme al artículo 1° de la presente ley y a fin de garantizar el goce de su salud integral, acceder a intervenciones quirúrgicas totales y parciales y/o tratamientos integrales hormonales para adecuar su cuerpo, incluida su genitalidad, a su identidad de género autopercibida, sin necesidad de requerir autorización judicial o administrativa." Gender Identity Law, No. 26.743, May 9, 2012 (Arg.). http://servicios.infoleg.gob.ar/infolegInternet/anexos/195000-199999/197860/norma.htm.

2. "Los tratamientos integrales hormonales"; "la intervención quirúrgica total o parcial"; "se requerirá, únicamente, el consentimiento informado de la persona."

3. This of course stands in marked contrast to the forms of gender-affirming care that are offered without lengthy surveillance to nontrans- people and people who are intersex, as discussed in the Introduction.

4. The history of how these protocols emerged and how various clinics adopted them is one that is primarily preserved through institutional memory. The story I tell here is the one I understand best based on formal and informal documents and discussions with those who have worked in these clinics, but details about the diffusion of consent-driven care are difficult to trace. Nevertheless, it was clear that the 1990s and the first decade of the 2000s marked a series of fruitful conversations and exchanges among activists, advocates, and care providers about shifting away from gatekeeping models of care.

5. A crucial part of the story of consent-driven care—one to which I cannot adequately attend in this book, given the bounds of its analysis—relates to the landscape of emergent HIV treatment and prevention paradigms. One of the major drivers of consent-driven hormone provision to poor trans- women in San Francisco had a great deal to do with concerns about HIV transmission. Specifically, the 1990s saw early research on high rates of HIV prevalence and incidence among trans- women of color engaging in sex work economies in urban centers throughout the world—often in terms that are rather shockingly out of step and out of touch with the ways that these individuals would understand or describe themselves (for example, an oft-cited article by K. W. Elifson and colleagues [1993] refers to trans- women as

"male transvestites"). Ironically, these articles often speak to the need for "tailored intervention efforts" (Elifson et al. 1993) that might lessen trans- people's alienation from sites of health-care provision. For Tom Waddell Health Center, reduced barriers in the provision of hormones were part of this tailoring. As the *Transgender Tuesdays* (Freeman and Walters-Koh 2012) documentary about the clinic claims in its tagline, "They came for the hormones and stayed for the health care." "Staying for the health care" was related to the urgent priority and desire on the part of care providers, the city, and the region to contain HIV infection rates through what health-care providers call "patient engagement." Relaxing barriers to hormone provision may have been in part a response to calls for trans- depathologization, but it was certainly not the sole reason for the adoption of consent-driven care. Nevertheless, in the years that followed, the clinic's protocols around consent-driven hormone provision took on a life of their own, apart from the contingent conditions of emergence related to concern around HIV transmission rates.

Notably, the fact that Tom Waddell Health Center formally adopted consent-driven protocols as a clinic run by the San Francisco Department of Public Health meant that other clinics within that system could adopt this approach with relative ease. This is how Dimensions, a San Francisco clinic for queer and trans- youth, was able to adopt a consent-driven model in 1998, even for care provision among those under eighteen. While the provision of hormones at Dimensions also required parental consent (technically making this an *assent* model for minors), the clinic also served emancipated minors, unhoused youth, and others living without guardianship. For these youth, a consent-driven model without parental consent was the clinic's general standard. Furthermore, during the 1990s and early 2000s, very few care providers were willing to prescribe hormones—even as part of a consent-driven model—to people who identified as genderqueer or nonbinary rather than specifically male-to-female (MTF) or female-to-male (FTM) (in the dominant parlance of the time). Dimensions presented an early exception to this exclusion. Currently, an increasing number of United States–based clinics prescribe hormones to nonbinary patients.

6. As Joanne Meyerowitz (2002) describes, trans- therapeutics in the midcentury until the 1980s in the United States were provided mainly by university-based gender centers. These programs were defined by their gatekeeping practices and, as Jules Gill-Peterson (2018) notes, by their exclusion of Black, Indigenous, and other people of color, as well as poor people and people with disabilities. These centers also produced research based on the patients they admitted, which itself had a racializing and class-stratifying effect on how transness was represented and how care provision was implemented. The introduction of consent-

driven care thus converged with the (extraordinarily limited) expansion of clinical trans- therapeutics to poor trans- people.

7. N. Y. Comp. Codes R. & Regs. tit. 18, § (2016).

8. In this manner, informed-consent processes are intimately linked to providers' desire for protection via care standards. For more on malpractice concerns and standards of care in trans- medicine, see Velocci 2021; shuster 2021.

9. Talia's reference to "harm reduction" is also a crucial health infrastructure, at least in the United States, that partially forms the conditions of emergence for consent-driven care. As G. Alan Marlatt and Katie Witkiewitz (2010, 591) describe, harm reduction is "a pragmatic approach to reduce the harmful consequences of alcohol and drug use or other high-risk activities by incorporating several strategies that cut across the spectrum from safer use to managed use to abstinence." According to its proponents, this paradigm of public health involves a shift away from abstinence-based treatment models (especially for substance use) and away from the moralizing frames of reference that underpin the requirement for abstinence. As these approaches were adopted into dominant forms of public-health practice, proponents argued that care could take a less judgmental, patronizing, and criminalizing approach to supporting patients in cultivating the forms of wellness that made life livable, even as these might involve practices that biomedical knowledge has generally regarded as "unhealthy." Notably, sociologist and activist Michelle O'Brien (2013) explicitly links trans- health's entanglements with capitalism, "off-label" pharmaceutical use, and the criminalization of syringes that harm-reduction programs attempt to mitigate in her influential article (originally a zine), "Tracing This Body: Transsexuality, Pharmaceuticals, and Capitalism."

10. While there were few laws that regulated gender reclassification prior to 2012, some Argentines were able to access changes to legal names or gender classifications through judicial orders. However, these typically required proof of surgeries, which had been legally prohibited during the Juan Carlos Onganía dictatorship in 1967 through the Law of the Practice of Medicine, Dentistry, and Collaborated Activities (Law No. 17.132, Jan. 31, 1967 [Arg.]) except in the case of a judicial order. Petitions seeking judicial approval were lengthy and were rarely met with success; it wasn't until 1997 that a document change was approved (notably for a trans- man who maintained a sustained legal case) (Cabral and Viturro 2006; Farji Neer 2012; Hollar 2018).

11. The legal right to identity carries a particular importance in the milieu of Argentina after the Dirty War, during which agents of the Jorge Rafael Videla dictatorship "disappeared" thirty thousand people. The right to identity relates directly to children who were forcibly taken from

the disappeared and given to families that supported the dictatorship. This is one of the many links that join travesti and trans- activists with the Madres and the Abuelas de la Plaza de Mayo, as analyzed by Cole Rizki (2020).

12. "En el marco de toda consulta, entre el personal de salud y las personas usuarias, se ponen en juego relaciones de poder y de saberes que han sido valorados de manera desigual y asimétrica. El desafío es hacer de la consulta un encuentro que permita la construcción conjunta de saberes. Se trata de habilitar un espacio que reconozca los recursos de cuidado propios de cada persona. En este sentido, es necesario tener en cuenta las diversas experiencias y prácticas que muchas personas trans han desarrollado en relación con la construcción corporal, frente a su histórica expulsión del sistema sanitario. . . . La singularidad de cada persona hace de la consulta una situación original. Por ese motivo no debe pensársela como un espacio formado por momentos fijos e invariables, sino por instancias lo suficientemente flexibles que permitan ordenar la relación entre lxs integrantes del equipo de salud y las personas usuarias, sin determinarla. Estas instancias variables se articulan en base al vínculo y la comunicación, y parten de las demandas y necesidades de cada persona."

13. The content of the guide, though formally authored by the Ministry of Health, was compiled by social scientists who had worked on issues of sex and gender and were thus familiar with the ways in which activists were making claims. Various activist groups were also consulted directly about the guide. Several study participants observed wryly that parts of the guide had been taken quite directly from an activist-produced guide that had been in circulation prior to the 2015 publication of the Ministry of Health guide. Antonio also commented that the limitations of the document—particularly the fact that the medical guidelines were "very binary" and the introduction "very queer"—reflected "the consequences of taking the trans- people as a focal population but not as a community that can produce knowledge" (interview, July 25, 2015).

14. Such transnational advocacy about the importance of informed consent for the realization of human rights was also echoed by intersex rights advocacy and activist groups, which intersected at points with trans- advocacy work.

15. As discussed in chapter 1, WPATH has led the implementation on a global scale of a diagnostic, psychotherapeutically focused, and stringently gatekeeping model of care. However, they have increasingly presented these in recent iterations as "flexible guidelines" that need to be adapted to specific sites of care and population needs. It had been in this milieu that informed-consent models have been engaged and provisionally advanced as within the bounds of ethical practice in trans- therapeutics.

16. Of course, in my observations—especially in observing clinicians

discussing case studies about so-called difficult patients—this supposed leveling was at its most equitable when patient and provider shared worldviews, treatment narratives, and racialized, classed, and abled subject positions that facilitated ease of communication. This relates to other social scientific observations about commensurability, difference, and notions of "culture" in biomedical practice (see Taylor 2003).

17. Critics point to some of the various hypocrisies that emerge in this origin story about medical bioethics. Sheeva Sabati (2019) calls these "collective myths" that situate bioethical principles as responding to "cases of exceptional violence . . . within an otherwise neutral history of research." Alongside Harriet A. Washington (2006), Sabati points to the multitudinous abuses of people—generally Black, Indigenous, and other people of color, people with disabilities, people in state institutions, poor people, intersex and trans- people, and subjects interpellated as "third world"—regardless of the supposed protections of bioethics. These scholars focus specifically on research bioethics, but I would suggest these critiques also extend to clinical bioethics. Sabati (1057) also argues that such abuses are not aberrations but rather the norm of research—a sustained complicity in the production of inequity and subordination that involves the routine racialized/abled exclusion of some people from the category of "human" (see also Wynter 2003).

18. Jukka Varelius (2006, 377), for example, describes autonomy as "self-rule that is free from both controlling interference by others and from limitations, such as inadequate understanding, that prevent meaningful choice."

19. Patients' Rights Act, Law No. 26.529, Nov. 19, 2009 (Arg.).

20. A few Argentine study participants pointed out that the congressional hearings about the Gender Identity Law in 2012 concurred with hearings on a "dignified death" law enabling physician-assisted suicide in cases of terminal illness. While this also passed with broad congressional support, some suggested that the high-profile controversy it caused might have prevented a higher degree of negative attention from being focused on the Gender Identity bill. The Catholic Church in particular had organized against the euthanasia bill and strongly opposed its passage.

21. Emiliano Litardo (2013) points out that bioethics formed only one part of the equation that produced the requirement of informed consent alongside self-perceived need—the right to identity was also key. Argentina's recent history has led to an understanding of human rights as a material form of accountability against state-sanctioned authoritarianism rather than an abstract set of ideals (Brysk 1994; Sriram 2004). This precedent provided traction for notions of autonomy and consent to take meaningful shape in a way that symbolically foregrounded freedom from coercion over and above objectives of collaborative clinical relations.

22. For more on the coconstitutiveness of disability, race, gender, and

sexuality, see Erevelles 1996; Samuels 2014; Snorton 2017; Clare 2017. For more on the limits of the human, personhood, and racialized humanisms, see Jackson 2020; Weheliye 2014; Spillers 2003.

23. More generally, shuster found that providers embraced a "rhetoric of informed consent" while acting "to override trans people's decisions about their health and lives" (195).

24. In addition, as Jules Gill-Peterson (2018) shows, medical age of consent has only enfranchised (some) adults rather than teenagers or children to make decisions about their bodies—including the ability to *refuse* nontherapeutic "care" in the form of feminizing or masculinizing procedures for intersex conditions. Even for those above the age of consent, Charis Thompson (2005, 225) notes that informed-consent protocols "require freedoms from various kinds of subjective and situational vulnerability that simply cannot be assumed" in many scenarios. Furthermore, eugenicist involuntary sterilizations—routine prior to the uptake of informed-consent laws—still persist (Hernandez 1976). In fact, as the 1975 *Madrigal v. Quilligan* (No. CV 75-2057-JWC [1978]) case demonstrates, Chicana women in the United States were coerced and bribed into signing forms consenting to sterilizing surgeries—sometimes not realizing they had undergone hysterectomies until years later (Hernandez 1976). In cases such as these, informed-consent contracts were wielded as weapons that forcefully reasserted the coercive power of medical providers as they sought to protect themselves against legal liability without regard for patients' needs or desires.

25. These tensions in fact form a center of gravity for studies in medical anthropology and sociology and have generated a range of theories and critiques, including the invisibility of the "culture" of medicine (Taylor 2003), its structuring coloniality (Anderson 2008; Fanon 1965), failures of translation when it comes to modes of treatment or care (Garcia 2010; Stevenson 2014), and the paucity of power analyses in bioethics (Holloway 2011).

26. Importantly, Lugones is not suggesting that hegemonically intelligible actions can be equated with agentic action either. Even for "shareholders in power" (210), legibility of intentionality is conditioned on acting "into the hegemonic system's vein" and offers only an *illusory* notion that people are indeed authoring their actions (217).

27. In a virtual panel titled "Trans Care" (Malatino, Gill-Peterson, and Cvetkovich 2020), Hil Malatino and Jules Gill-Peterson were in conversation on precisely this point. As Gill-Peterson said poignantly and succinctly in this exchange, "Transphobia makes you want to pass."

28. Sylvia Rivera and Marsha P. Johnson are recent historical figures who were marginalized from mainstream gay liberation movements of the 1970s. They were involved in a multitude of liberation movements, as well

as antipoverty and antiprison politics. Much of their work was mobilized through a group they founded called Street Transvestite Action Revolutionaries (STAR), which organized and housed queer and trans- youth. Historical primary sources about Rivera and Johnson have been made available through work to publicize the archive undertaken by New York–based activist and artist Tourmaline (n.d., esp. posts dated 2012–2013).

29. This insight about the relation between care and distribution is indebted in part to a discussion that took place December 2, 2020, among working group members in the Beyond Care project in the Feminist Research Institute at UC Davis.

30. In National Decree 721/2020, President Alberto Fernández enacted the Labor Quota Law for Travestis and Trans People in the Public Sector (Cupo Laboral Travesti Trans en el sector público), which requires public employers to hire travestis and trans- people to make up 1 percent of the public-sector workforce. Some activists critique the law as a means of containing resistance, while others question the ways it is likely to reproduce racialized and classed inequities by opening up positions only to those travestis and trans- people who are already comparatively insulated from conditions of dispossession. Another critique involves the divisive issue of sex work. Several well-known Argentine travesti activists are self-identified sex-work abolitionists who claim that sex work can never be freely chosen in conditions of employment exclusion. Other activists argue that sex work should be protected rather than abolished or criminalized. However, the question of sex work as a means of survival absent other means of sustenance formed a backdrop for the activism and legal debates leading up to this decree. Furthermore, many activists have hailed the decree as a victory, particularly given its having been championed by the late travesti activist Amancay Diana Sacayán, about whom I wrote in chapter 3.

31. As Fisch insists, "Full self-determination in relation to all other people, whether these are manifested as individuals or as a collective, is the same as freedom from domination" (22). However, this freedom from what he calls "alien determination," or the exercise of one's will over another, depends centrally on the presumption that self-determination is intrinsic to all human existence (23–24).

32. As British legal scholar Marc Weller (2008, 24) points out, these have long been part of cosmopolitan international legal systems, but only recently have these become actionable.

33. This forms part of Joseph Massad's (2018) argument in his article "Against Self-Determination," in which he asserts that formal principles of self-determination were key to the consolidation of settler colonialism, particularly as it applies to Israeli colonization, settlement, and sustained occupation of Palestinian territories. Other critics point

to the problematic domestication of human rights through global markets driven by United States and European economies of extraction, colonization of thought or resistant politics, or reassertion of neoliberal or imperial politics (Baxi 2006; Slaughter 2007; Spivak 2005; Hua 2011).

34. One way in which such capacity is denied is through racialized and contingent admittance to the very status of "human," as Sylvia Wynter (1994), Aimé Césaire (2000), C. Riley Snorton (2017), and others point out. Colonized and enslaved subjects in particular, and Black, Indigenous, and other people of color more generally, have been persistently excluded by institutions of governance, bureaucracy, and medicine from recognition as fully human, often through the subordinating and dehumanizing assertions of racial science.

35. As Indigenous feminist scholar Joanne Barker (Lenape) (2015) asserts, self-determination and its connection to sovereignty are historically contingent, but when it comes to Indigenous knowledge and action, these make up what she calls "polity of the Indigenous." Within such polities, particularly relative to Indigenous feminisms, claims are "often figured through international legal frameworks to rearticulate Indigenous sovereignty and self-determination over Indigenous (women's) lands, bodies, and families. . . . It is not an embrace of imperialist narratives of reconciliation and healing, but of an empowerment of refusal and grounding." Anticolonial scholars such as Aimé Césaire (2000) and Michel-Rolph Trouillot (1995) similarly engage the political refusals inherent in self-determination, particularly in the extralegal sense expressed in uprisings and insurrections by colonized subjects. Nikhil Pal Singh (2005) and Alondra Nelson (2011) also describe a political but not formally legalistic orientation to self-determination through the long tradition of U.S. Black nationalism and self-defense—including but not limited to the Black Panther Party—that insists on marshalling the power to decide conditions of life free from white supremacy, coercion, violence, and state repression. While each of these groups operates from an awareness of the international codification of self-determination as a fundamental right, they also explicitly trouble the ways that national and international legal apparatuses fail to confront unfreedoms.

36. Dean Spade (2006) also acknowledges individualist/collectivist tensions in his mobilization of the term *gender self-determination.* He describes it as "a tool to express opposition to the coercive mechanisms of the binary gender system (everything from assignment of birth gender to gender segregation of bathrooms to targeting of trans people by police)" (235). He asserts that he uses the term "strategically" and with a cognizance of the individualizing logics of capitalism that movements can strive to overcome.

37. The original text appears in French. I have used the translation offered by Espineira and Bourcier (2016).

38. The notion of self-perceived need versus diagnostic qualification became legible in part against the backdrop of other legal interventions, such as the 2010 Right to Protect Mental Health (Law 26.657). Article 3 of this law stipulated that mental-health providers were not permitted to make diagnoses on the basis of political affiliation, "lack of conformity" with "moral, social, cultural, political or religious beliefs prevailing in the community where the person lives," or "choice or sexual identity." Law No. 26657, Dec. 3, 2010 [32041] B.O. 1 (Arg).

39. This also follows Michelle Murphy's (2012, 32) account of feminist care collectives, which describes a similar political gesture: "Feminist self help critically *diagnosed* and redirected the exercise of power as it moved through technical practices that invested reproductive health with new political dispositions."

40. *Objects* in this regard refers not just to *things* in the conventional sense but rather to "something that people . . . act toward and with. Its materiality derives from action, not from a sense of prefabricated stuff or 'thing'-ness" (Star 2010, 630). Star's theorizing follows science and technology studies thought in considering the productive knowledge-making action of humans and nonhumans in interaction, and her work on boundary objects is no exception.

41. As I mentioned in the Introduction, the health-care providers with whom I spoke tended to be unusually sympathetic to (and sometimes even involved in the work of) trans- health activists when compared to their colleagues and to dominant practices of health care. The providers in my study, for example, often shared collective notions of self-determination with activists rather than fully embracing the notions of autonomy advanced by bioethics. However, they also recognized that the institutionalization of trans- health likely required a less explicitly politicized and collectivist orientation to autonomy.

42. As C. Riley Snorton (2017), Cameron Awkward-Rich (2020), and Jules Gill-Peterson (2018) point out, such horizons of freedom are sharply stratified by histories and presents of racialized unfreedoms. Among activists, these histories likely produced very different orientations to future freedoms promised by self-determination.

43. Talia and Mark were two examples among interviewees. ICATH also inhabited both social worlds.

44. "Somos tuteladas, somos vistas como sujetas inferiorizadas, incapacitadas, no podemos decidir sobre nuestras propias vidas. Otros y otras deciden sobre nosotras, deciden sobre nuestros cuerpos. Nos dicen qué tener, qué no tener y cómo ser. Obviamente nosotras, como buenas feministas, desobedecemos todo."

45. During one of my meetings with a health-care provider who worked at a public health clinic, I was joined by an individual who worked for a nongovernmental organization working in trans- advocacy. The physician, assuming that she had access to representatives of state government, asked her no fewer than three times in our half-hour conversation if she could help with financing to cover the cost of hormones for the clinic. She insisted each time that she did not have such inroads but sympathized with what they both recognized was a scarcity of affordable hormones for prescribing to trans- and travesti patients in public clinics. She later mentioned to me that local organizations often broker access to the Argentine state to arrange for certain clinics to receive funding for otherwise unaffordable supplies of testosterone, estrogen, and antiandrogens.

46. "Invisibles para un derecho y una bioética demasiad satisfechos de su propio progresismo—el cual se ha limitado, hasta el presente, a considerar la situación de aquellos y aquellas incluidos en su version restringida del mundo, ignorando hasta la existencia de todas y todos los demás."

6. Extending Depathologization

1. "Por justica real, económica, política, y social."

2. The group that drafted that version of the Gender Identity Law that passed the congressional vote was an ad hoc coalition led largely by trans- and travesti activists and included leftist queer and allied activists and attorneys. The ad hoc committee referred to themselves as the National Front for the Gender Identity Law, or the Frente. Drafts of less comprehensive and less depathologizing versions had been submitted by more mainstream advocacy groups in past years, and versions proposed by legislators were even more stringently pathologizing, requiring proof of surgeries for legal gender reclassification (see Hollar 2018).

3. "Fue mensaje muy fuerte . . . por las institucionces policías, médicas, policiales, todos instituciones que sistimaticamente . . . se burlaron, nos golpearon, nos censuraron. . . . [Fue mensaje fuerte] porque tomamos la decisión de hacer cosas. Y que podemos hacer muchas otras cosas."

4. The film about Tom Waddell Health Center in San Francisco, *Transgender Tuesdays: A Clinic in the Tenderloin* (Freeman and Walters-Koh 2012), also traffics in this affective organization.

5. "Pensar en la salud como un derecho básico suele ser casi imposible para quienes no se amoldan a las estructuras heteronormadas que buscan regular sus cuerpos."

6. This is, of course, linked to various discourses within the institutions of health care, biomedicine, and biomedical ethics. For instance,

patient-centered care, family-centered care, and informed-consent paradigms all center the notions of choice, autonomy, and patient–provider collaboration. Yet *autonomy* is not conceived or defined identically by those engaging in practices that might fall under any of these rubrics.

7. While there is a strong antiprison movement in Argentina, the term *abolitionist* refers more directly to people who strive to abolish sex work (including several notable travestis). This warrants more reflection than I have space for in this study, but it raises some compelling questions for thinking through the continuities and discontinuities of different facets and implications of abolitionist frameworks.

8. *Queer* has a specific resonance in the United States, and this particularity at times undermines its expansive political aspirations given its failures in translation and circulation. As Cole Rizki (2019) describes in his review of Héctor Domínguez Ruvalcaba's 2016 text, *Translating the Queer,* there is contention among Latin Americanists over whether *queer* performs any counterhegemonic work when mobilized cross-hemispherically. There is little disagreement over whether its meaning remains stable in translation—there is consensus that it does not. Yet, whether scholars view it as a colonizing or metropolitanizing imposition or as a site for generative contestation remains contested in this debate.

9. Historian Nayan Shah (2019) also considers the coalition-generating potentials of "putting one's body on the line." Reflecting on the political potentials of *queer* advanced by Cohen, Shah discusses the audacious political tactic of the hunger strike. He describes how queer and trans- Latinx activists in Southern California resisted the expansion of queer- and trans- specific "pods" in immigration detention facilities—a development that Immigration and Customs Enforcement claimed facilitated "safety." Activists rejected this position, highlighting interconnections between immigration, prison abolition, and queer/trans- justice movements.

10. For more extensive discussions of neoliberal transformations and Argentina's resulting debt crisis, see Cavallero and Gago 2021; D'Avella 2019; Gago 2017. Briefly, Argentina's government under Perón had refused an invitation to join the International Monetary Fund (IMF), which Juan Perón understood as an imperialist organization. After the 1976 military coup installed Jorge Rafael Videla as president, the nation implemented neoliberal reforms with a vengeance. Privatization and deepening social and economic inequality grew significantly through the next several decades, culminating in the 2001 economic crisis, during which over half of the population fell below the poverty line and the nation defaulted on its debt.

11. *Republic of Argentina v. NML Capital, Ltd.,* 573 U.S. 134 (2014).

12. Argentina's eventual repayment occurred only after the nation's

election of Mauricio Macri. The administration of his predecessor, Cristina Fernández de Kirchner, had paid off remaining IMF debts in 2006 and restructured private debts. However, the administration dug in its heels when it came to private debt holders that refused restructuring (like Elliott Management's), claiming that the nation refused to compromise funding health care, education, housing, and employment to repay the full debt. Macri's decision to pay in full on this and other sovereign debts converged with a massive national disinvestment in all of these sectors.

13. Also present during this conversation was a New York–based NGO worker who was in Argentina to study the policy work of the Gender Identity Law. While she was critical of her position, the access that this afforded her was notable. For example, she had easily arranged a meeting with the Office of the Ministry of Health—this was something that, as an activist, Joaquín (and I, as a United States–based social scientist) had repeatedly attempted and failed to do.

14. In 2007, the HRC backed an employment antidiscrimination bill that protected lesbian, gay, and bisexual workers but not trans- workers. Activists have also criticized the organization for focusing most of its concern on gay marriage at the expense of other issues of equity, especially those that disproportionately affect trans- people, poor people, and Black, Indigenous, and other people of color. Its employees have referred to it as a "White Men's Club" (Villarreal 2015).

15. Peronismo, or Peronism, is a political ideology in Argentina that is difficult to summarize. It originated in the populist reign of Juan Domingo Perón, alongside Evita Perón, his wife, with pushes for nationalizing resources and introduced programs that were generally supportive of working-class politics. Peronismo's legacies are contested, however, with groups that advocate seemingly conflicting political priorities under its banner. The Partido Justicialista, or Justicialist Party, is the largest congressional party in the Argentine government since 1987. It contains major splits between leftist and conservative factions. Many left-wing and socialist-leaning activists align themselves with a Kirchnerist Peronismo, including some of the activists with whom I spoke. For more on Peronismo from an ethnographic perspective, see D'Avella 2019.

16. For an analysis of the racialized ableism of this conceptualization, see McRuer 2018.

17. I use the term *justice* here because it was the term I heard activists use most frequently in their work to imagine different configurations of distribution and power. However, I also want to note the trouble with the term, as Eve Tuck and K. Wayne Yang (2016) discuss in their article "What Justice Wants." Tuck and Yang describe justice as a "placeholder"

or as a "meeting ground for politics of solidarity" (10). Yet they articulate a desire for "elsewheres beyond justice" (6). While it may do important work, justice's abstractions and deferrals catch in the limits of coloniality and nation-state forms. They instead gravitate toward "terms that articulate their theories of change: rematriation, reparations, regeneration, sovereignty, self-determination, de-colonization, resurgence, the good life, futurisms" (10).

18. "Hay que tener coraje para ser mariposa en un mundo de gusanos capitalistas."

19. "Tensionaba un doble desplazamiento. En primer lugar, la polarización tradicional marxista de capital/trabajo y, en segundo lugar, la polarización feminista de varones/mujeres. . . . El antagonismo capital/género sugerido por Berkins no está encorsetado en la diferencia sexual . . . sino que opone la multitud alegórica de las mariposa al capital parasitario. El coraje de volverse mariposas advierte sobre la imposibilidad de un reconocimiento sin redistribución y restitución. Empuja la representación acabada a la coalición, la armonía del consenso a la sucesiva interferencia, el diálogo al conflicto político."

Conclusion

1. *Oxford English Dictionary Online,* s.v. "revision (*n.*)" (Oxford: Oxford University Press, 2023).

2. As Jasbir Puar (2017, 49–51) contends, the shift from pathologizing treatment to affirming modification could simply reflect one of the many adaptations of control societies. On its own, this shift does little to trouble the notions of stratified "deservingness" that enshrine some into the "charmed circle" of citizenship while doubling down on the exclusion of others. María Soledad Cutuli (2017) empirically explores how pathologization persists among poor travestis despite the Argentine state's formal depathologization of trans- and travesti subjectivities.

3. Referencing Paul Starr's (1982) exegesis of the rise of medical professional authority in the United States, Epstein and Timmermans (2021) focus on cultural authority as one of the two forms of medical authority that Starr discusses. Cultural authority involves the power to define reality, while social authority describes the power to control what actions are undertaken. Epstein and Timmermans argue that the phenomenon of cultural authority and its formation, modification, and maintenance require greater critical engagement.

4. See, for example, Amin 2018; Aizura 2018; cárdenas 2016; Gill-Peterson 2018; Puar 2017; Schuller 2018; Snorton 2017. In particular, Kadji Amin (2018), Jules Gill-Peterson (2018), and Kyla Schuller (2018) caution against a celebratory orientation to plasticity through their

historical readings of sexological texts, within which the plasticity of sex is treated as an exemplification of a racialized abstraction of whiteness. For critiques of health and embodied plasticity through critiques of capital, see also O'Brien 2013.

5. One particular surgeon, for example, celebrated the ways she honed her (proprietary) genital surgery techniques by operating not only on trans- women but also on nontrans- women who were seeking reversals for ritual genital cutting.

6. *Bell & Anor v. Tavistock and Portman NHS Foundation Trust* (2020), EWHC 3274 (England and Wales).

7. *Bell & Anor v. Tavistock and Portman NHS Foundation Trust* (2021), EWCA Civ. 1363 (England and Wales).

8. "El proceso de reforma y revisión de la CIE-10 representa una oportunidad histórica para el activismo trans comprometido con la despatologización como lucha emancipatoria–aunque los términos mismos de esa emancipación estén también en disputa."

9. "La subversión del orden medicalizado de los cuerpos."

10. "Que Aparezca Tehuel: Favor de compartir como si fuese cis."

Bibliography

Abogad*s por los Derechos Sexuales. 2016. "Foto Colectiva de #ReconocerEsReparar en el Congreso | Abogad*s por los Derechos Sexuales." *Abosex* (blog), November 23, 2016. https://abosex.wordpress.com/2016/11/23/foto-colectiva-de-reconoceresreparar-en-el-congreso/.

Adler-Bolton, Beatrice, and Artie Vierkant. 2022. *Health Communism.* New York: Verso Press.

Aguiló, Ignacio. 2018. *The Darkening Nation.* Chicago: University of Chicago Press.

Aizura, Aren Z. 2018. *Mobile Subjects: Transnational Imaginaries of Gender Reassignment.* Durham, N.C.: Duke University Press.

Álvarez, Sonia E. 1999. "Advocating Feminism: The Latin American Feminist NGO 'Boom.'" *International Feminist Journal of Politics* 1 (2): 181–209.

Álvarez, Sonia E., Jeffrey W. Rubin, Millie Thayer, Gianpaolo Baiocchi, and Agustín Laó-Montes, eds. 2017. *Beyond Civil Society: Activism, Participation, and Protest in Latin America.* Durham, N.C.: Duke University Press.

Amar, Paul. 2013. *The Security Archipelago: Human-Security States, Sexuality Politics, and the End of Neoliberalism.* Durham, N.C.: Duke University Press.

Amin, Kadji. 2018. "Glands, Eugenics, and Rejuvenation in Man into Woman: A Biopolitical Genealogy of Transsexuality." *TSQ: Transgender Studies Quarterly* 5 (4): 589–605. https://doi.org/10.1215/23289252-7090059.

Anderson, Warwick. 2008. *Colonial Pathologies: American Tropical Medicine, Race, and Hygiene in the Philippines.* Durham, N.C.: Duke University Press.

APA (American Psychiatric Association). 1980. *Diagnostic and Statistical Manual of Mental Disorders-III.* 3rd ed. Washington, D.C.: American Psychiatric Association Publishing.

APA (American Psychiatric Association). 1987. *Diagnostic and Statistical Manual of Mental Disorders-III-R.* 3rd ed. Rev ed. Washington, D.C.: American Psychiatric Association Publishing.

APA (American Psychiatric Association). 1994. *Diagnostic and Statistical Manual of Mental Disorders-IV.* Washington, D.C.: American Psychiatric Association Publishing.

APA (American Psychiatric Association). 2000. *Diagnostic and Statistical Manual of Mental Disorders-IV-TR.* 4th ed. Text rev. Washington, D.C.: American Psychiatric Association Publishing.

APA (American Psychiatric Association). 2013. *Diagnostic and Statistical Manual of Mental Disorders-5.* Washington, D.C.: American Psychiatric Association.

Appadurai, Arjun. 1996. *Modernity at Large: Cultural Dimensions of Globalization.* Minneapolis: University of Minnesota Press.

Appadurai, Arjun. 2012. "Why Enumeration Counts." *Environment and Urbanization* 24 (2): 639–41.

Applebaum, Paul S., Charles W. Lidz, and Alan Meisel. 1987. *Informed Consent: Legal Theory and Clinical Practice.* New York: Oxford University Press.

Arondekar, Anjali. 2009. *For the Record: On Sexuality and the Colonial Archive in India.* Durham, N.C.: Duke University Press.

Audre Lorde Project. n.d. "About ALP." Accessed November 6, 2007. https://alp.org/about.

Auyero, Javier. 2012. *Patients of the State.* Durham, N.C.: Duke University Press.

Awkward-Rich, Cameron. 2020. "I Wish I Knew How It Would Feel to Be Free." *Paris Review,* June 11, 2020. https://www.theparisreview.org/blog/2020/06/11/i-wish-i-knew-how-it-would-feel-to-be-free/.

Awkward-Rich, Cameron. 2022. *The Terrible We: Thinking with Trans Maladjustment.* Durham, N.C.: Duke University Press.

Baird, Vanessa. 2013. "Trans Revolutionary." *New Internationalist,* June 1, 2013. https://newint.org/features/2013/06/01/argentina-transgender-rights.

Baker, Kellan, and Andrew Cray. 2013. "Why Gender-Identity Nondiscrimination in Insurance Makes Sense." Center for American Progress. May 2, 2013. https://www.americanprogress.org/issues/lgbt/reports/2013/05/02/62214/why-gender-identity-nondiscrimination-in-insurance-makes-sense/.

Baral, Stefan D., Tonia Poteat, Susanne Strömdahl, Andrea L. Wirtz, Thomas E. Guadamuz, and Chris Beyrer. 2013. "Worldwide Burden of HIV in Transgender Women: A Systematic Review and Meta-Analysis." *Lancet: Infectious Diseases* 13 (3): 214–22. https://doi.org/10.1016/S1473-3099(12)70315-8.

Barder, Alexander D. 2013. "American Hegemony Comes Home: The Chilean Laboratory and the Neoliberalization of the United States." *Alternatives: Global, Local, Political* 38 (2): 103–21.

Barker, Joanne. 2015. "Indigenous Feminisms." In *The Oxford Handbook of Indigenous People's Politics,* edited by José Antonio Lucero, Dale Turner, and Donna Lee VanCott. Online ed. Oxford: Oxford Academic. https://doi.org/10.1093/oxfordhb/9780195386653.013.007.

Barker, K. K. 1998. "A Ship upon a Stormy Sea: The Medicalization of Pregnancy." *Social Science & Medicine* 47 (8): 1067–76. https://doi.org/10.1016/s0277-9536(98)00155-5.

Bassi, Serena, and Greta LaFleur. 2022. "Introduction: TERFs, Gender-Critical Movements, and Postfascist Feminisms." *TSQ: Transgender Studies Quarterly* 9 (3): 311–33. https://doi.org/10.1215/23289252-9836008.

Batza, Katie. 2018. *Before AIDS: Gay Health Politics in the 1970s.* Philadelphia: University of Pennsylvania Press.

Baxi, Upendra. 2006. *The Future of Human Rights.* 2nd ed. Oxford: Oxford University Press.

Beauchamp, Toby. 2019. *Going Stealth: Transgender Politics and U.S. Surveillance Practices.* Durham, N.C.: Duke University Press.

Beauchamp, Tom L., and James F. Childress. 2001. *Principles of Biomedical Ethics.* New York: Oxford University Press.

Beck, Ulrich. 1992. *Risk Society: Towards a New Modernity.* Translated by Mark Ritter. London: Sage.

Bellacasa, Maria Puig de la. 2011. "Matters of Care in Technoscience: Assembling Neglected Things." *Social Studies of Science* 41 (1): 85–106.

Ben, Pablo, and Omar Acha. 2001. "The Construction of Sex, Gender, Ethnicity, and Childhood in the Biopolitics of Archivos. Argentina, 1902–1912." *Journal of Latin American Cultural Studies* 10 (March): 83–102. https://doi.org/10.1080/13569320020030060.

Benjamin, Ruha. 2018. "Black AfterLives Matter: Cultivating Kinfulness as Reproductive Justice." In *Making Kin Not Population,* edited by Adele E. Clarke and Donna Haraway, 41–65. Chicago: Prickly Paradigm Press.

Berger, Peter L., and Thomas Luckmann. 2011. *The Social Construction of Reality: A Treatise in the Sociology of Knowledge.* New York: Open Road Media.

Berkins, Lohana. 2007a. *Cumbia, copeteo, y lágrimas: Informe nacional sobre la situación de las travestis, transexuales y transgéneros.* Buenos Aires: Asociación de Lucha por la Identidad Travesti-Transexual.

Berkins, Lohana. 2007b. "Travestis: Una identidad política." *e-misférica* 4 (2): https://hemisphericinstitute.org/es/emisferica-42/4-2-review-essays/lohana-berkins.html.

Berkins, Lohana. 2015. "El travesticidio también es femicidio." *Página 12,* June 12, 2015. https://www.pagina12.com.ar/diario/suplementos/las12/13-9791-2015-06-12.html.

Berkins, Lohana, and Josefina Fernández, eds. 2005. *La gesta del nombre propio.* Buenos Aires: Madres de Plaza de Mayo.

Berlant, Lauren. 2011. *Cruel Optimism.* Durham, N.C.: Duke University Press.

Bernal, Victoria, and Inderpal Grewal, eds. 2014. *Theorizing NGOs: States, Feminisms, and Neoliberalism.* Durham, N.C.: Duke University Press.

Berne, Patricia, Aurora Levins Morales, David Langstaff, and Sins Invalid. 2018. "Ten Principles of Disability Justice." *WSQ: Women's Studies Quarterly* 46 (1): 227–30. https://doi.org/10.1353/wsq.2018.0003.

Bernstein, Elizabeth. 2018. *Brokered Subjects: Sex, Trafficking, and the Politics of Freedom.* Chicago: University of Chicago Press.

Berwick, Donald, Thomas Nolan, and Joseph Whittington. 2008. "The Triple Aim: Care, Health, and Cost." *Health Affairs* 27 (3): 759–69.

Bhanji, Nael. 2011. "TRANS/SCRIPTIONS: Homing Desires, (Trans)Sexual Citizenship, and Racialized Bodies." In *Transgender Migrations: The Bodies, Borders, and Politics of Transition,* edited by Trystan T. Cotten, 157–75. New York: Routledge.

Bierria, Alisa. 2014. "Missing in Action: Violence, Power, and Discerning Agency." *Hypatia* 29 (1): 129–45. https://doi.org/10.1111/hypa.12074.

Blumer, Herbert. 1986. *Symbolic Interactionism: Perspective and Method.* Berkeley: University of California Press.

Bockting, Walter, Beatrice Robinson, Autumn Benner, and Karen Scheltema. 2004. "Patient Satisfaction with Transgender Health Services." *Journal of Sex & Marital Therapy* 30 (4): 277–94. https://doi.org/10.1080/00926230490422467.

Boellstorff, Tom, Mauro Cabral, Micha Cárdenas, Trystan Cotten, Eric A. Stanley, Kalaniopua Young, and Aren Z. Aizura. 2014. "Decolonizing Transgender: A Roundtable Discussion." *TSQ: Transgender Studies Quarterly* 1 (3): 419–39. https://doi.org/10.1215/23289252-2685669.

Bolsonaro, Jair. 2019. "Speech by Brazil's President Jair Bolsonaro at the Opening of the 74th United Nations General Assembly–New York, September 24, 2019." Ministério das Relações Exteriores. https://www.gov.br/mre/en/content-centers/speeches-articles-and-interviews/president-of-the-federative-republic-of-brazil/speeches/speech-by-brazil-s-president-jair-bolsonaro-at-the-opening-of-the-74th-united-nations-general-assembly-new-york-september-24-2019-photo-alan-santos-pr.

Bonita, R., R. Beaglehole, and T. Kjellström. 2006. *Basic Epidemiology.* 2nd ed. Geneva: World Health Organization.

Borgogno, Ignacio Gabriel Ulises, and REDLACTRANS. 2009. "La transfobia en el america latina y el caribe: Un estudio en el marco de REDLACTRANS." Buenos Aires: REDLACTRANS.

Bowker, Geoffrey C., and Susan Leigh Star. 1999. *Sorting Things Out: Classification and Its Consequences.* Cambridge, Mass.: MIT Press.

Branigin, Anne, and N. Kirkpatrick. 2022. "Anti-trans Laws Are on the Rise. Here's a Look at Where—and What Kind." *Washington Post*, October 14, 2022. https://www.washingtonpost.com/lifestyle/2022/10/14/anti-trans-bills/.

Breilh, Jaime. 2008. "Latin American Critical ('Social') Epidemiology: New Settings for an Old Dream." *International Journal of Epidemiology* 37 (4): 745–50. https://doi.org/10.1093/ije/dyn135.

Bridges, Khiara M. 2011. *Reproducing Race: An Ethnography of Pregnancy as a Site of Racialization.* Berkeley: University of California Press.

Briggs, Laura. 2002. *Reproducing Empire: Race, Sex, Science, and U.S. Imperialism in Puerto Rico.* Berkeley: University of California Press.

Brown, Phil. 1993. "When the Public Knows Better: Popular Epidemiology Challenges the System." *Environment: Science and Policy for Sustainable Development* 35 (8): 16–41. https://doi.org/10.1080/00139157.1993.9929114.

Bruno, Isabelle, Emmanuel Didier, and Tommaso Vitale. 2014. "Statactivism: Forms of Action between Disclosure and Affirmation." *Open Journal of Sociopolitical Studies* 7 (2): 198–220. Available at https://papers.ssrn.com/abstract=2466882.

Brysk, Alison. 1994. *The Politics of Human Rights in Argentina: Protest, Change, and Democratization.* Stanford, Calif.: Stanford University Press.

Burke, Mary. 2011. "Resisting Pathology: GID and the Contested Terrain of Diagnosis in the Transgender Health Movement." In *Sociology of Diagnosis,* edited by P. J. McGann, David J. Hutson, and Barbara Katz Rothman, 183–210. Bingley, U.K.: Emerald Group Publishing.

Cabral, Mauro. 2007. "Post Scriptum." In *Cumbia, copeteo, y lágrimas: Informe nacional sobre la situación de las travestis, transexuales y transgéneros,* edited by Lohana Berkins, 143–48. Buenos Aires: Asociación de Lucha por la Identidad Travesti-Transexual.

Cabral, Mauro. 2010. "Autodeterminación y libertad." *Página 12,* October 22, 2010. https://www.pagina12.com.ar/diario/suplementos/soy/1-1675-2010-10-22.html.

Cabral, Mauro. 2012. "Gender Identity Law in Argentina." Sexuality Policy Watch. May 7, 2012. https://sxpolitics.org/around-the-world-257/7544.

Cabral, Mauro, ed. 2009. *Interdicciones: Escrituras de la intersexualidad en castellano.* Córdoba: Anarrés Editorial.

Cabral, Mauro, and Paula Viturro. 2006. "(Trans)Sexual Citizenship in Contemporary Argentina." In *Transgender Rights,* edited by Paisley Currah, Richard M. Juang, and Shannon Minter, 262–73. Minneapolis: University of Minnesota Press.

Cabral Grinspan, Mauro. 2017. "Trans Depathologization: A Sexual Rights Issue." *Journal of Sexual Medicine* 14 (5): e267–68. https://doi.org/10.1016/j.jsxm.2017.04.304.

Callen-Lorde Community Health Center. 2000. "Protocols for the Provision of Hormone Therapy." New York: Callen-Lorde Community Health Center.

Callen-Lorde Community Health Center. 2014. "Protocols for the Provision of Hormone Therapy (Updated)." New York: Callen-Lorde Community Health Center. https://static1.squarespace.com/static/5ac6a3e825bf0250fa23d6cb/t/5beceba240ec9a141594abe7/1542253481054/Callen-Lorde-TGNC-Hormone-Therapy-Protocols-2018.pdf.

Caminos, Luciana. 2018. "#24M Santa Fe: Reparación histórica para trans perseguidas en dictadura." *Agencia Presentes,* March 24, 2018. http://agenciapresentes.org/2018/03/24/santa-fe-reparacion-historica-para-trans-perseguidas-en-dictadura/.

Campanile, Carl. 2011a. "Cuomo Chops Off Sex-Change Funds." *New York Post,* January 20, 2011. https://nypost.com/2011/10/01/cuomo-chops-off-sex-change-funds/.

Campanile, Carl. 2011b. "Let Taxpayers Foot Sex-Op Bill: Panel." *New York Post,* September 29, 2011. https://nypost.com/2011/09/29/let-taxpayers-foot-sex-op-bill-panel/.

Campos, Ricardo, and Enric Novella. 2017. "La Higiene Mental Durante El Primer Franquismo: De La Higiene Racial a La Prevención de La Enfermedad Mental (1939–1960)." *Dynamis* 37 (1). https://scielo.isciii.es/scielo.php?script=sci_arttext&pid=S0211-95362017000100004.

Capicüa. 2014. "Aportes Para Pensar La Salud de Personas Trans: Actualizando El Paradigma de Derechos Humanos En Salud." Buenos Aires: Capicüa. https://www.scribd.com/document/286831450/Capicua-Guia-Sobre-Salud-Trans.

cárdenas, micha. 2016. "Pregnancy: Reproductive Futures in Trans of Color Feminism." *TSQ: Transgender Studies Quarterly* 3 (1–2): 48–57. https://doi.org/10.1215/23289252-3334187.

Carpenter, Leonore, and R. Barrett Marshall. 2017. "Walking While Trans: Profiling of Transgender Women by Law Enforcement, and the Problem of Proof." *William & Mary Journal of Women and the Law* 24 (1): 5–38.

Cartwright, Ryan Lee. 2021. *Peculiar Places: A Queer Crip History of White Rural Nonconformity.* Chicago: University of Chicago Press.

Case, Laura K., and Vilayanur S. Ramachandran. 2012. "Alternating Gender Incongruity: A New Neuropsychiatric Syndrome Providing Insight into the Dynamic Plasticity of Brain-Sex." *Medical Hypotheses* 78 (5): 626–31. https://doi.org/10.1016/j.mehy.2012.01.041.

Castelli Rodríguez, Luisina. 2020. "Hacerse presente. Personas con discapacidad, feminismos y acción política." *RELIES: Revista del Laboratorio Iberoamericano para el Estudio Sociohistórico de las Sexualidades* 3 (May): 86–105. https://doi.org/10.46661/relies.4924.

Cavallero, Lucí, and Verónica Gago. 2021. *A Feminist Reading of Debt.* London: Pluto Press.

Cavar, Sarah, and Alexandre Baril. 2021. "Blogging to Counter Epistemic Injustice: Trans Disabled Digital Micro-resistance." *Disability Studies Quarterly* 41 (2): https://doi.org/10.18061/dsq.v41i2.7794.

CELIV (Centro de Estudios Latinoamericanos sobre Inseguridad y Violencia). 2020. "Población privada de libertad en Argentina: un análisis comparado en perspectiva temporal temporal 2013–2019." Caseros, Argentina: La Universidad de Tres de Febrero.

Centro Cultural Tierra Violeta. 2014. "Community Event Announcement for Seminario Sobre Despatologización." Buenos Aires: Centro Cultural Tierra Violeta.

Césaire, Aimé. 2000. *Discourse on Colonialism.* New York: Monthly Review Press.

Chakrabarty, Dipesh. 2001. *Provincializing Europe: Postcolonial Thought and Historical Difference.* New ed. Princeton, N.J.: Princeton University Press.

Charlton, James I. 2000. *Nothing about Us without Us: Disability Oppression and Empowerment.* Berkeley: University of California Press.

Chatterjee, Partha. 2004. *The Politics of the Governed: Reflections on Popular Politics.* New York: Columbia University Press.

Cheng, Sealing. 2010. *On the Move for Love: Migrant Entertainers and the U.S. Military in South Korea.* Philadelphia: University of Pennsylvania Press.

Chiang, Howard. 2021. *Transtopia in the Sinophone Pacific.* New York: Columbia University Press.

Clare, Eli. 1999. *Exile and Pride: Disability, Queerness, and Liberation.* Cambridge, Mass.: South End Press.

Clare, Eli. 2017. *Brilliant Imperfection: Grappling with Cure.* Durham, N.C.: Duke University Press.

Clarke, Adele E. 2005. *Situational Analysis: Grounded Theory after the Postmodern Turn.* Thousand Oaks, Calif.: SAGE.

Clarke, Adele E. 2010. "From the Rise of Medicine to Biomedicalization: U.S. Healthscapes and Iconography, Circa 1890–Present." In *Biomedicalization: Technoscience, Health, and Illness in the U.S.,* edited by Adele E. Clarke, Laura Mamo, Jennifer Ruth Fosket, Jennifer R. Fishman, and Janet K. Shim, 104–46. Durham, N.C.: Duke University Press.

Clarke, Adele E., Carrie Friese, and Rachel Washburn, eds. 2016. *Situational Analysis in Practice: Mapping Research with Grounded Theory.* New York: Routledge.

Clarke, Adele E., and Joan H. Fujimura. 1992. *The Right Tools for the Job: At Work in Twentieth-Century Life Sciences.* Princeton, N.J.: Princeton University Press.

Clarke, Adele E., Laura Mamo, Jennifer Ruth Fosket, Jennifer R. Fishman, and Janet K. Shim. 2010. *Biomedicalization: Technoscience, Health, and Illness in the U.S.* Durham, N.C.: Duke University Press.

Clarke, Adele E., and Virginia L. Olesen. 1999. *Revisioning Women, Health, and Healing: Feminist, Cultural, and Technoscience Perspectives.* New York: Routledge.

Clarke, Adele E., Janet K. Shim, Laura Mamo, Jennifer Ruth Fosket, and Jennifer R. Fishman. 2010. "Biomedicalization: Technoscientific Transformations of Health, Illness, and U.S. Biomedicine." In *Biomedicalization: Technoscience, Health, and Illness in the U.S.,* edited by Adele E. Clarke, Laura Mamo, Jennifer Ruth Fosket, Jennifer R. Fishman, and Janet K. Shim, 47–87. Durham, N.C.: Duke University Press.

Cohen, Cathy. 1997. "Punks, Bulldaggers, and Welfare Queens: The Radical Potential of Queer Politics?" *GLQ: A Journal of Lesbian and Gay Studies* 3 (4): 437–65.

Cole, Stephen R., Michael G. Hudgens, M. Alan Brookhart, and Daniel Westreich. 2015. "Risk." *American Journal of Epidemiology* 181 (4): 246–50. https://doi.org/10.1093/aje/kwv001.

Colectivo Situaciones. 2005. "Something More on Research Militancy: Footnotes on Procedures and (In)Decisions." Translated by Sebastian Touza and Nate Holdren. *Ephemera: Theory & Politics in Organization* 5 (4): 602–14.

Colen, Shellee. 1995. "'Like a Mother to Them': Stratified Reproduction and West Indian Childcare Workers and Employers in New York." In *Conceiving the New World Order: The Global Politics of Reproduction,* edited by Faye D. Ginsburg and Rayna R. Reiter, 78–102. Berkeley: University of California Press.

Conti, Diana. 2016. Víctimas de Violencia Institucional Por Motivo de Identidad de Género. Régimen Reparatorio. 2526-D-2016. https://www.hcdn.gob.ar/proyectos/textoCompleto.jsp?exp=2526-D-2016&tipo=LEY.

Cooper, Hannah L. F., and Mindy Fullilove. 2016. "Editorial: Excessive Police Violence as a Public Health Issue." *Journal of Urban Health* 93 (1): 1–7. https://doi.org/10.1007/s11524-016-0040-2.

Cooper, Melinda. 2017. *Family Values: Between Neoliberalism and the New Social Conservatism.* New York: Zone Books.

CORREPI. n.d. Coordinadora Contra la Represión Policial e Institucional. http://www.correpi.org/.

Corrigan, Oonagh. 2003. "Empty Ethics: The Problem with Informed Consent." *Sociology of Health & Illness* 25 (7): 768–92.

"The Counted: Tracking People Killed by Police in the United States." n.d. *Guardian.* https://www.theguardian.com/us-news/series/counted-us-police-killings.

Crenshaw, Kimberlé. 1989. “Demarginalizing the Intersection of Race and Sex: A Black Feminist Critique of Antidiscrimination Doctrine, Feminist Theory, and Antiracist Politics.” *University of Chicago Legal Forum* 140, 139–67.

Creswell, John W. 2006. *Qualitative Inquiry and Research Design: Choosing among Five Approaches.* 2nd ed. Thousand Oaks, Calif.: Sage Publications.

Critical Resistance. n.d. “What Is the PIC? What Is Abolition?” *Critical Resistance* (blog). Accessed September 1, 2022. https://criticalresistance.org/mission-vision/not-so-common-language/.

Critical Resistance and Incite! 2003. “Critical Resistance-Incite! Statement on Gender Violence and the Prison-Industrial Complex.” *Social Justice* 30, no. 3 (93): 141–50.

Cruz, Taylor M. 2020. “Perils of Data-Driven Equity: Safety-Net Care and Big Data’s Elusive Grasp on Health Inequality.” *Big Data & Society* 7 (1): https://doi.org/10.1177/2053951720928097.

Cruz, Taylor M., and Emily Allen Paine. 2021. “Capturing Patients, Missing Inequities: Data Standardization on Sexual Orientation and Gender Identity across Unequal Clinical Contexts.” *Social Science & Medicine* 285 (September): https://doi.org/10.1016/j.socscimed.2021.114295.

Currah, Paisley. 2020. “Can We Stop Talking about Transphobia Already?” Presented at the QPW#10, virtual, August 27, 2020. YouTube video, Queer Politics, “QPW#10 Paisley Currah,” 58:28. https://www.youtube.com/watch?v=LrWs8r_1WtA.

Currah, Paisley. 2022. *Sex Is as Sex Does: Governing Transgender Identity.* New York: NYU Press.

Currah, Paisley, and Lisa Jean Moore. 2009. “‘We Won’t Know Who You Are’: Contesting Sex Designations in New York City Birth Certificates.” *Hypatia* 24 (3): 113–35.

Currah, Paisley, and Susan Stryker. 2015. Introduction to *TSQ: Transgender Studies Quarterly* 2 (1): 1–12. https://doi.org/10.1215/23289252-2848859.

Currie, Morgan, Britt S. Paris, Irene Pasquetto, and Jennifer Pierre. 2016. “The Conundrum of Police Officer-Involved Homicides: Counter-Data in Los Angeles County.” *Big Data & Society* 3 (2): https://doi.org/10.1177/2053951716663566.

Cutuli, María Soledad. 2011. “El Escándalo. Modos de Estar, Negociar, Resistir y Demandar. El Caso de Las Travestis y Transexuales Del Área Metropolitana de Buenos Aires.” In *Etnografía de Tramas Políticas Colectivas: Estudios En Argentina y Brasil,* edited by M. Grimberg, M. Macedo Ernandez, and V. Manzano. Buenos Aires: Antropofagia/FFyL-UBA.

Cutuli, María Soledad. 2012. "Resisting, Demanding, Negotiating, and Being: The Role of Scandals in the Everyday Lives of Argentinean Travestis." *Jindal Global Law Review* 4 (1): 71–88.

Cutuli, María Soledad. 2013. "'Maricas' and 'Travestis': Rethinking Shared Experiences." *Sociedad y Economía* 24 (June): 183–204.

Cutuli, María Soledad. 2015. "Travesti Associations, State Policies, and NGOs: Resistance and Collective Action in Buenos Aires, Argentina." *Sexualities* 18 (3): 297–309.

Cutuli, María Soledad. 2017. "La Travesti Permitida y La Narcotravesti: Imágenes Morales En Tensión." *Cadernos Pagu* 50: https://doi.org/10.1590/18094449201700500003.

D'Avella, Nicholas. 2019. *Concrete Dreams: Practice, Value, and Built Environments in Post-Crisis Buenos Aires.* Illustrated edition. Durham, N.C.: Duke University Press.

Davis, Angela Y. 2003. *Are Prisons Obsolete?* New York: Seven Stories Press.

Davy, Zowie, Anniken Sørlie, and Amets Suess Schwend. 2018. "Democratising Diagnoses? The Role of the Depathologisation Perspective in Constructing Corporeal Trans Citizenship." *Critical Social Policy* 38 (1): 13–34. https://doi.org/10.1177/0261018317731716.

Dean, Mitchell. 1998. "Risk, Calculable and Incalculable." *Soziale Welt* 49 (1): 25–42.

Degener, Theresia. 2017. "A New Human Rights Model of Disability." In *The United Nations Convention on the Rights of Persons with Disabilities: A Commentary,* edited by Valentina Della Fina, Rachele Cera, and Giuseppe Palmisano, 41–59. Cham, Switzerland: Springer International Publishing.

Delgado, Richard, and Jean Stefancic. 2001. *Critical Race Theory: An Introduction.* New York: NYU Press.

De Mauro Rucovsky, Martín. 2019. "The *Travesti* Critique of the Gender Identity Law in Argentina." Translated by Ian Russell. *TSQ: Transgender Studies Quarterly* 6 (2): 223–38. https://doi.org/10.1215/23289252-7348510.

Department of Health, New York State. 2013. "New York State Prevention Agenda 2013–2018: Priorities, Focus Areas, Goals, and Objectives, 1/25/2013." New York State Department of Public Health. January 25, 2013. https://www.health.ny.gov/prevention/prevention_agenda/2013-2017/tracking_indicators.htm.

Department of Health, New York State. 2015. "New York State Medicaid Updates Regulations." *New York State Medicaid Update* 31 (3), March 2015. http://www.health.ny.gov/health_care/medicaid/program/update/2015/2015-03.htm.

Derrida, Jacques. 1978. *Writing and Difference.* Translated by Alan Bass. Chicago: University of Chicago Press.

DHHS (Department of Health and Human Services). 1981. "Health Technology Assessment Reports." DHHS Publication No. (PHS) 84–3370. Rockville, Md.: U.S. Dept. of Health and Human Services, Public Health Service, Office of the Assistant Secretary for Health.

Dilts, Andrew. 2012. "Incurable Blackness: Criminal Disenfranchisement, Mental Disability, and the White Citizen." *Disability Studies Quarterly* 32 (3): https://doi.org/10.18061/dsq.v32i3.3268.

DiPietro, PJ. 2016. "Decolonizing Travesti Space in Buenos Aires: Race, Sexuality, and Sideways Relationality." *Gender, Place & Culture* 23 (5): 677–93. https://doi.org/10.1080/0966369X.2015.1058756.

Domínguez Ruvalcaba, Héctor. 2016. *Translating the Queer: Body Politics and Transnational Conversations.* London: Zed Books.

Drescher, Jack. 2010. "Queer Diagnoses: Parallels and Contrasts in the History of Homosexuality, Gender Variance, and the Diagnostic and Statistical Manual." *Archives of Sexual Behavior* 39 (2): 427–60. https://doi.org/10.1007/s10508-009-9531-5.

Drescher, Jack. 2013. "Gender Identity Diagnoses: History and Controversies." In *Gender Dysphoria and Disorders of Sex Development: Progress in Care and Knowledge,* edited by Baudewijntje P. C. Kreukels, Thomas D. Steensma, and Annelou L. C. de Vries, 137–50. New York: Springer. https://doi.org/10.1007/978-1-4614-7441-8_7.

Drescher, Jack. 2020. "Queer Diagnoses Parallels and Contrasts in the History of Homosexuality, Gender Variance, and the Diagnostic and Statistical Manual (DSM) Review and Recommendations Prepared for the DSM-V Sexual and Gender Identity Disorders Work Group." *FOCUS* 18 (3): 308–35. https://doi.org/10.1176/appi.focus.18302.

Drescher, Jack, Peggy Cohen-Kettenis, and Sam Winter. 2012. "Minding the Body: Situating Gender Identity Diagnoses in the ICD-11." *International Review of Psychiatry* 24 (6): 568–77. https://doi.org/10.3109/09540261.2012.741575.

Du Bois, W. E. B. 1903. *The Souls of Black Folk.* Cambridge: Cambridge University Press.

Duggan, Lisa. 2003. *The Twilight of Equality? Neoliberalism, Cultural Politics, and the Attack on Democracy.* Boston: Beacon Press.

Dutta, Aniruddha. 2012. "An Epistemology of Collusion: Hijras, Kothis, and the Historical (Dis)Continuity of Gender/Sexual Identities in Eastern India." *Gender & History* 24 (3): 825–49. https://doi.org/10.1111/j.1468-0424.2012.01712.x.

Dutta, Aniruddha. 2013. "Legible Identities and Legitimate Citizens: The Globalization of Transgender and Subjects of HIV-AIDS Prevention in Eastern India." *International Feminist Journal of Politics* 15 (4): 494–514. https://doi.org/10.1080/14616742.2013.818279.

Dutta, Aniruddha, and Raina Roy. 2014. "Decolonizing Transgender in

India: Some Reflections." *TSQ: Transgender Studies Quarterly* 1 (3): 320–37. https://doi.org/10.1215/23289252-2685615.

Edelman, Elijah Adiv. 2011. "'This Area Has Been Declared a Prostitution Free Zone': Discursive Formations of Space, the State, and Trans 'Sex Worker' Bodies." *Journal of Homosexuality* 58 (6–7): 848–64. https://doi.org/10.1080/00918369.2011.581928.

Edwards, Erika Denise. 2020. *Hiding in Plain Sight: Black Women, the Law, and the Making of a White Argentine Republic.* Tuscaloosa: University of Alabama Press.

Edwards, Nadine. 2005. *Birthing Autonomy: Women's Experiences of Planning Home Births.* New York: Routledge.

Ehrenreich, Barbara, and Deirdre English. 1973. *Complaints and Disorders: The Sexual Politics of Sickness.* New York: Feminist Press at CUNY.

Eisfeld, Justus. 2014. "International Statistical Classification of Diseases and Related Health Problems." *TSQ: Transgender Studies Quarterly* 1 (1–2): 107–10. https://doi.org/10.1215/23289252-2399740.

Elena, Eduardo. 2011. *Dignifying Argentina: Peronism, Citizenship, and Mass Consumption.* Pittsburgh: University of Pittsburgh Press.

Elifson, K. W., J. Boles, E. Posey, M. Sweat, W. Darrow, and W. Elsea. 1993. "Male Transvestite Prostitutes and HIV Risk." *American Journal of Public Health* 83 (2): 260–62. https://doi.org/10.2105/AJPH.83.2.260.

Enke, Finn. 2012. "The Education of Little Cis: Cisgender and the Discipline of Opposing Bodies." In *Transfeminist Perspectives in and beyond Transgender and Gender Studies,* edited by Finn Enke, 60–78. Philadelphia: Temple University Press.

Epstein, Steven. 1996. *Impure Science: AIDS, Activism, and the Politics of Knowledge.* Berkeley: University of California Press.

Epstein, Steven. 2021. "Cultivated Co-production: Sexual Health, Human Rights, and the Revision of the ICD." *Social Studies of Science* 51 (5): 657–82. https://doi.org/10.1177/03063127211014283.

Epstein, Steven, and Stefan Timmermans. 2021. "From Medicine to Health: The Proliferation and Diversification of Cultural Authority." *Journal of Health and Social Behavior* 62 (3): 240–54. https://doi.org/10.1177/00221465211010468.

Erevelles, Nirmala. 1996. "Disability and the Dialectics of Difference." *Disability & Society* 11 (4): 519–38. https://doi.org/10.1080/09687599627570.

Erevelles, Nirmala. 2011. *Disability and Difference in Global Contexts: Enabling a Transformative Body Politic.* New York: Palgrave Macmillan.

Erevelles, Nirmala. 2015. "Race." In *Keywords for Disability Studies,* edited by Rachel Adams, Benjamin Reiss, and David Serlin, 145–47. New York: New York University Press.

Espineira, Karine, and Sam Bourcier. 2016. "Transfeminism: Something

Else, Somewhere Else." *TSQ: Transgender Studies Quarterly* 3 (May): 84–94. https://doi.org/10.1215/23289252-3334247.

Ewald, François. 1991. "Insurance Risk." In *The Foucault Effect: Studies in Governmentality,* edited by Graham Burchell, Colin Gordon, and Peter Miller, 197–210. London: University of Chicago Press.

Ewald, François. 2020. *The Birth of Solidarity: The History of the French Welfare State.* Edited by Melinda Cooper. Translated by Timothy Scott Johnson. Durham, N.C.: Duke University Press.

Fanon, Frantz. 1965. *A Dying Colonialism.* New York: Grove Press.

Farji Neer, Anahí. 2012. "Producción Generizada de Los Cuerpos En El Discurso Jurídico Argentino. Análisis de Tres Fallos Correspondientes al Período 1970–2010." *Revista Sociedad y Equidad* no. 3: 1–22.

Farji Neer, Anahí. 2017. *Travestismo, transexualidad y transgeneridad en los discursos del estado Argentino: Desde los edictos policiales hasta la Ley de Identidad de Género.* Buenos Aires: Teseo y Universidad de Buenos Aires Sociales.

Farji Neer, Anahí. 2018. "Los/as profesionales de la salud frente a la Ley de Identidad de Género argentina. Tensiones entre el saber experto y el cuidado integral." *Physis: Revista de Saúde Coletiva* 28 (3). https://www.redalyc.org/journal/4008/400858445018/html/.

Farmer, Paul, Arthur Kleinman, Jim Kim, and Matthew Basilico, eds. 2013. *Reimagining Global Health: An Introduction.* Berkeley: University of California Press.

Ferguson, Roderick A. 2004. *Aberrations in Black: Toward a Queer of Color Critique.* Minneapolis: University of Minnesota Press.

Fernandes-Taylor, Sara, and Joan R. Bloom. 2011. "Post-Treatment Regret among Young Breast Cancer Survivors." *Psycho-Oncology* 20 (5): 506–16. https://doi.org/10.1002/pon.1749.

Fernández, Josefina. 2004. *Cuerpos Desobedientes: Travestismo E Identidad de Genero.* Buenos Aires: Edhasa.

Fernández, Josefina. 2005. "Travestismo y violencia policial." In *La gesta del nombre propio,* edited by Lohana Berkins and Josefina Fernández, 39–65. Buenos Aires: Madres de Plaza de Mayo.

Fernández, Josefina. 2020. *La Berkins: Una combatiente de frontera.* Buenos Aires: Penguin Random House/Grupo Editorial Argentina.

Fernández Romero, Francisco. 2020. "Walking While Travesti: Direct and Indirect Criminalization in Public Space." Thinking Trans // Trans Thinking Conference, Austin, Texas.

Fernández Romero, Francisco. 2021. "'We Can Conceive Another History': Trans Activism around Abortion Rights in Argentina." *International Journal of Transgender Health* 22 (1–2): 126–40. https://doi.org/10.1080/26895269.2020.1838391.

Finchelstein, Federico. 2014. *The Ideological Origins of the Dirty War:*

Fascism, Populism, and Dictatorship in Twentieth Century Argentina. New York: Oxford University Press.

Fisch, Jörg. 2015. *The Right of Self-Determination of Peoples: The Domestication of an Illusion.* New York: Cambridge University Press.

Fisk, Norman M. 1974. "Editorial: Gender Dysphoria Syndrome—The Conceptualization That Liberalizes Indications for Total Gender Reorientation and Implies a Broadly Based Multi-dimensional Rehabilitative Regimen." *Western Journal of Medicine* 120 (5): 386–91.

Fitzsimmons, Tim. 2018. "'Transsexualism' Removed from World Health Organization's Disease Manual." *NBC News,* June 20, 2018, sec. Out Health and Wellness. https://www.nbcnews.com/feature/nbc-out/transsexualism-removed-world-health-organization-s-disease-manual-n885141.

Fleming, Mark, Janet Shim, Irene Yen, Meredith Van Natta, Christoph Hanssmann, and Nancy Burke. 2019. "Caring for 'Super-Utilizers': Neoliberal Social Assistance in the Safety-Net." *Medical Anthropology Quarterly* 33 (2): 173–90. https://doi.org/10.1111/maq.12481.

FM En Tránsito. 2016. "Denuncian el vaciamiento del consultorio inclusivo LGBT de Morón." *Cooperativa de Trabajo para la Comunicación Social,* October 4, 2016. https://comunicacionsocial.org.ar/denuncian-el-vaciamiento-del-consultorio-inclusivo-lgbt-de-moron/.

Foucault, Michel. 1990. *The History of Sexuality: An Introduction.* New York: Vintage Books.

Foucault, Michel. 2003. *"Society Must Be Defended": Lectures at the Collège de France, 1975–1976.* Translated by David Macey. New York: Picador.

Freeman, Mark, and Nathaniel Walters-Koh, dir. 2012. *Transgender Tuesdays: A Clinic in the Tenderloin.* San Francisco: Little Red Dots. DVD.

Frickel, Scott, Sahra Gibbon, Jeff Howard, Joanna Kempner, Gwen Ottinger, and David J. Hess. 2010. "Undone Science: Charting Social Movement and Civil Society Challenges to Research Agenda Setting." *Science, Technology, & Human Values* 35 (4): 444–73. https://doi.org/10.1177/0162243909345836.

Frieder, K., and M. Romero. 2014. "Ley de Identidad de Género y Acceso al Cuidado de La Salud de Las Personas Trans En Argentina." Buenos Aires: Fundación Huésped and Asociación de Travestis, Transexuales y Transgéneros de Argentina (ATTTA). https://www.huesped.org.ar/wp-content/uploads/2018/03/Aristegui-Zalazar_2014_Ley-de-Identidad-de-Genero-y-acceso-a-la-salud-en-poblacion-trans.pdf.

Friedman, Elisabeth Jay, and Constanza Tabbush. 2016. "#NiUnaMenos: Not One Woman Less, Not One More Death!" *NACLA,* November 1, 2016. https://nacla.org/news/2016/11/01/niunamenos-not-one-woman-less-not-one-more-death.

Fukui, Elliott, and Christoph Hanssmann. 2022. "Aftercare & Catharsis: Cultivating the Trans Arts of Living." *Feminist Formations* 34 (3): 200–212.

Fundación Huésped. 2014. "Campaña 'Expectativas.'" Fundación Huésped. May 16, 2014. https://www.huesped.org.ar/noticias/campana-expectativas/.

Gago, Verónica. 2017. *Neoliberalism from Below: Popular Pragmatics and Baroque Economies.* Translated by Liz Mason-Deese. Durham, N.C.: Duke University Press.

Gago, Verónica, Ni Una Menos, Ramsey McGlazer, Verónica Carchedi, and Liz Mason-Deese. 2018. "Critical Times/The Earth Trembles." *Critical Times* 1 (1): 158–77. https://doi.org/10.1215/26410478-1.1.158.

Galtung, Johan. 1969. "Violence, Peace, and Peace Research." *Journal of Peace Research* 6 (3): 167–91.

Garcia, Angela. 2010. *The Pastoral Clinic: Addiction and Dispossession along the Rio Grande.* Berkeley: University of California Press.

Garretón, Manuel Antonio. 2002. "La transformación de la acción colectiva en América Latina." *Revista de la CEPAL* 2002 (76): 7–24. https://doi.org/10.18356/92d9a65f-es.

GATE (Global Action for Trans Equality). 2011. *It's Time for Reform: A Report on the GATE Experts Meeting.* The Hague, Netherlands, November 16–18, 2011. Archived at https://globaltransaction.files.wordpress.com/2012/05/its-time-for-reform.pdf.

Gehi, Pooja S., and Gabriel Arkles. 2007. "Unraveling Injustice: Race and Class Impact of Medicaid Exclusions of Transition-Related Health Care for Transgender People." *Sexuality Research & Social Policy* 4 (4): 7–35. https://doi.org/10.1525/srsp.2007.4.4.7.

Giddens, Anthony. 1990. *The Consequences of Modernity.* Stanford, Calif.: Stanford University Press.

Gill-Peterson, Jules. 2018. *Histories of the Transgender Child.* Minneapolis: University of Minnesota Press.

Gill-Peterson, Jules. 2021. "When Did We Become Cis?" *Sad Brown Girl* (blog). July 4, 2021. https://sadbrowngirl.substack.com/p/when-did-we-become-cis.

Gilman, Sander L. 1985. *Difference and Pathology: Stereotypes of Sexuality, Race, and Madness.* Ithaca, N.Y.: Cornell University Press.

Gilmore, Ruth Wilson. 2007. *Golden Gulag: Prisons, Surplus, Crisis, and Opposition in Globalizing California.* Berkeley: University of California Press.

GLAAD and Sylvia Rivera Law Project. 2013a. "Healthcare for All: Give Trans People Access to the Care They Need." November 15, 2013. YouTube video, 2:07. https://www.youtube.com/watch?v=kfzfUzU_574&list=PLoihXOaL4AoU_sTH9eF37SEpygDD2n1xK&index=2.

GLAAD and Sylvia Rivera Law Project. 2013b. "Healthcare Professional

Calls for Care for All." November 15, 2013. YouTube video, 2:41. https://www.youtube.com/watch?v=hHTD-JfLeHo&list=PLoihXOaL4AoU_sTH9eF37SEpygDD2n1xK&index=3.

GLAAD and Sylvia Rivera Law Project. 2013c. "A Parent Calls for Healthcare for All." November 15, 2013. YouTube video, 2:23. https://www.youtube.com/watch?v=gXtohkK1vQk&list=PLoihXOaL4AoU_sTH9eF37SEpygDD2n1xK&index=2.

Glaser, Barney G., and Anselm L. Strauss. 1967. *The Discovery of Grounded Theory: Strategies for Qualitative Research.* New Brunswick, N.J.: Aldine Transaction.

Goffman, Erving. 1986. *Stigma: Notes on the Management of Spoiled Identity.* New York: Touchstone.

Goldberg, David Theo. 2009. *The Threat of Race: Reflections on Racial Neoliberalism.* Malden, Mass.: Wiley-Blackwell.

Gollan, Daniel. 2016. "Cobertura Universal Con Menos Acceso." *Página 12,* August 5, 2016, sec. Opinion. https://www.pagina12.com.ar/diario/sociedad/3-306060-2016-08-05.html.

Gonsalves, Tara. 2020. "Gender Identity, the Sexed Body, and the Medical Making of Transgender." *Gender & Society* 34 (6): 1005–33. https://doi.org/10.1177/0891243220965913.

Gorton, R. Nick. 2013. "Transgender as Mental Illness: Nosology, Social Justice, and the Tarnished Golden Mean." In *The Transgender Studies Reader 2,* edited by Susan Stryker and Aren Aizura, 644–52. New York: Routledge.

Gorz, André. 1967. *Strategy for Labor: A Radical Proposal.* Boston: Beacon Press.

Gould, Deborah B. 2009. *Moving Politics: Emotion and ACT UP's Fight against AIDS.* Chicago: University of Chicago Press.

Gourevitch, Marc N., Lesley H. Curtis, Maureen S. Durkin, Angela Fagerlin, Annetine C. Gelijns, Richard Platt, Belinda M. Reininger, Judith Wylie-Rosett, Katherine Jones, and William M. Tierney. 2019. "The Emergence of Population Health in US Academic Medicine: A Qualitative Assessment." *JAMA Network Open* 2 (4): https://doi.org/10.1001/jamanetworkopen.2019.2200.

Grant, Jaime M., Lisa A. Mottet, Justin Tanis, Jack Harrison, Jody L. Herman, and Mara Keisling. 2011. "Injustice at Every Turn: A Report of the National Transgender Discrimination Survey." Washington, DC: National Center for Transgender Equality and National Gay and Lesbian Task Force. https://transequality.org/sites/default/files/docs/resources/NTDS_Report.pdf.

Gray, Mary L. 2009. *Out in the Country: Youth, Media, and Queer Visibility in Rural America.* New York: NYU Press.

Green, Erica, Katie Benner, and Robert Pear. 2018. "'Transgender' Could

Be Defined Out of Existence under Trump Administration." *New York Times,* October 21, 2018, sec. Politics. https://www.nytimes.com/2018/10/21/us/politics/transgender-trump-administration-sex-definition.html.

Green, Kai M., and Treva Ellison. 2014. "Tranifest." *TSQ: Transgender Studies Quarterly* 1 (1–2): 222–25. http://doi.org/10.1215/23289252-2400082.

Grewal, Inderpal, and Caren Kaplan, eds. 1994. *Scattered Hegemonies: Postmodernity and Transnational Feminist Practices.* Minneapolis: University of Minnesota Press.

Grubbs, Vanessa. 2017. *Hundreds of Interlaced Fingers: A Kidney Doctor's Search for the Perfect Match.* New York: Amistad.

Gupta, Kristina. 2019. *Medical Entanglements: Rethinking Feminist Debates about Healthcare.* New Brunswick, N.J.: Rutgers University Press.

Gutiérrez, María Alicia. 2005. "La imagen del cuerpo." In *La gesta del nombre propio,* edited by Lohana Berkins and Josefina Fernández, 71–91. Buenos Aires: Madres de Plaza de Mayo.

Haas, Jennifer S., Kathryn A. Phillips, Laurence C. Baker, Dean Sonneborn, and Charles E. McCulloch. 2003. "Is the Prevalence of Gatekeeping in a Community Associated with Individual Trust in Medical Care?" *Medical Care* 41 (5): 660–68.

Hall, Stuart. 1997. "Subjects in History: Making Diasporic Identities." In *The House That Race Built: Original Essays by Toni Morrison, Angela Y. Davis, Cornel West, and Others on Black Americans and Politics in America Today,* edited by Wahneema Lubiano, 289–300. New York: Random House.

Hanssmann, Christoph. 2016. "Passing Torches?: Feminist Inquiries and Trans-Health Politics and Practices." *TSQ: Transgender Studies Quarterly* 3 (1–2): 120–36.

Haraway, Donna J. 1990. "Situated Knowledges: The Science Question in Feminism and the Privilege of Partial Perspective." In *Simians, Cyborgs, and Women: The Reinvention of Nature,* 183–201. New York: Routledge.

Hare, Lauren, Pascal Bernard, Francisco J. Sánchez, Paul N. Baird, Eric Vilain, Trudy Kennedy, and Vincent R. Harley. 2009. "Androgen Receptor Repeat Length Polymorphism Associated with Male-to-Female Transsexualism." *Biological Psychiatry* 65 (1): 93–96. https://doi.org/10.1016/j.biopsych.2008.08.033.

Haritaworn, Jin. 2015. *Queer Lovers and Hateful Others: Regenerating Violent Times and Places.* London: Pluto Press.

Haritaworn, Jin, Adi Kuntsman, and Silvia Posocco. 2013. "Introduction: Murderous Inclusions." *International Feminist Journal of Politics* 15 (4): 445–52.

Harris, Cheryl I. 1993. "Whiteness as Property." *Harvard Law Review* 106 (8): 1707–91.

Hartmann, Christopher. 2016. "Postneoliberal Public Health Care Reforms: Neoliberalism, Social Medicine, and Persistent Health Inequalities in Latin America." *American Journal of Public Health* 106 (12): 2145–51. https://doi.org/10.2105/AJPH.2016.303470.

Health Care for the Homeless Clinicians' Network. 2002. "The Rationale for Hormone Therapy in Primary Care." *Healing Hands: Health Care for the Homeless Clinicians' Network Newsletter,* June 2022.

Health Liberation Now! n.d. "Welcome to Health Liberation Now!" Accessed September 1, 2022. https://healthliberationnow.com/.

Hein, Jan. 2020. "Europeanized Places, Europeanized People: The Discursive Construction of Argentina." *Journal of Postcolonial Linguistics* 2: 28–45.

Hernandez, Antonia. 1976. "Chicanas and the Issue of Involuntary Sterilization: Reforms Needed to Protect Informed Consent." *Chicano Law Review* 3 (3): 3–37.

Herring, Scott. 2010. *Another Country: Queer Anti-Urbanism.* New York: NYU Press.

Hess, David J. 2016. *Undone Science: Social Movements, Mobilized Publics, and Industrial Transitions.* Cambridge, Mass.: MIT Press.

Hevia, Martín, and Daniela Schnidrig. 2014. "Autonomy, Consent and Medical Confidentiality: Patients' Rights in Argentina." *Law and Business Review of the Americas* 20 (4): 515–36.

Heyes, Cressida, and J. R. Latham. 2018. "Trans Surgeries and Cosmetic Surgeries: The Politics of Analogy." *TSQ: Transgender Studies Quarterly* 5 (2): 174–89. https://doi.org/10.1215/23289252-4348617.

Hogle, Linda F. 2019. "Accounting for Accountable Care: Value-Based Population Health Management." *Social Studies of Science* 49 (4): 556–82. https://doi.org/10.1177/0306312719840429.

Hollar, Julie. 2018. "The Political Mediation of Argentina's Gender Identity Law: LGBT Activism and Rights Innovation." *Journal of Human Rights* 17 (4): 453–69. https://doi.org/10.1080/14754835.2018.1450739.

Holloway, Karla F. C. 2011. *Private Bodies, Public Texts: Race, Gender, and a Cultural Bioethics.* Durham, N.C.: Duke University Press.

Hooker, Juliet. 2017. *Theorizing Race in the Americas: Douglass, Sarmiento, Du Bois, and Vasconcelos.* New York: Oxford University Press.

HoSang, Daniel Martinez, Oneka LaBennett, and Laura Pulido, eds. 2012. *Racial Formation in the Twenty-First Century.* Berkeley: University of California Press.

Hua, Julietta. 2011. *Trafficking Women's Human Rights.* Minneapolis: University of Minnesota Press.

Human Rights Campaign. 2006. *Corporate Equality Index 2006: A Report*

Card on Gay, Lesbian, Bisexual and Transgender Equality in Corporate America.* https://assets2.hrc.org/files/assets/resources/CorporateEqualityIndex_2006.pdf?_ga=2.6383030.508139212.1681225680-564636146.1681225680.

ICATH (Informed Consent for Access to Trans Health). n.d. "Informed Consent for Access to Trans Health (ICATH)." Accessed July 3, 2016. http://www.icath.org/.

Institute of Medicine. 2011. *The Health of Lesbian, Gay, Bisexual, and Transgender People: Building a Foundation for Better Understanding.* Washington, D.C.: National Academies Press. http://www.ncbi.nlm.nih.gov/pubmed/22013611.

International Gay and Lesbian Human Rights Commission. 2005. "Institutional Memoir of the 2005 Institute for Trans and Intersex Activist Training." Accessed April 20, 2023. https://iglhrc.org/sites/default/files/367-1.pdf.

Irving, Dan. 2008. "Normalized Transgressions: Legitimizing the Transsexual Body as Productive." *Radical History Review* 100: 38.

Irving, Dan. 2009. "The Self Made Man as Risky Business: A Critical Examination of Gaining Recognition for Trans Rights through Economic Discourse." *Temple Political and Civil Rights Law Review* 18 (2): 375–95.

Jackson, Zakiyyah Iman. 2020. *Becoming Human: Meaning and Matter in an Antiblack World.* New York: NYU Press.

Jain, S. Lochlann. 2013. *Malignant: How Cancer Becomes Us.* Berkeley: University of California Press.

Jarrín, Carmen Alvaro. 2016. "Untranslatable Subjects: Travesti Access to Public Health Care in Brazil." *TSQ: Transgender Studies Quarterly* 3 (3–4): 357–75. https://doi.org/10.1215/23289252-3545095.

Johnson, Austin. 2018. "Rejecting, Reframing, and Reintroducing: Trans People's Strategic Engagement with the Medicalisation of Gender Dysphoria." *Sociology of Health & Illness* 41 (November). https://doi.org/10.1111/1467-9566.12829.

Joly, Eduardo. 2010. "Salud Integral de Las Personas Con Discapacidad." Presentation delivered at the Congress de países del Mercosur (Southern Common Market) on Bioethics and Human Rights. Department of Medicine, University of Buenos Aires. December 3, 2010. https://www.rumbos.org.ar/_files/ugd/7d0edb_5af1131465264e1288be3817093f1e34.pdf.

Jordan-Young, Rebecca M. 2010. *Brain Storm: The Flaws in the Science of Sex Differences.* Cambridge, Mass.: Harvard University Press.

Jost-Creegan, Kelsey M. 2017. "Debts of Democracy: Framing Issues and Reimagining Democracy in Twenty-First Century Argentine Social Movements." *Harvard Human Rights Journal* 30. https://harvardhrj

.com/wp-content/uploads/sites/14/2020/06/30_Jost-Creegan_Debts-of-Democracy.pdf.

Kaba, Mariame. 2021. *We Do This 'Til We Free Us: Abolitionist Organizing and Transforming Justice.* Chicago: Haymarket Books.

Kafer, Alison. 2013. *Feminist, Queer, Crip.* Bloomington: Indiana University Press.

Kamens, Sarah R. 2011. "On the Proposed Sexual and Gender Identity Diagnoses for DSM-5: History and Controversies." *Humanistic Psychologist* 39 (1): 37–59. https://doi.org/10.1080/08873267.2011.539935.

Kara, Sheherezade. 2017. "Gender Is Not an Illness: How Pathologizing Trans People Violates International Human Rights Law." Global Action for Trans Equality (GATE). https://otdchile.org/wp-content/uploads/2017/12/Gender-is-not-an-illness-GATE-.pdf.

Kawachi, I., S. V. Subramanian, and N. Almeida-Filho. 2002. "A Glossary for Health Inequalities." *Journal of Epidemiology and Community Health* 56 (9): 647–52. https://doi.org/10.1136/jech.56.9.647.

Kelley, Robin D. G. 2008. *Yo' Mama's Disfunktional! Fighting the Culture Wars in Urban America.* Boston: Beacon Press.

Kelly, Mary Louise. 2021. "Cecilia Gentili on the Repeal of N.Y.'s 'Walking While Trans' Anti-loitering Law." *NPR,* February 4, 2021, sec. Law. https://www.npr.org/2021/02/04/964172284/cecilia-gentili-on-the-repeal-of-n-y-s-walking-while-trans-anti-loitering-law.

Kennedy, Edward M. 2007. "Public Health: An Essential Commitment to the Nation." *Journal of Public Health Management and Practice* 13 (2): 93–94. https://doi.org/10.1097/00124784-200703000-00002.

Khanna, Akshay, Priyashri Mani, Zachary Patterson, Maro Pantazidou, and Maysa Shqerat. 2013. "The Changing Faces of Citizen Action: A Mapping Study through an 'Unruly' Lens." *IDS Working Papers* 2013 (423): 1–70. https://doi.org/10.1111/j.2040-0209.2013.00423.x.

Kindig, David, and Greg Stoddart. 2003. "What Is Population Health?" *American Journal of Public Health* 93 (3): 380–83.

Kirk, Stuart A., and Herb Kutchins. 1992. *The Selling of DSM: The Rhetoric of Science in Psychiatry.* New York: Transaction Publishers.

Kismödi, Eszter, Mauro Cabral, and Jack Byrne. 2016. "Transgender Health Care and Human Rights." In *Principles of Transgender Medicine and Surgery,* edited by Randi Ettner, Stan Monstrey, and Eli Coleman, 379–401. New York: Routledge.

Knorr Cetina, Karin. 1999. *Epistemic Cultures: How the Sciences Make Knowledge.* Cambridge, Mass.: Harvard University Press.

Koyama, Emi. 2003. "The Transfeminist Manifesto." In *Catching a Wave: Reclaiming Feminism for the 21st Century,* 244–59. Boston: Northeastern University Press.

Krueger, Richard B., Geoffrey M. Reed, Michael B. First, Adele Marais,

Eszter Kismödi, and Peer Briken. 2017. "Proposals for Paraphilic Disorders in the International Classification of Diseases and Related Health Problems, Eleventh Revision (ICD-11)." *Archives of Sexual Behavior* 46 (5): 1529–45. https://doi.org/10.1007/s10508-017-0944-2.

Kuhn, Roger. 2021. "Two-Spirit Love: Toward an Inclusion of Sexual Sovereignty and Erotic Survivance." PhD diss., California Institute of Integral Studies. https://www.proquest.com/openview/01c9fc4929f0d4a3c5c1b61b15ea2924/1?pq-origsite=gscholar&cbl=18750&diss=y.

Kukla, Rebecca, Miriam Kuppermann, Margaret Little, Anne Drapkin Lyerly, Lisa M Mitchell, Elizabeth M. Armstrong, and Lisa Harris. 2009. "Finding Autonomy in Birth." *Bioethics* 23 (1): 1–8. https://doi.org/10.1111/j.1467-8519.2008.00677.x.

Kulick, Don. 1998. *Travesti: Sex, Gender, and Culture among Brazilian Transgendered Prostitutes.* Chicago: University of Chicago Press.

La Información. 2016. "El 80% de las transexuales de América Latina mueren antes de los 35 años." *La Información,* February 25, 2016, sec. Sociedad. https://www.lainformacion.com/asuntos-sociales/fallecimiento-y-muerte/el-80-de-las-transexuales-de-america-latina-mueren-antes-de-los-35-anos_js6B8Atjsg2OXOQcnQxvu2/.

Lakoff, Andrew. 2006. *Pharmaceutical Reason: Knowledge and Value in Global Psychiatry.* Cambridge: Cambridge University Press.

Lamble, Sarah. 2008. "Retelling Racialized Violence, Remaking White Innocence: The Politics of Interlocking Oppressions in Transgender Day of Remembrance." *Sexuality Research & Social Policy* 5 (1): 24–42.

Laraña, Enrique, Hank Johnston, and Joseph R. Gusfield, eds. 1994. *New Social Movements: From Ideology to Identity.* Philadelphia: Temple University Press.

Latham, J. R. 2017. "Making and Treating Trans Problems: The Ontological Politics of Clinical Practices." *Studies in Gender and Sexuality* 18 (1): 40–61. https://doi.org/10.1080/15240657.2016.1238682.

Latour, Bruno. 1987. *Science in Action: How to Follow Scientists and Engineers through Society.* Cambridge, Mass.: Harvard University Press.

Lewis, Vek. 2010. *Crossing Sex and Gender in Latin America.* New York: Palgrave Macmillan.

Lewis, Vek, and Dan Irving. 2017. "Strange Alchemies: The Trans- Mutations of Power and Political Economy." *TSQ: Transgender Studies Quarterly* 4 (1): 4–15. https://doi.org/10.1215/23289252-3711493.

Liboiron, Max. 2021. *Pollution Is Colonialism.* Durham, N.C.: Duke University Press.

Link, Bruce G., and Jo Phelan. 1995. "Social Conditions as Fundamental Causes of Disease." *Journal of Health and Social Behavior* 35 (January): 80–94.

Litardo, Emiliano. 2013. "Los Cuerpos Desde Ese Otro Lado: La Ley de

Identidad de Género En Argentina." *Meritum, Revista de Direito Da Universidade FUMEC* 8 (2). http://www.fumec.br/revistas/meritum/article/view/2168.

Llaveria Caselles, Eric. 2021. "Epistemic Injustice in Brain Studies of (Trans)Gender Identity." *Frontiers in Sociology* 6. https://www.frontiersin.org/article/10.3389/fsoc.2021.608328.

Loder, Charisse M., Leah Minadeo, Laura Jimenez, Zakiya Luna, Loretta Ross, Nancy Rosenbloom, Caren M. Stalburg, and Lisa H. Harris. 2020. "Bridging the Expertise of Advocates and Academics to Identify Reproductive Justice Learning Outcomes." *Teaching and Learning in Medicine* 32 (1): 11–22. https://doi.org/10.1080/10401334.2019.1631168.

Logroño, Sol. 2019. "Health on the Move: Social Movements and Popular Health in La Plata, Argentina." *Ciência & Saúde Coletiva* 24 (12): 4579–86. https://doi.org/10.1590/1413-812320182412.25152019.

Long Chu, Andrea. 2018. "My New Vagina Won't Make Me Happy." *New York Times,* Opinion, November 24, 2018.

Löwy, Ilana. 2011. "Historiography of Biomedicine: 'Bio,' 'Medicine,' and In Between." *Isis* 102 (1): 116–22.

Loyd, Jenna. 2017. "Obamacare and Sovereign Debt: Race, Reparations, and the Haunting of Premature Death." In *Subprime Health: Debt and Race in U.S. Medicine,* edited by Nadine Ehlers and Leslie R. Hinkson, 55–82. Minneapolis: University of Minnesota Press.

Lugones, María. 2003. *Pilgrimages/Peregrinajes: Theorizing Coalition against Multiple Oppressions.* Lanham, Md.: Rowman & Littlefield.

Lugones, María. 2007. "Heterosexualism and the Colonial/Modern Gender System." *Hypatia* 22 (1): 186–209.

Lugones, María. 2010. "Decolonial Feminism." *Hypatia* 25 (4): 742–59.

Luna, Florencia, and Arleen L. F. Salles. 2006. "Latin American Bioethics: Some Reflections." In *Bioethics and Vulnerability: A Latin American View,* edited by Florencia Luna, Peter Herissone-Kelly, and Laura Pakter, 9–17. Kenilworth, U.K.: Rodopi.

Luna, Zakiya. 2009. "From Rights to Justice: Women of Color Changing the Face of US Reproductive Rights Organizing." *Societies without Borders* 4 (3): 343–65. https://doi.org/10.1163/187188609X12492771031618.

Luna, Zakiya. 2020. *Reproductive Rights as Human Rights: Women of Color and the Fight for Reproductive Justice.* New York: NYU Press.

Lynne, Alyssa. 2021. "Paired Double Consciousness: A Du Boisian Approach to Gender and Transnational Double Consciousness in Thai Kathoey Self-Formation." *Social Problems* 68 (2): 250–66. https://doi.org/10.1093/socpro/spaa073.

Machado, Cristiani Vieira. 2018. "Health Policies in Argentina, Brazil, and Mexico: Different Paths, Many Challenges." *Ciência & Saúde Coletiva* 23 (7): 2197–212.

Machina, Mark J., and Kip Viscusi, eds. 2014. *Handbook of the Economics of Risk and Uncertainty.* Vol. 1. Amsterdam: North-Holland.

Magness, Josh. 2018. "Transgender Asylum-Seeker Who Died in ICE Custody Was Physically Abused, Autopsy Says." *Miami Herald,* November 27, 2018. https://www.miamiherald.com/latest-news/article222239810.html.

Malatino, Hil. 2019. *Queer Embodiment: Monstrosity, Medical Violence, and Intersex Experience.* Lincoln: University of Nebraska Press.

Malatino, Hil. 2022. *Side Affects: On Being Trans and Feeling Bad.* Minneapolis: University of Minnesota Press.

Malatino, Hil, Jules Gill-Peterson, and Ann Cvetkovich. 2020. "Trans Care: A Critical Conversation." Penn State University, December 2, 2020. Rock Ethics Institute, December 4, 2020, YouTube video, 1:28:06, https://www.youtube.com/watch?v=T9cYstwdhTA.

Mamo, Laura. 2010. "Fertility, Inc.: Consumption and Subjectification in U.S. Lesbian Reproductive Practices." In *Biomedicalization: Technoscience, Health, and Illness in the U.S.,* edited by Adele E. Clarke, Laura Mamo, Jennifer Ruth Fosket, Jennifer R. Fishman, and Janet K. Shim, 173–96. Durham, N.C.: Duke University Press.

Mapping Police Violence. n.d. "Mapping Police Violence Report." Accessed April 29, 2023. https://www.mappingpoliceviolence.org.

Marlatt, G. Alan, and Katie Witkiewitz. 2010. "Update on Harm-Reduction Policy and Intervention Research." *Annual Review of Clinical Psychology* 6 (1): 591–606. https://doi.org/10.1146/annurev.clinpsy.121208.131438.

Martin, Emily. 1987. *The Woman in the Body: A Cultural Analysis of Reproduction.* Boston: Beacon Press.

Martínez, Juliana, and Salvador Vidal-Ortiz. 2021. "Travar el saber: Travesti-Centred Knowledge-Making and Education." *Bulletin of Latin American Research* 40 (5): 665–78.

Marx, Karl. 1971. *On Revolution.* New York: McGraw-Hill.

Massad, Joseph. 2018. "Against Self-Determination." *Humanity Journal* 9 (2): 161–91. https://doi.org/10.1353/HUM.2018.0010.

Máximo, Matías. 2016. "Argentina gritó 'basta de travesticidios.'" *LATAM* (blog). July 4, 2016. https://distintaslatitudes.net/argentina-grito-basta-travesticidios.

Mbembe, Achille. 2003. "Necropolitics." *Public Culture* 15 (1): 11–40. https://doi.org/10.1215/08992363-15-1-11.

McAlevey, Jane F. 2016. *No Shortcuts: Organizing for Power in the New Gilded Age.* New York: Oxford University Press.

McKillop, Matt, and Vinu Ilakkuvan. 2019. "The Impact of Chronic Underfunding on America's Public Health System: Trends, Risks, and Recommendations." Washington, D.C.: Trust for America's

Health. https://collections.nlm.nih.gov/catalog/nlm:nlmuid-101751510-pdf.

McReynolds-Pérez, Julia. 2017. "No Doctors Required: Lay Activist Expertise and Pharmaceutical Abortion in Argentina." *Signs: Journal of Women in Culture and Society* 42 (4): 349–75. https://doi.org/10.1086/688183.

McRuer, Robert. 2018. *Crip Times: Disability, Globalization, and Resistance.* New York: NYU Press.

Metzl, Jonathan M., and Anna Kirkland. 2010. *Against Health: How Health Became the New Morality.* New York: NYU Press.

Meyer, David S., and Nancy Whittier. 1994. "Social Movement Spillover." *Social Problems* 41 (2): 277–98. https://doi.org/10.2307/3096934.

Meyerowitz, Joanne. 2002. *How Sex Changed: A History of Transsexuality in the United States.* Cambridge, Mass.: Harvard University Press.

Mingus, Mia. 2015. "Medical Industrial Complex Visual." *Leaving Evidence* (blog). February 6, 2015. https://leavingevidence.wordpress.com/2015/02/06/medical-industrial-complex-visual/.

Minter, Shannon Price. 2018. "Transgender Family Law." *Family Court Review* 56 (3): 410–22. https://doi.org/10.1111/fcre.12357.

Miranda, Marisa A. 2018. "Late Eugenics in Argentina and Its Family Stereotype, Second Half of the Twentieth Century." *História, Ciências, Saúde-Manguinhos* 25 (suppl. 1): 33–50. https://doi.org/10.1590/S0104-59702018000300003.

Mitchell, David, and Sharon Snyder. 2003. "The Eugenic Atlantic: Race, Disability, and the Making of an International Eugenic Science, 1800–1945." *Disability & Society* 18 (7): 843–64. https://doi.org/10.1080/0968759032000127281.

Mogul, Joey L., Andrea J. Ritchie, and Kay Whitlock. 2011. *Queer (In) Justice: The Criminalization of LGBT People in the United States.* Boston: Beacon Press.

Motta, Sara C. 2019. "Feminising Our Revolutions." *Soundings* 71 (April): 15–27. https://doi.org/10.3898/SOUN.71.01.2019.

Muñoz, José Esteban. 2009. *Cruising Utopia: The Then and There of Queer Futurity.* New York: New York University Press.

Murphy, Michelle. 2012. *Seizing the Means of Reproduction: Entanglements of Feminism, Health, and Technoscience.* Durham, N.C.: Duke University Press.

Murphy, Michelle. 2017. *The Economization of Life.* Durham, N.C.: Duke University Press.

Mustafa, Zubeida. 1971. "The Principle of Self-Determination in International Law." *International Lawyer* 5 (3): 479–87.

Nadasen, Premilla. 2004. *Welfare Warriors: The Welfare Rights Movement in the United States.* New York: Routledge.

Namaste, Viviane K. 2000. *Invisible Lives: The Erasure of Transsexual and Transgendered People.* Chicago: University of Chicago Press.

Namaste, Viviane. 2011. *Sex Change, Social Change: Reflections on Identity, Institutions, and Imperialism.* Toronto: Canadian Scholars' Press.

Narayan, Sasha Karan, Rayisa Hontscharuk, Sara Danker, Jess Guerriero, Angela Carter, Gaines Blasdel, Rachel Bluebond-Langner et al. 2021. "Guiding the Conversation: Types of Regret after Gender-Affirming Surgery and Their Associated Etiologies." *Annals of Translational Medicine* 9 (7): 605. https://doi.org/10.21037/atm-20-6204.

Nelson, Alondra. 2011. *Body and Soul: The Black Panther Party and the Fight against Medical Discrimination.* Minneapolis: University of Minnesota Press.

Nepon, Ezra Berkley. 2016. *Dazzle Camouflage: Spectacular Theatrical Strategies for Resistance and Resilience.* Philadelphia: Ezra Berkley Nepon.

New York State Department of Health. 2011. "Medicaid Redesign Team (MRT) Health Disparities Work Group: Final Recommendations." New York: New York State Department of Health. https://www.health.ny.gov/health_care/medicaid/redesign/docs/health_disparities_report.pdf.

Nye, Coleman. 2012. "Cancer Previval and the Theatrical Fact." *TDR/The Drama Review* 56 (4 (216)): 104–20. https://doi.org/10.1162/DRAM_a_00217.

OAS (Organization of American States). 2014. "An Overview of Violence against LGBTI Persons in the Americas: A Registry Documenting Acts of Violence between January 1, 2013 and March 31, 2014." Washington, D.C.: Organization of American States. http://www.oas.org/en/iachr/media_center/preleases/2014/153a.asp.

O'Brien, Michelle. 2013. "Tracing This Body: Transsexuality, Pharmaceuticals, and Capitalism." In *The Transgender Studies Reader 2,* edited by Susan Stryker and Aren Z. Aizura, 56–65. New York: Routledge.

Office of the Attorney General. 2014. "A.G. Schneiderman Announces Settlement with Health Care Company That Provided Substandared Service to Jail Inmates in 13 NY Counties." September 25, 2014. New York State Office of the Attorney General Press Release Archive.

Office of the National Coordinator for Health Information and Technology. 2015. "Health Information Technology Certification Criteria, 170.315 (a) (5) Demographics." Accessed April 29, 2023. https://www.healthit.gov/test-method/demographics.

O'Hagan, Ellie. 2018. "Back the Gender Recognition Act Reform. It's the Feminist Thing to Do." *Guardian,* October 19, 2018, sec. Opinion. https://www.theguardian.com/commentisfree/2018/oct/19/gender-recognition-act-feminist-self-identification-consultation.

Ong, Aihwa. 2006. *Neoliberalism as Exception: Mutations in Citizenship and Sovereignty.* Durham, N.C.: Duke University Press.

Orgullo Disca. n.d. "Orgullo Disca: Rebelión Feminista." Accessed March 20, 2022. https://rebelionfeminista.org/2020/07/28/orgullo-disca/.

O'Riordan, Kate. 2012. "The Life of the Gay Gene: From Hypothetical Genetic Marker to Social Reality." *Journal of Sex Research* 49 (4): 362–68.

OUTrans. n.d. "Les Transféminismes." OUTrans (website). Accessed April 25, 2023. https://outrans.org/ressources/articles/transfeminismes/.

Palmeiro, Cecilia. 2018. "The Latin American Green Tide: Desire and Feminist Transversality." *Journal of Latin American Cultural Studies* 27 (4): 561–64. https://doi.org/10.1080/13569325.2018.1561429.

Palmeiro, Cecilia. 2020. "Ni Una Menos and the Politics of Translation." *Spheres: Journal for Digital Cultures* no. 6: 1–7. http://spheres-journal.org/ni-una-menos-and-the-politics-of-translation/.

Pandemonium, Eire. 2020. "Discapacidad y Rebeldía: Nos hemos cansado de tutelaje." *Rebelión Feminista* (blog). December 1, 2020. https://rebelionfeminista.org/2020/12/01/discapacidad-y-rebeldia-nos-hemos-cansado-de-tutelaje/.

Paradise, Julia, and Kaiser Family Foundation. 2015. "Medicaid Moving Forward." Kaiser Family Foundation. March 9, 2015. https://www.kff.org/report-section/medicaid-moving-forward-tables/.

Patel, Geeta. 2017. *Risky Bodies & Techno-Intimacy: Reflections on Sexuality, Media, Science, Finance.* Seattle: University of Washington Press.

Pearce, Ruth. 2018. *Understanding Trans Health.* Bristol: Policy Press.

Pearce, Ruth, Sonja Erikainen, and Ben Vincent. 2020. "TERF Wars: An Introduction." *Sociological Review* 68 (4): 677–98. https://doi.org/10.1177/0038026120934713.

Pellegrino, Edmund. 1986. "Rationing Health Care: The Ethics of Medical Gatekeeping." *Journal of Contemporary Health Law & Policy* 2 (1): 23–46.

Pérez, Moira, and Blas Radi. 2020. "Gender Punitivism: Queer Perspectives on Identity Politics in Criminal Justice." *Criminology & Criminal Justice* 20 (5): 523–36. https://doi.org/10.1177/1748895820941561.

Perlongher, Néstor. 2004. "Príncipe y plebeyo." Reprinted in *Página 12,* November 7, 2004.

Phillips-Fein, Kim. 2017. *Fear City: New York's Fiscal Crisis and the Rise of Austerity Politics.* New York: Metropolitan Books.

Pickerill, Jenny, and John Krinsky. 2012. "Why Does Occupy Matter?" *Social Movement Studies* 11 (3–4): 279–87. https://doi.org/10.1080/14742837.2012.708923.

Piepzna-Samarasinha, Leah Lakshmi. 2018. *Care Work: Dreaming Disability Justice.* Vancouver: Arsenal Pulp Press.

Pierce, Joseph M., María Amelia Viteri, Diego Falconí Trávez, Salvador Vidal-Ortiz, and Lourdes Martínez-Echazábal. 2021. "Introduction: *Cuir*/Queer Américas: Translation, Decoloniality, and the Incommensurable." *GLQ: A Journal of Lesbian and Gay Studies* 27 (3): 321–27. https://doi.org/10.1215/10642684-8994028.

Pis Diez, Nayla María. 2019. "La marea verde/violeta, lo popular y el contexto: Una reconstrucción y algunos elementos sobre el movimiento feminista en Argentina." *Libertas* 19 (2): 342–61. https://doi.org/10.34019/1980-8518.2019.v19.28896.

Pitts, Andrea J. 2018. "Examining Carceral Medicine through Critical Phenomenology." *IJFAB: International Journal of Feminist Approaches to Bioethics* 11 (2): 14–35.

Pitts-Taylor, Victoria. 2016. *The Brain's Body: Neuroscience and Corporeal Politics.* Durham, N.C.: Duke University Press.

Planey, Arianna. 2021. "Disability and Access to Healthcare." Fordham University Center for Ethics Education, October 19, 2021. Zoom panel.

Plemons, Eric. 2010. "Envisioning the Body in Relation: Finding Sex, Changing Sex." In *The Body Reader: Essential Social and Cultural Readings,* edited by Lisa Jean Moore and Mary Kosut, 317–28. New York: NYU Press.

Plemons, Eric. 2017. *The Look of a Woman: Facial Feminization Surgery and the Aims of Trans- Medicine.* Durham, N.C.: Duke University Press.

Poteat, Tonia, Andrea L. Wirtz, Anita Radix, Annick Borquez, Alfonso Silva-Santisteban, Madeline B. Deutsch, Sharful Islam Khan, Sam Winter, and Don Operario. 2015. "HIV Risk and Preventive Interventions in Transgender Women Sex Workers." *Lancet* 385 (9,964): 274–86. https://doi.org/10.1016/S0140-6736(14)60833-3.

Prison Insider. 2020. "Argentina: 'The System Filters Complaints.'" *Prison Insider* (blog). September 29, 2020. https://www.prison-insider.com/en/articles/argentine-le-systeme-filtre-les-plaintes.

Professionals Concerned with Gender Diagnoses in the DSM. 2010. "Statement on Gender Incongruence in Adults in the DSM-5." March 30, 2010. Archived at: https://web.archive.org/web/20100503020556/http:/gidconcern.wordpress.com/statement-on-gender-incongruence-in-adults-and-adolescents-in-the-dsm-5/.

Programa Nacional de Salud Sexual y Procreación Responsable. 2015. "Atención de la salud integral de personas trans: Guía para equipos de salud." Buenos Aires: Presidencia de la Nación: Ministerio de Salud.

Puar, Jasbir. 2007. *Terrorist Assemblages: Homonationalism in Queer Times.* Durham, N.C.: Duke University Press.

Puar, Jasbir. 2017. *The Right to Maim: Debility, Capacity, Disability.* Durham, N.C.: Duke University Press.

Pyne, Jake. 2014. "Gender Independent Kids: A Paradigm Shift in Approaches to Gender Non-conforming Children." *Canadian Journal of Human Sexuality* 23 (1): 1–8. https://doi.org/10.3138/cjhs.23.1.CO1.

Quijano, Aníbal. 2000. "Coloniality of Power, Eurocentrism, and Latin America." *Nepantla* 1 (3): 533–80.

Radford, Jill, and Diana E. H. Russell. 1992. *Femicide: The Politics of Woman Killing.* Woodbridge, Conn.: Twayne.

Radi, Blas. 2020. "Reproductive Injustice, Trans Rights, and Eugenics." *Sexual and Reproductive Health Matters* 28 (1). https://doi.org/10.1080/26410397.2020.1824318.

Radi, Blas, and Alejandra Sardá-Chandiramani. 2016. "Travesticidio/Transfemicidio: Coordenadas Para Pensar Los Crimenes de Travestis y Mujeres Trans En Argentina." Boletín Del Observatorio de Género. Buenos Aires. https://www.aacademica.org/blas.radi/14.pdf.

Ramos, Marco A. 2013. "Psychiatry, Authoritarianism, and Revolution: The Politics of Mental Illness during Military Dictatorships in Argentina, 1966–1983." *Bulletin of the History of Medicine* 87 (2): 250–78. https://doi.org/10.1353/bhm.2013.0029.

Rao, Devi M. 2009. "'Making Medical Assistance Available': Enforcing the Medicato Act's Availability Provision through § 1983 Litigation." *Columbia Law Review* 109 (6): 1440–81.

Raymond, Janice G. 1979. *The Transsexual Empire: The Making of the She-Male.* Boston: Beacon Press.

Reagon, Bernice Johnson. 1983. "Coalition Politics: Turning the Century." In *Home Girls: A Black Feminist Anthology,* edited by Barbara Smith, 356–68. New York: Kitchen Table, Women of Color Press.

Redacción La Tinta. 2019. "El avance de consultorios inclusivos." November 6, 2019. https://latinta.com.ar/2019/11/el-avance-de-consultorios-inclusivos/.

Redacción Marcha. 2020. "Lohana Berkins: 'Las travestis tenemos la capacidad de engendrar otra historia,' 2010 Speech at the Seminario Internacional 'Derecho al aborto, una deuda de la democracia.'" *Marcha,* May 25, 2020. https://www.marcha.org.ar/lohana-berkins-las-travestis-tenemos-la-capacidad-de-engendrar-otra-historia/.

Reddy, Chandan. 2011. *Freedom with Violence: Race, Sexuality, and the US State.* Durham, N.C.: Duke University Press.

REDI. n.d. "Red por los Derechos de las Personas con Discapacidad (REDI)." Accessed October 29, 2020. http://www.redi.org.ar/.

Regier, Darrel A., Emily A. Kuhl, and David J. Kupfer. 2013. "The DSM-5: Classification and Criteria Changes." *World Psychiatry* 12 (2): 92–98. https://doi.org/10.1002/wps.20050.

Riggs, Damien W., and Clare Bartholomaeus. 2018. "Fertility Preserva-

tion Decision Making amongst Australian Transgender and Non-binary Adults." *Reproductive Health* 15 (1): 181. https://doi.org/10.1186/s12978-018-0627-z.
Ritchie, Andrea. 2017. *Invisible No More: Police Violence against Black Women and Women of Color.* Boston: Beacon Press.
Rizki, Cole. 2019. "Latin/x American Trans Studies: Toward a Travesti-Trans Analytic." *TSQ: Transgender Studies Quarterly* 6 (2): 145–55. https://doi.org/10.1215/23289252-7348426.
Rizki, Cole. 2020. "'No State Apparatus Goes to Bed Genocidal Then Wakes Up Democratic': Fascist Ideology and Transgender Politics in Post-Dictatorship Argentina." *Radical History Review* no. 138: 82–107. https://doi.org/10.1215/01636545-8359271.
Roberts, Dorothy. 1997. *Killing the Black Body: Race, Reproduction, and the Meaning of Liberty.* New York: Vintage.
Robinson, Cedric. 1983. *Black Marxism: The Making of the Black Radical Tradition.* Chapel Hill: University of North Carolina Press.
Rosendo, Ernestina, Gonzalo Beladrich, Rodrigo Remis Santin, Victoria Cejas, Pedro Bianchi, Carlos Díaz, Juan Maddoni, Saskia Ivana Aufenacker, and Paula Grisolía. 2016. "Representaciones sociales sobre la población trans en estudiantes de psicología." *Anuario de Investigación USAL* no. 2 (April). https://p3.usal.edu.ar/index.php/anuario investigacion/article/view/3606.
Ross, Loretta. 2006. "Understanding Reproductive Justice: Transforming the Pro-choice Movement." *Off Our Backs* 36 (4): 14–19.
Ross, Loretta, and Rickie Solinger. 2017. *Reproductive Justice: An Introduction.* Oakland: University of California Press.
Sabati, Sheeva. 2019. "Upholding 'Colonial Unknowing' through the IRB: Reframing Institutional Research Ethics." *Qualitative Inquiry* 25 (9–10): 1056–64. https://doi.org/10.1177/1077800418787214.
Sabsay, Leticia. 2016. *The Political Imaginary of Sexual Freedom: Subjectivity and Power in the New Sexual Democratic Turn.* London: Springer.
Saldivia Menajovsky, Laura. 2018. "La bioética despatologizadora del derecho a la identidad de género." In *Bioética laica: vida, muerte, género, reproducción y familia,* edited by Pauline Capdevielle and María de Jesús Medina Arellano, 137–53. México: Instituto de Investigaciones Jurídicas (UNAM).
Salessi, Jorge. 1995. *Medicos Maleantes y Maricas: Higiene, Criminología y Homosexualidad en la Construcción de la Nación Argentina.* Rosario, Argentina: Beatriz Viterbo Editora.
Samuels, Ellen. 2014. *Fantasies of Identification: Disability, Gender, Race.* New York: NYU Press.
Savcı, Evren. 2021. *Queer in Translation: Sexual Politics under Neoliberal Islam.* Durham, N.C.: Duke University Press.
Schevers, Ky. 2021. "Feeling Regret about My Detransition and Past

Activism." *Medium,* June 28, 2021. https://kyschevers.medium.com/feeling-regret-about-my-detransition-and-past-activism-db958d541085.

Schneider, Erik. 2018. "Trans-Children: Between Normative Power and Self-Determination." In *Normed Children: Effects of Gender and Sex Related Normativity on Childhood and Adolescence,* edited by Erik Schneider and Christel Baltes-Löhr, 167–88. Bielefeld, Germany: Transcript.

Schrader, Stuart, and Facundo Chavez Penillas. 2012. "Crisis, Class, and Disability in Argentina: Red Por Los Derechos de Las Personas Con Discapacidad." *Disability Studies Quarterly* 32 (3). https://doi.org/10.18061/dsq.v32i3.3274.

Schuller, Kyla. 2018. *The Biopolitics of Feeling: Race, Sex, and Science in the Nineteenth Century.* Durham, N.C.: Duke University Press.

Schuller, Kyla. 2021. *The Trouble with White Women: A Counterhistory of Feminism.* New York: Bold Type Books.

Schulz, Sarah. 2018. "The Informed Consent Model of Transgender Care: An Alternative to the Diagnosis of Gender Dysphoria." *Journal of Humanistic Psychology* 58 (1). https://journals.sagepub.com/doi/full/10.1177/0022167817745217.

Schweik, Susan M. 2009. *The Ugly Laws: Disability in Public.* New York: NYU Press.

Scott, James C. 1999. *Seeing like a State: How Certain Schemes to Improve the Human Condition Have Failed.* New Haven, Conn.: Yale University Press.

Sedgwick, Eve Kosofsky. 1991. "How to Bring Your Kids Up Gay." *Social Text* 29: 18–27. https://doi.org/10.2307/466296.

Sekuler, Todd. 2013. "Convivial Relations between Gender Non-conformity and the French Nation-State." *L'Esprit Créateur* 53 (1): 15–30. https://doi.org/10.1353/esp.2013.0010.

Sengoopta, Chandak. 2000. *Otto Weininger: Sex, Science, and Self in Imperial Vienna.* Chicago: University of Chicago Press.

Shah, Nayan. 2019. "Putting One's Body on the Line." *GLQ: A Journal of Lesbian and Gay Studies* 25 (1): 183–87. https://doi.org/10.1215/10642684-7275446.

Sherwin, Susan. 1992. *No Longer Patient: Feminist Ethics and Health Care.* Philadelphia: Temple University Press.

Shim, Janet K. 2010. "The Stratified Biomedicalization of Heart Disease: Expert and Lay Perspectives on Racial and Class Inequality." In *Biomedicalization: Technoscience, Health, and Illness in the U.S.,* edited by Adele E. Clarke, Laura Mamo, Jennifer Ruth Fosket, Jennifer R. Fishman, and Janet K. Shim, 218–41. Durham, N.C.: Duke University Press.

Shim, Janet K. 2014. *Heart-Sick: The Politics of Risk, Inequality, and Heart Disease.* New York: NYU Press.

Short, Susan E., and Stefanie Mollborn. 2015. "Social Determinants and

Health Behaviors: Conceptual Frames and Empirical Advances." *Current Opinion in Psychology* 5 (October): 78–84. https://doi.org/10.1016/j.copsyc.2015.05.002.

shuster, stef. 2019. "Performing Informed Consent in Transgender Medicine." *SSM Social Science & Medicine* 226: 190–97.

shuster, stef. 2021. *Trans Medicine: The Emergence and Practice of Treating Gender.* New York: NYU Press.

Siegel, Reva. 1997. "Why Equal Protection No Longer Protects: The Evolving Forms of Status-Enforcing State Action." *Stanford Law Review* 49 (5): 1111. https://doi.org/10.2307/1229249.

Silliman, Jael, Marlene Gerber Fried, Loretta Ross, and Elena Gutierrez. 2004. *Undivided Rights: Women of Color Organizing for Reproductive Justice.* Cambridge, Mass.: South End Press.

Simonetto, Patricio, and Marce Butierrez. 2022. "The Archival Riot: *Travesti*/Trans* Audiovisual Memory Politics in Twenty-First-Century Argentina." *Memory Studies* 16 (2): 280–95. https://doi.org/10.1177/17506980211073099.

Singer, T. Benjamin. 2006. "From the Medical Gaze to Sublime Mutations: The Ethics of (Re)Viewing Non-normative Body Images." In *The Transgender Studies Reader,* edited by Susan Stryker and Stephen Whittle, 601–20. New York: Routledge.

Singer, T. Benjamin. 2015. "The Profusion of Things: The 'Transgender Matrix' and Demographic Imaginaries in US Public Health." *TSQ: Transgender Studies Quarterly* 2 (1): 58–76.

Singh, Jennifer. 2016. *Multiple Autisms: Spectrums of Advocacy and Genomic Science.* Minneapolis: University of Minnesota Press.

Singh, Nikhil Pal. 2005. *Black Is a Country: Race and the Unfinished Struggle for Democracy.* Cambridge, Mass.: Harvard University Press.

Sins Invalid. 2019. *Skin, Tooth, and Bone: The Basis of Movement Is Our People (A Disability Justice Primer).* Oakland: Sins Invalid. https://www.sinsinvalid.org/disability-justice-primer.

Sins Invalid. n.d. "Sins Invalid." Accessed October 29, 2020. https://www.sinsinvalid.org.

SisterSong. n.d. "SisterSong: Women of Color Reproductive Justice Collective." https://www.sistersong.net.

Sitrin, Marina, ed. 2006. *Horizontalism: Voices of Popular Power in Argentina.* Oakland, Calif.: AK Press.

Skidmore, Emily. 2011. "Constructing the 'Good Transsexual': Christine Jorgensen, Whiteness, and Heteronormativity in the Mid-Twentieth-Century Press." *Feminist Studies* 37 (2): 270–300.

Slaughter, Joseph R. 2007. *Human Rights, Inc: The World Novel, Narrative Form, and International Law.* New York: Fordham University Press.

Smith, Lindsay Adams. 2016. "Identifying Democracy: Citizenship, DNA, and Identity in Postdictatorship Argentina." *Science, Technology, & Human Values* 41 (6): 1037–62.

Snorton, C. Riley. 2017. *Black on Both Sides: A Racial History of Trans Identity.* Minneapolis: University of Minnesota Press.

Snorton, C. Riley, and Jin Haritaworn. 2013. "Necropolitics: A Transnational Reflection on Violence, Death, and the Trans of Color Afterlife." In *Transgender Studies Reader 2,* edited by Susan Stryker and Aren Z. Aizura, 66–76. New York: Routledge.

Somerville, Siobhan B. 2000. *Queering the Color Line: Race and the Invention of Homosexuality in American Culture.* Durham, N.C.: Duke University Press.

Sosa, Cecilia. 2021. "Mourning, Activism, and Queer Desires: Ni Una Menos and Carri's Las hijas del fuego." *Latin American Perspectives* 237 (48): 137–54.

Spade, Dean. 2006. "Compliance Is Gendered: Struggling for Gender Self-Determination in a Hostile Economy." In *Transgender Rights,* edited by Paisley Currah, Richard M. Juang, and Shannon Price Minter, 217–41. Minneapolis: University of Minnesota Press.

Spade, Dean. 2010. "Medicaid Policy & Gender-Confirming Healthcare for Trans People: An Interview with Advocates." *Seattle Journal for Social Justice* 8 (2): 497–514.

Spade, Dean. 2015. *Normal Life: Administrative Violence, Critical Trans Politics, and the Limits of Law.* Rev. and expanded ed. Durham, N.C.: Duke University Press.

Spade, Dean. 2020. *Mutual Aid: Building Solidarity during This Crisis (and the Next).* New York: Verso Books.

Spade, Dean, Gabriel Arkles, Phil Duran, and Pooja Gehi. 2009. "Medicaid Policy & Gender-Confirming Healthcare for Trans People: An Interview with Advocates." *Seattle Journal for Social Justice* 8: 497.

Spillers, Hortense J. 2003. *Black, White, and in Color: Essays on American Literature and Culture.* Chicago: University of Chicago Press.

Spinelli, Hugo Guillermo. 2004. "La violencia como problema de salud pública: El terrorismo de Estado en Argentina 1976–1981." In *Salud Colectiva Cultura, Instituciones, Subjetividad Epidemiología, Gestión y Políticas,* edited by Hugo Guillermo Spinelli, 49–67. Buenos Aires: Lugar Editorial.

Spivak, Gayatri Chakravorty. 1999. *A Critique of Postcolonial Reason: Toward a History of the Vanishing Present.* Cambridge, Mass.: Harvard University Press.

Spivak, Gayatri Chakravorty. 2005. "Use and Abuse of Human Rights." *Boundary 2* 32 (1): 131–89. https://doi.org/10.1215/01903659-32-1-131.

Sriram, Chandra Lekha. 2004. *Confronting Past Human Rights Violations: Justice vs Peace in Times of Transition.* London: Cass.

Stanley, Eric A. 2014. "Gender Self-Determination." *TSQ: Transgender*

Studies Quarterly 1 (1–2): 89–91. https://doi.org/10.1215/23289252-2399695.

Star, Susan Leigh. 1989. *Regions of the Mind: Brain Research and the Quest for Scientific Certainty.* Stanford, Calif.: Stanford University Press.

Star, Susan Leigh. 1993. "Cooperation without Consensus in Scientific Problem Solving: Dynamics of Closure in Open Systems." In *CSCW: Cooperation or Conflict?,* edited by S. Easterbrook, 93–105. London: Springer.

Star, Susan Leigh. 1999. "The Ethnography of Infrastructure." *American Behavioral Scientist* 43 (3): 377–91. https://doi.org/10.1177/00027649921955326.

Star, Susan Leigh. 2002. "Infrastructure and Ethnographic Practice: Working on the Fringes." *Scandinavian Journal of Information Systems* 14 (2): 107–22.

Star, Susan Leigh. 2010. "This Is Not a Boundary Object: Reflections on the Origin of a Concept." *Science, Technology, & Human Values* 35 (5): 601–17.

Star, Susan Leigh, and James R. Griesemer. 1989. "Institutional Ecology, 'Translations' and Boundary Objects: Amateurs and Professionals in Berkeley's Museum of Vertebrate Zoology, 1907–39." *Social Studies of Science* 19 (3): https://doi.org/10.1177/030631289019003001.

Star, Susan Leigh, and Karen Ruhleder. 1996. "Steps toward an Ecology of Infrastructure: Design and Access for Large Information Spaces." *Information Systems Research* 7 (1): 111–34.

Starr, Paul. 1982. *The Social Transformation of American Medicine.* New York: Basic Books.

Stein, Dan J., Peter Szatmari, Wolfgang Gaebel, Michael Berk, Eduard Vieta, Mario Maj, Ymkje Anna de Vries et al. 2020. "Mental, Behavioral, and Neurodevelopmental Disorders in the ICD-11: An International Perspective on Key Changes and Controversies." *BMC Medicine* 18 (1): 21. https://doi.org/10.1186/s12916-020-1495-2.

Stepan, Nancy. 1991. *The Hour of Eugenics: Race, Gender, and Nation in Latin America.* Ithaca, N.Y.: Cornell University Press.

Stern, Alexandra. 2005. *Eugenic Nation: Faults and Frontiers of Better Breeding in Modern America.* Berkeley: University of California Press.

Stevenson, Lisa. 2014. *Life beside Itself: Imagining Care in the Canadian Arctic.* Berkeley: University of California Press.

Stoler, Ann Laura. 1995. *Race and the Education of Desire: Foucault's History of Sexuality and the Colonial Order of Things.* Durham, N.C.: Duke University Press.

Stone, Sandy. 1992. "The 'Empire' Strikes Back: A Posttranssexual Manifesto." *Camera Obscura* 10 (2): 150–76. https://doi.org/10.1215/02705346-10-2_29-150.

Stop Trans Pathologization. 2012. "Stop Trans Pathologization."

Archived on TGEU website. Accessed May 4, 2023. https://tgeu.org/stp-2012/#stp-docu-2.

Strangio, Chase. 2012. "Debating 'Gender Identity Disorder' and Justice for Trans People." *HuffPost,* December 5, 2012. https://www.huffpost.com/entry/gender-identity-disorder-dsm_b_2247081.

Strauss, Anselm L., and Juliet M. Corbin. 1998. *Basics of Qualitative Research: Techniques and Procedures for Developing Grounded Theory.* Thousand Oaks, Calif.: Sage Publications.

Stryker, Susan, Paisley Currah, and Lisa Jean Moore. 2008. "Introduction: Trans-, Trans, or Transgender?" *WSQ: Women's Studies Quarterly* 36 (3): 11–22. https://doi.org/10.1353/wsq.0.0112.

Subramaniam, Banu. 2014. *Ghost Stories for Darwin: The Science of Variation and the Politics of Diversity.* Champaign: University of Illinois Press.

Suess, Amets. 2015. "Trans Depathologization Perspectives and Public Health Frameworks: Intersections and Alliances." *European Journal of Public Health* 25 (suppl. 3). https://doi.org/10.1093/eurpub/ckv173.013.

Suess, Amets, Karine Espineira, and Pau Crego Walters. 2014. "Depathologization." *TSQ: Transgender Studies Quarterly* 1 (1–2): 73–77. https://doi.org/10.1215/23289252-2399650.

Suess Schwend, Amets. 2020. "Trans Health Care from a Depathologization and Human Rights Perspective." *Public Health Reviews* 41 (1): 3. https://doi.org/10.1186/s40985-020-0118-y.

Sutton, Barbara. 2007. "Poner El Cuerpo: Women's Embodiment and Political Resistance in Argentina." *Latin American Politics and Society* 49 (3): 129–62. https://doi.org/10.1111/j.1548-2456.2007.tb00385.x.

Sutton, Barbara. 2020. "Intergenerational Encounters in the Struggle for Abortion Rights in Argentina." *Women's Studies International Forum* 82 (September). https://doi.org/10.1016/j.wsif.2020.102392.

Swarr, Amanda Lock, and Richa Nagar, eds. 2010. *Critical Transnational Feminist Praxis.* Albany: SUNY Press.

Sylvia Rivera Law Project. 2008. *"It's War in Here": A Report on the Treatment of Transgender and Intersex People in New York State Men's Prisons.* New York: Sylvia Rivera Law Project.

Sylvia Rivera Law Project. 2013. "Eliminating the Medicaid Exclusion for Transition-Related Care in NYS: Good Public Health, the Right Thing to Do, and Ultimately a Cost-Saving Measure." Sylvia Rivera Law Project. https://srlp.org/wp-content/uploads/2012/08/Health-Costs-Final-Memo.pdf.

Sylvia Rivera Law Project. 2014. "Trans Healthcare Infographic from SRLP and GLAAD!" July 24, 2014. Sylvia Rivera Law Project. http://srlp.org/new-trans-healthcare-infographic-from-srlp-and-glaad/.

Sylvia Rivera Law Project. 2017a. *"It's War in Here": Republication of the 2008 Report on the Treatment of Transgender and Intersex People in New York State Men's Prisons.* New York: Sylvia Rivera Law Project.

Sylvia Rivera Law Project. 2017b. "Tell New York to Remove Barriers to Gender-Affirming Healthcare." Sylvia Rivera Law Project. https://srlp.org/tell-new-york-to-remove-barriers-to-gender-affirming-healthcare/.

TallBear, Kim. 2014. "Standing with and Speaking as Faith: A Feminist-Indigenous Approach to Inquiry." *Journal of Research Practice* 10 (2): N17–N17.

Tanenbaum, Sandra. 2017. "Can Payment Reform Be Social Reform? The Lure and Liabilities of the 'Triple Aim.'" *Journal of Health Politics, Policy, and Law* 42 (1): 53–71.

Tanis, Justin. 2016. "The Power of 41%: A Glimpse into the Life of a Statistic." *American Journal of Orthopsychiatry* 86 (4): 373–77. https://doi.org/10.1037/ort0000200.

Tarzibachi, Eugenia. 2017. *Cosa de Mujeres: Menstruación, género y poder.* Buenos Aires: Sudamericana.

Taylor, Janelle S. 2003. "Confronting 'Culture' in Medicine's 'Culture of No Culture.'" *Academic Medicine Academic Medicine* 78 (6): 555–59.

Theumer, Emmanuel. 2018. "El coraje de ser mariposas, la resistencia." *La Tinta,* November 8, 2018. https://latinta.com.ar/2018/11/coraje-ser-mariposas-resistencia/.

Theumer, Emmanuel. 2020. "The Self-Perceived Gender Identity." *Interventions* 22 (4): 498–513. https://doi.org/10.1080/1369801X.2020.1749708.

Thomas, Ralph. 2006. "State Tries to Rule Out Aid for Sex-Change Surgery." *Seattle Times,* August 7, 2006, sec. Local News.

Thomas, William I., and Dorothy Swaine Thomas. 1970. "Situations Defined as Real Are Real in Their Consequences." In *Social Psychology through Symbolic Interaction,* edited by Gregory P. Stone and Harvey A. Faberman, 54–155. Waltham, Mass.: Xerox Publishers.

Thompson, Charis. 2005. *Making Parents: The Ontological Choreography of Reproductive Technologies.* Cambridge, Mass.: MIT Press.

Thompson, Hale M. 2016. "Patient Perspectives on Gender Identity Data Collection in Electronic Health Records: An Analysis of Disclosure, Privacy, and Access to Care." *Transgender Health* 1 (1): 205–15. https://doi.org/10.1089/trgh.2016.0007.

Thompson, Hale, and Lisa King. 2015. "Who Counts as 'Transgender'? Epidemiological Methods and a Critical Intervention." *TSQ: Transgender Studies Quarterly* 2 (1): 148–59. https://doi.org/10.1215/23289252-2848913.

Tom Waddell Health Center. 2001. "Protocols for Hormonal Reassignment of Gender from Tom Waddell Health Center." San Francisco: Tom Waddell Health Center.

Tom Waddell Health Center. 2013. "Protocols for the Hormonal Reassignment of Gender (Updated)." San Francisco: Tom Waddell Health Center. https://www.sfdph.org/dph/comupg/oservices/medsvs/hlthctrs/transgendprotocols122006.pdf.

Tourmaline. n.d. *The Spirit Was . . .* (blog). https://thespiritwas.tumblr.com.

Towle, Evan B., and Lynn M. Morgan. 2002. "Romancing the Transgender Native: Rethinking the Use of the 'Third Gender' Concept." *GLQ: A Journal of Lesbian and Gay Studies* 8 (4): 469–97. https://doi.org/10.1215/10642684-8-4-469.

TransJustice. 2006. "Trans Action for Social and Economic Justice: Statements by TransJustice, A Project of the Audre Lorde Project." In *The Color of Violence: The Incite! Anthology*, 227–30. Cambridge, Mass.: South End Press.

Traps. n.d. "MANIFESTO: Demonstration against the WPATH—For Trans Bodily Autonomy and Transfeminist Solidarity." Traps MTL. Accessed September 19, 2022. https://www.trapsmtl.com/mission.

Travers, Ann. 2019. *The Trans Generation: How Trans Kids (and Their Parents) Are Creating a Gender Revolution.* New York: NYU Press.

Trouillot, Michel-Rolph. 1995. *Silencing the Past: Power and the Production of History.* Boston: Beacon Press.

TSER (Trans Student Educational Resource). 2016. "Why We Used Trans* and Why We Don't Anymore—Trans Student Educational Resources." Accessed June 1, 2020. http://www.transstudent.org/asterisk.

Tuck, Eve, and K. Wayne Yang. 2012. "Decolonization Is Not a Metaphor." *Decolonization: Indigeneity, Education & Society* 1 (1): 1–40.

Tuck, Eve, and K. Wayne Yang. 2016. "What Justice Wants." *Critical Ethnic Studies* 2 (2): 1. https://doi.org/10.5749/jcritethnstud.2.2.0001.

Turda, Marius, and Aaron Gillette. 2014. *Latin Eugenics in Comparative Perspective.* London: Bloomsbury Publishing.

Turner, Janice. 2020. "Keira Bell: 'I Couldn't Sit by While So Many Others Made the Same Mistake,'" *Times,* December 1, 2020, sec. News. https://www.thetimes.co.uk/article/keira-bell-i-couldnt-sit-by-while-so-many-others-made-the-same-mistake-gb03n3mlr.

Tyler, Imogen, and Tom Slater. 2018. "Rethinking the Sociology of Stigma." *Sociological Review* 66 (4): 721–43. https://doi.org/10.1177/0038026118777425.

Urquhart, Evan. 2021. "Detransition Movement Debunked: Former Leader Ky Schevers on Why the Anti-trans Group Is like the Ex-Gays." *Slate,* February 1, 2021. https://slate.com/human-interest/2021/02/detransition-movement-star-ex-gay-explained.html.

Valentine, David. 2007. *Imagining Transgender: An Ethnography of a Category.* Durham, N.C.: Duke University Press.

Valentine, David. 2012. "Sue E. Generous: Toward a Theory of Non-transexuality." *Feminist Studies* 38 (1): 185–211.

Van Eijk, Marieke. 2017. "Insuring Care: Paperwork, Insurance Rules, and Clinical Labor at a U.S. Transgender Clinic." *Culture, Medicine, and Psychiatry: An International Journal of Cross-Cultural Health Research* 41 (4): 590–608. https://doi.org/10.1007/s11013-017-9529-8.

Varelius, Jukka. 2006. "The Value of Autonomy in Medical Ethics." *Medicine, Health Care, and Philosophy* 9 (3): 377–88. https://doi.org/10.1007/s11019-006-9000-z.

Vargas, Chris, and Eric A. Stanley, dirs. 2015. *Criminal Queers.* Homotopia Film.

Velasco Garrido, Marcial, Annette Zentner, and Reinhard Busse. 2011. "The Effects of Gatekeeping: A Systematic Review of the Literature." *Scandinavian Journal of Primary Health Care* 29 (1): 28–38. https://doi.org/10.3109/02813432.2010.537015.

Velocci, Beans. 2021. "Standards of Care: Uncertainty and Risk in Harry Benjamin's Transsexual Classifications." *TSQ: Transgender Studies Quarterly* 8 (4): 462–80.

Villarreal, Yezmin. 2015. "5 Most Disappointing Things We Learned about HRC's 'White Men's Club.'" *Advocate,* June 4, 2015. https://www.advocate.com/human-rights-campaign-hrc/2015/06/04/5-most-disappointing-things-we-learned-about-hrcs-white-mens-cl.

Viteri, María Amelia. 2017. "Intensiones: Tensions in Queer Agency and Activism in Latino América." *Feminist Studies* 43 (2): 405–17. https://doi.org/10.1353/fem.2017.0028.

Ward, Deborah E. 2009. *The White Welfare State: The Racialization of U.S. Welfare Policy.* Ann Arbor: University of Michigan Press.

Washington, Harriet A. 2006. *Medical Apartheid: The Dark History of Medical Experimentation on Black Americans from Colonial Times to the Present.* New York: Doubleday.

Wayar, Marlene. 2007. "La Visibilidad de lo Invisible." In *Cumbia, copeteo, y lágrimas: Informe nacional sobre la situación de las travestis, transexuales y transgéneros,* edited by Lohana Berkins, 43–54. Buenos Aires: Asociación de Lucha por la Identidad Travesti-Transexual.

Wayar, Marlene. 2012. "¿Qué pasó con la T?" *Página 12,* May 11, 2012, sec. SOY. https://www.pagina12.com.ar/diario/suplementos/soy/1-2436-2012-05-11.html.

Wayar, Marlene. 2018. *Travesti: Una Teoría Lo Suficientemente Buena.* Buenos Aires: Muchas Nueces.

Weber, Max. 1978. *Economy and Society.* Berkeley: University of California Press.

Weed, Lawrence L. 1970. *Medical Records, Medical Education, and Patient Care: The Problem-Oriented Record as a Basic Tool.* Cleveland: Press of Case Western Reserve University.

Weheliye, Alexander G. 2014. *Habeas Viscus: Racializing Assemblages, Biopolitics, and Black Feminist Theories of the Human.* Durham, N.C.: Duke University Press.

Welfare Warriors Research Collaborative. 2010. "A Fabulous Attitude: Low-Income LGBTGNC People Surviving and Thriving on Love, Shelter, and Knowledge." New York: Queers for Economic Justice. Available at Candid Issue Lab, January 1, 2010, https://search.issuelab.org/resource/a-fabulous-attitude-low-income-lgbtgnc-people-surviving-and-thriving-on-love-shelter-and-knowledge.html.

Welker-Hood, Kristen. 2014. "Underfunding and Undervaluing the Public Health Infrastructure: Reinforcing the Haves and the Have-Nots in Health." *Public Health Nursing* 31 (6): 481–83. https://doi.org/10.1111/phn.12165.

Weller, Marc. 2008. *Escaping the Self-Determination Trap.* Boston: Martinus Nijhoff.

White, Alexandria. 2020. "Citi Launches 'True Name' Feature with Mastercard to Allow Trans and Non-binary People to Use Their Chosen Name." *CNBC,* October 19, 2020, sec. Latest. https://www.cnbc.com/select/citi-mastercard-launch-true-name-for-lgbtq-community/.

WHO (World Health Organization). n.d. "Gender Incongruence and Transgender Health in the ICD." World Health Organization, Frequently Asked Questions. Accessed April 29, 2023. https://www.who.int/standards/classifications/frequently-asked-questions/gender-incongruence-and-transgender-health-in-the-icd#.

WHO (World Health Organization). 1975. *ICD-9: International Statistical Classification of Diseases and Related Problems.* Geneva: World Health Organization.

WHO (World Health Organization). 1992. *ICD-10: International Classification of Diseases.* Geneva: World Health Organization.

WHO (World Health Organization). 2004. *ICD-10: International Statistical Classification of Diseases and Related Health Problems.* 2nd ed. Geneva: World Health Organization.

WHO (World Health Organization). 2018. "Mental Health ATLAS 2017." Geneva: World Health Organization. https://www.who.int/publications-detail-redirect/9789241514019.

WHO (World Health Organization). 2019. *ICD-11: International Classification of Diseases.* https://icd.who.int/en.

Willems, D. 2001. "Balancing Rationalities: Gatekeeping in Health Care." *Journal of Medical Ethics* 27 (1): 25–29. https://doi.org/10.1136/jme.27.1.25.

Williams, Callum, and Mahiben Maruthappu. 2013. "'Healthconomic Crises': Public Health and Neoliberal Economic Crises." *American Journal of Public Health* 103 (1): 7–9. https://doi.org/10.2105/AJPH.2012.300956.

Williams, Cristan. 2014. "Fact Checking Janice Raymond: The NCHCT Report." TransAdvocate. September 18, 2014. https://www.transadvocate.com/fact-checking-janice-raymond-the-nchct-report_n_14554.htm.

Williams, Raymond. 1954. *Preface to Film.* London: Film Drama.

Williams, Raymond. 1983. *Keywords: A Vocabulary of Culture and Society.* London: Fontana Press.

Willse, Craig. 2015. *The Value of Homelessness: Managing Surplus Life in the United States.* Minneapolis: University of Minnesota Press.

Winters, Kelley. 2011. "The Proposed Gender Dysphoria Diagnosis in the DSM-5." *GID Reform Weblog by Kelley Winters* (blog). June 7, 2011. https://gidreform.wordpress.com/2011/06/07/the-proposed-gender-dysphoria-diagnosis-in-the-dsm-5/.

WPATH (World Professional Association for Transgender Health). 2011. *WPATH Standards of Care for the Health of Transsexual, Transgender, and Gender Nonconforming People.* 7th ed.

Wynter, Sylvia. 1994. "'No Humans Involved': An Open Letter to My Colleagues." *Knowledge on Trial* 1 (1): 42–73.

Wynter, Sylvia. 2003. "Unsettling the Coloniality of Being/Power/Truth/Freedom: Towards the Human, After Man, Its Overrepresentation: An Argument." *CR: The New Centennial Review* 3 (3): 257–337. https://doi.org/10.1353/ncr.2004.0015.

Yogyakarta Principles. 2007. *The Yogyakarta Principles: The Application of International Human Rights Law in Relation to Sexual Orientation and Gender Identity.* http://www.yogyakartaprinciples.org/.

Yogyakarta Principles. 2010. "An Activist's Guide to The Yogyakarta Principles." http://ypinaction.org/content/activists_guide.

Yogyakarta Principles. 2017. "Yogyakarta Principles Plus 10." https://yogyakartaprinciples.org/principles-en/yp10/.

Young, Iris Marion. 2011. *Responsibility for Justice.* Oxford: Oxford University Press.

Zachs, Maxwell, Carla Antonelli, Vladimir Luxuria, Kim Schicklang, Jenna Talackova, and Rochelle Gregorie. 2012. "We Are Trans* Not Sick!!" Change.Org. October 20, 2012. https://www.change.org/p/world-health-organisation-who-we-are-trans-not-sick.

Zubiaurre-Elorza, Leire, Carme Junque, Esther Gómez-Gil, Santiago Segovia, Beatriz Carrillo, Giuseppina Rametti, and Antonio Guillamon. 2013. "Cortical Thickness in Untreated Transsexuals." *Cerebral Cortex* 23 (12): 2855–62. https://doi.org/10.1093/cercor/bhs267.

Index

Page numbers in italics refer to figures.

ableism: and austerity politics (racialized), 324n16; criminalization and, 147–49; depathologization activists and, 107; eugenic, 106; pathologization and, 60–61, 65; racialized, 59; of trans- activists, 245; transphobia and, 69–70
abolitionist frameworks, 240, 242, 323n7
abortions: in Argentina, 62–63, 118, 205, 232, 237, 252, 296n11, 303n1; embodied autonomy and, 239; restrictions on, 187; in the U.S., 239
Abuelas de la Plaza de Mayo, 131, 306n26, 307n34, 315n11. *See also* Madres de la Plaza de Mayo
activism, disability. *See* disability activism
activism, feminist: health care, 28, 49, 56, 58–59, 76; transnational, 97; travestis and, 117, 119. *See also* feminist movements
activism, grassroots, 4, 21, 146, 154, 162, 165–67, 178, 308n2
activism and activists: antiausterity, 259; antigatekeeping, 39, 72, 185; Black and Indigenous, 62; gay and lesbian, 57, 229–30; gay and lesbian depathologization, 48, 255; Green Tide, 48, 62–63; HIV/AIDS, 3, 26, 243, 256; Indian, 139; Indigenous, 62; involved in Ministry of Health guide, 316n13; transfeminine, 1; transmasculine, 305n14; women of color, 61
activist providers, 75, 298n27
activists, coalitional depathologization: analyzing trans- health within political economy, 238–39; extending depathologization, 43, 48, 109, 230–31, 235–36, 239–41, 245, 258, 268–69; gatekeeping and, 227; horizontal modes of action, 241–43; and issues of debt, 37, 249–53; self-determination and, 210
activists, depathologization: and debts of democracy, 249; diagnoses and, 34, 47–48, 80, 104–8; dreams of, 255; gatekeeping and, 216; illness-care conundrum and, 48, 57; largely focused on health and medicine, 28; self-determination and, 39–40; shaping trans- health, 31; transnational, 43–44, 93–95; trans- therapeutics and, 50, 54, 250
activists, reproductive justice, 59, 62–63, 296n12
activists, trans- and travesti: bill for reparations for, 129–30; collaboration, 221; debt and,

253; the disappeared and, 315n11; epidemiological biographies and, 38; Gender Identity Law and, 41, 249, 322n2; growth of activism in Buenos Aires, 24; neoliberalism and, 39; open to coalitions, 229–30, 244; population health and, 141; reproductive justice activists and, 62–63

activists, trans- health: autonomy and, 203, 218, 219; bioethical frameworks and, 227; boundary objects and, 219; care without pathology in practice, 189; challenging hierarchical frameworks of biomedical care, 12; collective self-determination and, 208–11; compared to advocates, 21; consent-driven care and, 190, 191, 199, 203, 221, 223, 226; critique Labor Quota Law, 319n30; desire to level the power relations, 199; developed politicized diagnosis to contest pathologization, 256; different from mainstream LGBQ activism, 234; epidemiological biographies and, 38; erasure of trans- lives and, 207; focus on material redistribution, 39; general demographics of, 22; informed consent and, 205, 217, 219, 221; interviewed by author, 20–21; medical paternalism and, 226; Medicare and, 287n45; readily contribute to determining trans- health practice, 31; resisting pathologization, 8; self-determination and, 188–89, 216, 218, 223–24; self-perceived need and, 224–25; study sites and methods, 20–21; transfeminist care and, 198, 228; working-class struggle of, 235

activists, travesti: collective forms of redress and, 131; "Expectativas" campaign and, 118–21; focus on material redistribution, 39; Gender Identity Law and, 74–75; informal economies and, 24; in Pride march, 126–27. *See also* activists, trans- and travesti

activists in Argentina, trans- health: epidemiological biographies of, 116–20, 132–33, 137–38, 140; focus on state violence and criminalization, 112–14, 129–30, 133, 137, 140–43; statistical collectivization of, 134–35, 139, 141, 143. *See also* activists, travesti

activists in New York, trans- health: addressing economic risk, 153, 174–75, 179–82; campaign to reframe trans- health, 146–47; economized epidemiological biographies and, 147–48, 172–74, 179, 182; in Medicaid campaign videos, 176–78; Medicaid exclusion and, 148–50, 154–55, 158–71; statistical collectivization and, 147, 149

Adams v. Federal Bureau of Prisons, 298n26

Adán (physician), 197, 236–37

Adler-Bolton, Beatrice, 290n67

"administrative violence," 164, 290n63, 302n29, 307n32

advocates, trans- health: addressing economic risk, 148–49, 174, 180; assert claim to social belonging and financialized care, 182–83; autonomy and, 203; bioethical frameworks and, 227; bridging care, 201; campaign to reframe trans- health, 146–47; care without pathology in practice, 189; challenging hierarchical frameworks of biomedical care, 12; collaboration of poverty lawyers and, 163; collaborative care and, 199; compared to activists, 21; consent-driven care and, 190, 191, 203, 223, 226; constrained informed consent and, 205; economic productivity of trans- people and, 180–81; economized epidemiological biographies and, 147–48, 162, 179; harm of denying trans- therapeutics, 153–54; health risks and, 153, 164; interviewed by author, 20–21; in Medicaid campaign videos, 176–78; Medicaid exclusion, 171; Medicaid exclusion and, 148–49, 150, 154–55, 158–59, 160–61, 163, 165–71; medical paternalism and, 226; readily contribute to determining trans- health practice, 31; scarcity of affordable hormones and, 322n45; self-determination and, 218, 223–24; self-perceived need and, 224–25; statistical collectivization and, 134, 147, 149, 153, 182; *Yogyakarta Principles* drafted by, 188

Affordable Care Act (ACA), 25–26, 53–54, 69, 138, 151, 157, 161, 270, 287n46, 294n4. *See also* Section 1557 of Affordable Care Act

African Americans, 234, 238. *See also* Black people

"Against Self-Determination" (article), 319n33

agency: bioethics asserts importance of, 205; counterhegemonic forms of, 208; hegemonic, 206–7, 215; individual, 206; insurgent, 208, 221; transformative, 208, 215, 221

aggregation of health outcomes, 114, 134, 136–37, 151–52

aggregative slippages, 140

aggression: misogynistic, 143; physical, 122–23, 126

Aizura, Aren Z., 35, 284n21, 292n75

Alfonsín, Raúl, 130

Alliance Defending Freedom, 7

Amanda (advocate and attorney), 66–67, 70–71, 73–74, 91–92, 158–62, 165, 216–18, 224, 227, 261

amendment to end Medicaid exclusion, 158. *See also* Medicaid

American Medical Association (AMA), 298n24

American Psychiatric Association (APA), 9, 57, 78, 83, 88, 91, 94, 289n55

American Public Health Association, 298n24

Ana (travesti activist), 229–32, 235–38, 244, 249, 252, 261

anthropologists view of gender nonnormativity, 86, 289n59, 300n9

anti-Blackness, 31, 106, 283n19

anticolonialism, 13, 212, 215, 260, 284n21, 320n35

antidiscrimination: ACA included provision for, 161; bill for employment, 324n14; as first of the Triple Aims, 154, 177; materially focused objectives instead of, 39, 136–38, 270

antidiscrimination rules (Title IX), 287n46, 287n47

antigatekeeping approaches and activism, 39, 72, 75, 185, 217, 228

anti-immigrant legislation, 291n71

anti-imperialism, 39, 62–64, 245, 248

antiprison movements, 215, 323n7

antitrans- legislation and politics, 7, 9–10, 283n17

Antonio (transnational advocate), 94, 96–97, 105–6, 225, 243–45, 247–50, 261, 316n13

Anya (advocate and activist), 58, 158–65, 203, 217, 243–44, 261

Aramburu, Pedro Eugenio, 121

Archives of Criminology, Forensic Medicine, and Psychiatry, 86

Argentina: Argentina, 230; austerity measures in, 54, 62; awareness of *ICD* revisions, 96; Buenos Aires as study site, 23; constitutional law in, 205; criminalization and trans- health care in, 71; Derecho a la Protección de la Salud Mental

(Right to Protect Mental Health), 301n25; eugenics in, 29; femicides in, 303n1; Green Tide in, 62–63, 108; health-care coverage in, 54–55, 96; health-care reform in, 297n17; histories of racialization in, 304n3; human rights in, 225; Lacanian psychodynamic focus in, 29; mental health in, 94; Patients' Rights Act in, 205; psychiatric regimes in, 30; public hospital system in, 4; repays NML Capital Ltd., 246–48, 323n12; RJ movements in, 59, 62–63; shift to consent-driven care, 195; travesticides in, 111. *See also* Gender Identity Law (Argentina)
Association for the Fight for Transvestite and Transsexual Identity (Asociación Lucha por la Identidad Travesti-Transexual), 118
"at risk" populations, 152
attorney advocates, 146, 150
attorneys, trans- health: Medicaid and, 154; Medicaid coverage for nontrans- people and, 154
Audre Lorde Project, 162–63, 310n16
austerity: in Argentina, 7, 54, 124, 237, 297n17, 307n29, 323n12; characterizing trans- health as too expensive, 35; deservingness of care and, 36, 71, 139, 222; disability and, 245, 291n68; economic violence of, 62; "free rider" and, 248; during Macri administration, 7, 54, 237, 307n29; Medicaid and, 71, 147–48, 156–59, 167, 174–75, 180, 249–50; political resistance to, 42, 62, 66, 180, 211, 222, 227, 230–31, 239, 245, 250, 255, 259, 270, 291n68; politics of, 7, 35–36, 39, 42, 54, 66, 71, 124, 147–48, 156, 162, 167, 174–75; restricting self-determination, 211; shift in health-care management and, 151; in the U.S., 147, 151, 156–58, 211
autonomy: activists and providers shared understanding of, 219; bioethics and, 317n21; bodily, 188, 195–96, 206, 210–11, 218; as boundary object, 226; collective rather than individual, 207; defined, 204, 213, 317n18, 322n6; embodied, 222, 239; individual bodily, 63, 66; individual right to care and, 217; informed consent and, 219; in medical situations, 60; patient, 191, 199, 201, 203; self-determination and, 208, 211, 218
Auyero, Javier, 237
Awkward-Rich, Cameron, 32, 321n42

Barker, K. K., 60
barriers, administrative, 137, 307n32
Bell, Keira, 263, 264
Benjamin, Harry, 297n19, 300n14
Benjamin, Ruha, 143
Berkins, Lohana, 49, 111, 118–20, 123, 125, 131, 133, 138–39, 141, 222, 245, 251–52, 303n1, 305n11
Berkins, La (Fernández), 305n11
Beth (nurse practitioner), 94, 107
Beyond Care project, 319n29
Biden administration, 7, 26, 138
Bierria, Alisa, 208, 215
bioethics, medical: autonomy and, 218–19, 321n41; Catholicism and, 205; informed consent and, 189, 203–9, 227, 317n21; origins of, 317n17; trans- patients' narratives and, 206
biological indicators for transness, 101, 302n28
biomedical authority, 260, 271, 325n3
biomedical care, 11–12, 33, 49–50, 271
biomedical entrepreneurialism, 40, 292n75
biomedicalization, 292n75, 293n85, 294n2
biomedicine: pathologization and, 86–87, 107; privileged status

of, 224; site of collective struggle, 269; STS and, 17, 286n36; trans- activism shaped, 6; trans- health and, 48
biopolitics: feminist and trans-feminist, 223, 256; Foucauldian, 293n84; as organizing regime of power, 44, 69, 223, 256; and population, 135; racialized, 290n64; and technologies of health, 29, 41–44
biopower, 293n84
Black activism and feminism: and Black nationalism, 320n35; and Black Power, 62, 215; reproductive justice and, 61–62
Blackness, 23, 31, 86–87, 106, 291n71, 304n3
Black on Both Sides (Snorton), 241
Black Panther Party, 217, 320n35
Black people: exclusion of coverage for trans- therapeutics, 314n6; "human" status and, 320n34; a new welfare state for, 234; non-marital and matriarchal relations of, 157; racialized disparities in care of, 282n5; racialized gender and, 241; study participants, 22; trans-, 6, 87, 180, 184
Black women: enslaved, 86–87; erasure of Blackness and, 304n3; racialized medical care for child-bearing, 60–61; state violence and, 208; welfare-rights campaigns of, 157, 173, 311n20
Bocchio, Diego, 238
Bolsonaro, Jair, 9
Boucher, Roan, 211, 212, 221
boundary objects, 189, 219–20, 223, 226, 321n40
Bowers, Marci, 1
Brazil: sex-reassignment surgery in, 295n5; trans- therapeutics in, 295n7; travestis in, 285n26
Bridges, Khiara, 61
bridge to care and/or coverage: diagnostic classification as, 45, 53, 54, 64, 80, 106; endocrine disorder as, 103; gender dysphoria as a nonpathologizing, 91–92; *ICD*'s revisions and, 97–98, 99; work-arounds and, 100–104, 109–10
Buenos Aires: activism in, 64, 74, 112, 129; art exhibit in, 111; clinics, 197; conurbanos in, 231, 237; conversation on who deserves public forms of care, 4–5, 35–36; criminalization of sexual/gender nonnormativity, 71–72; epidemiological biographies in, 120; as ethnographic site of study, 16–17; implicit forms of racialized trans- health, 37; media campaign in, 113; municipal codes in, 121; prisons in, 74; public clinics in, 231; social movements in, 23; as study site, 23–24; therapy responses in, 288n54; travestis in, 24; treatment of travestis in, 121, 124, 131. *See also* epidemiological biographies
bureaucracies: of health reimbursement, 48; providers and, 102; state, 237; trans- people and, 104–5
Burke, Mary, 57

Cabral Grinspan, Mauro (or Mauro Cabral), 67, 188, 211, 227, 266, 290n61, 292n79, 305n14
Callen-Lorde Community Health Center, 190–91, 193, 198, 201, 220–21
Campanile, Carl, 166–67, 174, 181
cancer, 263–64
capitalism: racial, 231, 238, 252, 269, 291n70; travesti and trans- led struggles against, 245, 251–52
care: equity as part of Triple Aims, 153–54, 177; feminist and trans-feminist, 210, 217, 223; models of, 2, 8, 10, 70, 199, 219, 226,

313n4; refusal of, 203–4, 318n24; relations, 43, 47, 63, 75, 185, 189, 198–200, 223–24, 226, 231, 238, 252
care without pathology: horizontal modes of, 197–98, 242; meanings of, 32, 47, 50–51, 66, 75, 294n2; origins of, 28; political vision of, 76, 227, 253, 255, 258, 261; in practice, 192–203, 227
Casillas v. Daines, 160, 310n14
Catholicism, 29, 205, 291n71
Cavallero, Lucí, 250
Césaire, Aimé, 320nn34–35
Change.org petition, 59
Christian fundamentalists, 7, 10, 263, 264
cis, as a term, 283n16
Citibank trans-targeted advertising campaign, 183–84, 245, 312n27
citizenship claims, 113, 123, 136, 139, 142
civil rights claims, 142
Claire (trans- advocate), 67, 166, 167–68
Clare, Eli, 64, 65, 206
Clarissa (nurse practitioner), 77–78, 104
Clarke, Adele, 20, 257, 293n85, 294n2
classifications: diagnostic, 33–34, 80–82; evolution of trans- diagnoses, 88, 89–90, 300n15; as medium of power, 109; nonpsychiatric, 34; pathologizing, 84; in practice, 87, 300n13
classificatory revision of trans- health, 78–79, 108
classificatory systems, 31, 33, 87–88
class inequity, racialized, 18, 106, 121–22, 139, 288n53, 291n70, 296n11
clinics: community-based, 3; consent-driven care at, 191–92, 313n4; for LGBTQ+ patients, 26; model for comprehensive care in public, 231–32, 252; trans- focused, 3
Clinton administration, 156
coalition, Health Care for All!, 147, 154, 167–68, 171–72, 174, 178, 179, 180, 311n19
coalitional depathologization activists. *See* activists, coalitional depathologization
coalitional relationships, 48, 59, 63, 244
coalitions: legal, 163; working-class, 237, 242
coding, medical, 52–53, 59–60
coercion: collective, 207–8; freedom from, 210, 217, 218, 320n35
Cohen, Cathy, 235, 241, 253, 323n9
Cohen-Kettenis, Peggy, 92, 301n17
Colen, Shellee, 60
collective health movements and activism, 38, 113, 114, 130, 131, 215–16, 259
colonization: gender systems of, 84, 299n7; knowledge, 31, 106; pathologization and, 43; queerness and, 298n22; settler, 291n71, 319n33
comorbidities as obstruction to trans- health access, 103–4
Comunidad Homosexual Argentina, 196
consent, age of, 318n24
consent-driven care, 190–92, 195–97, 199–202, 208, 222–26, 258, 313n5, 314n6, 315n9
consultorios inclusivos, 232, 236–38, 252
conurbanos, 231, 237, 252, 286n33
conversion therapies, 57, 92, 188, 265
cooperation without consensus, 40, 50, 189, 219, 228
cooperatives, worker-owned, 36, 290n66
cosmetic surgeries, 68, 309n9
cost containment as a part of Triple Aims, 154, 177
counter-data action, 134, 140
coverage, health-care: in Argentina, 54–55, 96; depathologization

and need for, 45–46; *DSM* and, 87–88; gender dysphoria diagnosis for, 92; by Gender Identity Law, 41; *ICD* and, 87–88, 98–99, 100–101, 103; medically necessary procedures and, 55, 70; for nontrans- people, 11, 283n20; psychiatric diagnoses and, 51–53; for trans- people, 283n20; for trans- therapeutics, 38, 41; workarounds for, 80, 106
Cox, Laverne, 161
Crenshaw, Kimberlé, 81, 299n5
criminalization: endangering trans- life, 38; as historical extensions of colonial queerness, 298n22; as key term in journal articles, 115; legal, 70, 73, 75; of public space, 14, 30, 31, 106; race and queer, 298n21; racialized, 106, 210; racialized and sexualized, 307n32; of sexual/gender nonnormativity, 71–73; trans- health care, 70–71; transness and, 49; travesti and trans- led struggles against, 245; of travestis, 14, 24, 74–75, 128, 229
Criminal Queers (film), 209
Crip Times (McRuer), 291n68
critical race theory, 293n81
Cruz, Angela, 158
Cruz v. Zucker, 158–59, 161
Cumbia, copeteo, y lágrimas (Cumbia, drinks, and tears), 116, 120–22, 124, 125, 126, 128t, 130, 227
Cuomo administration, 145, 157–59, 161, 165, 166–67, 168, 171, 175
Currah, Paisley, 13, 270, 271

Darryl (nurse practitioner), 202
deaths, trans-, 217
deaths, travesti, 125–27
deaths, travesti and trans-, 136
de Bonafini, Hebe, 131
debts: in Argentina, 246–48, 250–51, 297n17, 323n10, 324n12; politics of, 37, 62, 69, 108–9, 158, 184, 200, 231, 249–52, 290n67; sovereign, 37, 231, 290n67
"debts of democracy," 139, 231, 249, 307n34
Declaration of Helsinki, 204
decolonial, as a term, 284n21
decolonial feminist inquiries, 17
decolonial trans- studies, 28
decriminalization: consent-driven care and, 199; in epidemiological studies, 139; institutionalize, 125; of judicial authority from transness, 31
dejudicialization, 196, 199
de la Torre, Tehuel, 129, 270–71
demedicalization, 27, 49, 50
democracy in Argentina, political, 130–31, 133, 139
demographics of study participants, 22
Department of Health and Human Services (DHHS), 155–56, 310n15
Department of Mental Health and Substance Abuse (WHO), 95
Department of Sexual and Reproductive Health and Research (WHO), 95
depathologization: about, 27, 48; activists and, 31; Amets Suess view on, 49; as anchoring concept, 257; autonomy and, 66; and broader conditions of trans- life, 258, 262; classificatory, 81; consent-driven care and, 199, 226; consultorios inclusivos and, 232; depsychopathologization and, 296n9; diagnostic, 80, 84, 97, 109; disability model and, 63–65; feminist movements and, 62–64; of feminized bodies, 58–59; in France, 289n60; institutionalization of, 219; interwoven with many systems of care, 267; and need for care coverage, 45–47; neoliberalism and, 39–40;

with other movements, 49, 57, 75–76; positions on, 11, 48–49; pregnancy model and, 59–61; self-determination and, 66, 211; seminar on, 266; transformative agency and, 208; in trans- health care, 8–9, 49–50, 57–58, 240; trans- therapeutics and, 50, 313n5
depathologization, coalitional, 211–13, 226, 230–40, 242, 249, 252–53, 258–59, 265, 268
depathologization activists. *See* activists, depathologization
depsychopathologization, 49, 56–57, 130, 296n9
Derecho a la Protección de la Salud Mental (Right to Protect Mental Health), 301n25
destigmatization: consent-driven care and, 199; of judicial authority from transness, 31
detransitioning, 263–65
diagnoses: to access health care, 50, 52–53, 55; changing the terms of, 79–81; coding, 34, 53, 60, 192; depathologized, 88; disability justice and, 65; and heterogeneity, 98–99; insurance reimbursement and mental health, 192; Medicaid discriminating on basis of, 160, 309n12; medical instead of psychiatric, 94–95, 107; mental health, 216; power and complexity of, 64; psychiatric, 2, 28, 47, 69–70, 106, 107–8; revising pathologizing psychiatric, 33; revisions of trans- health due to changes to, 267–68; trans-, 33–34; trans-sexualism as, 78; as workarounds, 80, 100, 102
Diagnostic and Statistical Manual (DSM). See *DSM (Diagnostic and Statistical Manual)*
diagnostic classifications, 29, 33–34, 52, 54, 80–82, 85, 101
dictatorships: Aramburu, 121; the disappeared and, 23, 306n26, 307n29, 315n11; Onganía, 315n10; as present force, 292n73; psychiatry and, 289n56; reparations and, 39, 129–30; travestis and trans- people detained during, 72; travestis endure state violence even after, 131; Videla, 118, 130
Dimensions (clinic), 313n5
Dirty War, 131, 306n26, 315n11
disabilities, people with: and coconstitutiveness with other forms of difference, 317n22; consent and, 206; coverage for, 102, 314n6; epidemiological biographies and, 304n4; eugenics and, 60–61; guardianship and, 64, 296n13; pathologization and, 64; racialized, 106; state bureaucracies and, 302n29; and trans- people similarly pathologized, 107
disability, 29, 106, 291n68
disability activism, 48–49, 56, 59, 63–66, 212, 255, 289n60
disability justice, 28, 239–40, 241, 256, 288n49
disability studies scholars, 205–6
disappeared, the, Argentina, 129, 306n26, 307n29, 315n11
discrimination: Affordable Care Act and, 53–54, 294n4; based on diagnosis, 154; gender identity, 25; health care, 123–24, 176; medical and employment, 182; police, 122, 126; sex, 310n15; state, 129
Disobedient Bodies/Cuerpos Desobedientes (Fernández), 119
distress-based model of diagnoses, 91, 93, 108, 143
distribution, economic, 211, 319n29
doctors, trans- health, 178
double bind, trans- people in, 71, 79, 191
double standard of gatekeeping, 67, 72
Drescher, Jack, 57, 92, 301n17

DSM (*Diagnostic and Statistical Manual*): changes to, 9, 257–58; gender dysphoria in, 51–52, 294n3, 300n14, 302n26; gender identity disorder in, 51–52, 294n3, 296n10, 302n26; *ICD* and, 289n55; privatization of care and, 30; revision of, 33–34, 92–94, 96, 99, 108; trans- diagnoses in, 78, 87–88, 192; version 5, 83, 90, 92, 300n16; version III, 88–89; version II-R, 89; version IV, 88, 89, 92; versions studied by author, 83, 299n6
Du Bois, W. E. B., 143
Duggan, Lisa, 235, 243
Dutta, Aniruddha, 139

Echazú, Nadia, 118, 120
economic distribution, 37, 211, 319n29
economic justice, 241
"economization of life," 180, 312n23
economized epidemiological biographies, 39, 144, 147–50, 162, 175, 177, 180
Elifson, K. W., 313n5
"Eliminating the Medicaid Exclusion for Transition-Related Care in NYS" (fact sheet), 150, 162, 164–65, 167, 174–75, 179, 311n21
Elliott Management, 246, 323n12
employment, 1, 24, 39, 132, 142, 177, 182, 211, 229, 270, 310n16. *See also* labor exclusions
employment antidiscrimination bill, 294n4, 324n14
endocrine disorders, 52, 80, 98, 100–103, 192–93, 294n3
Enke, Finn, 283n16
enslavement: and exclusion from personhood, 320n34; and medicine, 86–87; regimes in the U.S., 84, 86, 291n71, 293n84; and "ungendering," 86–87
epidemiological biographies: about, 38, 112–13, 116; *Cumbia, copeteo, y lágrimas* (Cumbia, drinks, and tears), 116, 120–22, 124, 125, 126, 128t, 130, 227; differences between New York and Buenos Aires, 308n2; disability and, 304n4; draw on unrepresented sample, 140; "A Fabulous Attitude," 172; focused on material relief, 136–38, 140–41; *La gesta del nombre propio* (The struggle for one's own name), 116–17, 119–22, 125–26, *127*; life expectancy and, 129–30; population health and, 131–34, 179; reparations bill cites, 130; self-enumeration in, 139; state securitization and, 304n5
epidemiological biographies, economized, 39, 144, 147–50, 162, 175, 177, 180. *See also* "Eliminating the Medicaid Exclusion for Transition-Related Care in NYS" (fact sheet)
epidemiology, 114–16, 132
ethnographic data, 16–17
ethnographic study sources, 20–22
eugenic pathologization, 59, 60–61, 63, 65, 66, 85–86, 135
eugenics: in Argentine ideology, 288n53; normalization of, 31; passive, 296n12; practices, 188; racialized, 28, 66, 291n71; theory, 29
euthanasia, 205, 317n20
"Everyone Needs Access to Safe, Reliable Healthcare" (infographic), 150, 169
"Expectativas" media campaign, 113, 116, 117–19, 128, 135
experimentation, 85, 86–87, 282n13
Experts Meeting at GATE, 98–99
exploitation, racialized, 62, 63
extending depathologization. *See* activists, coalitional depathologization

"Fabulous Attitude, A" (study), 150, 172–74, 179, 311n19

fact sheet on eliminating Medicaid exclusion, 150, 162, 164–65, 167, 174–75, 179, 311n21
fascism, Argentine, 131, 291n71, 292n73
femicides, 250, 303n1
feminist biopolitics. *See* biopolitics
feminist care collectives, 321n39
feminist coalition politics, 242–43
feminist movements: abortion and, 296n11; in Argentina, 230; health care, 3, 26; in Ireland, 187; Latin American, 62; transnational, 255. *See also* activism and activists
feminists, gender-critical, 9. *See also* trans-exclusionary radical feminists (TERFs)
feminist self-help health practice, 256
feminist strikes, 250, 256
Feminist STS, 17–18, 32, 135
Ferguson, Roderick, 234–35
Fernández, Alberto, 8, 243, 319n30
Fernández, Josefina, 49, 71, 119–20, 141, 245, 305n11
Fernández de Kirchner, Cristina, 24, 297n17, 298n21, 323n12
Fernández Romero, Francisco, 62
financial costs of trans- health, 35–36, 200–201
financing systems, health-care, 34–35, 104
Fisch, Jörg, 214, 319n31
Fisk, Norman, 300n16
Foucault, Michel, 135, 293n84
France, depathologizing trans- health, 289n60
fraudulence claims, 52, 69, 80, 299n3, 308n5
freeze-frame policy in prisons, 74, 298n26
Frente de Liberación Homosexual, 196
Frente Nacional por la Ley de Identidad de Género (the National Front for the Gender Identity Law), 41
Fundación Rumbos (organization), 64
fundamentalists, Christian, 7, 10, 263, 264
furia travesti, 134, 259
Furia Travesti (art exhibit), 111, 116, 266

Gago, Verónica, 250
gatekeeping: medical, 41, 48, 67–68, 188–90, 195, 216, 220–28, 297n17; model of care, 190–92, 201, 313n4, 316n15; trans- health, 47, 49, 55–56, 66, 67–69, 70, 72, 297n17
gay and lesbian demedicalization and depsychopathologization projects, 27, 49, 56–57
gay and lesbian organizations, mainstream, 229–30, 247, 322n2
gay liberation movements, 57, 318n28
gay marriage, 229, 324n14
gender: and coconstitutiveness with other forms of difference, 317n22; criminalization of, 30; defined, 85; hierarchies, 67; identity, 25–26, 54, 85, 138, 188, 294n4, 306n24, 310n15; ideology, 9, 263; listed on forms, 104; markers, 2–3, 281n6; nonnormativity, 8, 40, 121, 172, 207, 291n71; normativity, 69–70; police profiling by, 71; reclassification, 2, 24, 30–31, 41, 71, 79, 195, 292n79, 315n10; as a term, 9–10
gender-affirming care: expense of, 4–6, 282n5; at hospital systems, 3; lifting of Medicaid exclusion for, 42, 302n26; Medicare and, 161; for minors, 281n9; to nontrans- people, 11–12; provided by Gender Identity Law, 7–8; technologies of, 15; for trans- and nontrans people, 11–12, 283n20

gender centers, university-based, 314n6
gender-confirming procedures, 285n31, 295n6, 308n4
gender dysphoria, 170, 193
Gender Dysphoria, 34, 51–52, 88, 90–93, 101, 294n3, 300n14, 300n16, 302n26
Gender Identity Disorder (GID): added to *DSM,* 78, 296n10; coverage based on diagnosis of, 2, 34, 51–52; in *DSM,* 91; in *DSM* and *ICD,* 87; in *DSM-IV,* 88; Medicaid and diagnosis of, 294n3, 302n26; on medical record in perpetuity, 92
Gender Identity Law (Argentina): antidiagnostic provisions of, 83, 88, 96–97, 108, 258; binary infrastructure of, 292n79; coalitional activists work on, 113, 229, 231–32, 244, 249, 322n2; consent-driven care and, 190, 195–99; depathologization and, 9, 290n61; distinct from Brazil's provisions, 295n5; epidemiological biographies and, 38, 129; euthanasia bill hearings concurred with, 317n20; fears of reversal of, 7–8; fourfold approach to, 31, 74–75; gay- and lesbian-led groups and, 247; illness–care conundrum and, 46; limits of, 296n12; medicalization or nonmedicalization, 261; organizing that preceded, 211; provisions of, 2–3, 41–42, 187–88, 270; referred to travestis, transexuales, and transgéneros, 128; requirements prior to, 24, 55–56, 67, 79; Right to Protect Mental Health Law prior to, 292n77; self-perceived need and, 54–55, 216, 225
gender identity laws in other countries, 292n78
Gender Incongruence, 34, 78, 88, 90, 95, 99
"Gender Is Not an Illness," 188
gender self-determination. *See* self-determination
genital surgeries, 2, 55, 79, 326n5
genitourinary disorders, 98
genocide, 291n71
gesta del nombre propio, La (The struggle for one's own name), 116–17, 119–22, 125–26, *127*
GID Reform Advocates, 92
Gill-Peterson, Jules, 45, 85, 282n13, 283n16, 314n6, 318n24, 318n27, 321n42
Giuliani, Rudy, 26
"Give Trans People Access to the Care They Need" (video), 150
GLAAD, 145, 150, 167–70, 180, 311n18
Glaser, Barney G., 19
Global Action for Trans Equality (GATE), 45–46, 49, 59, 72, 95, 97–98, 188, 199, 294n1
Global North: anthropologists based in, 86; ethnographic sites of study in, 17; as mythologized center of knowledge, 17; paradigms of diagnostic pathologization in, 97; providers based in, 290n61; researchers based in, 19, 230; as a term, 18; transness and, 284n21; trans- people's self-view in, 300n10; use of trans*, 15, 285n27; well-funded NGOs in, 247
Global South: debt vulturism in, 247; ethnographic sites of study in, 17; gender expression in, 86; movement-building, 97; social movements in, 37; as a source of data not theory, 19; as a term, 18; travesti and trans- people, 237; use of trans*, 14–15; whitening regimes in, 291n71
Goldberg, David Theo, 37, 291n70
Golden, Marty, 145

Gondolín hotel (Buenos Aires), 36, 246, 290n65
Gorton, R. Nick, 93, 106
grassroots organizing. *See* activism, grassroots
Green Tide (Marea Verde) feminist movement, 28, 48, 62–63, 108–9, 239, 253, 288n49
Griesemer, James R., 189, 219
Grillo, Tirre, 213–14
grounded theory, 18–19, 286n34
guardianship, 64, 296n13
guide, published by Ministry of Health, 197–98, 316n13
Guimaraes García, Florencia Agustina, 111–12, 116, 137, 266
Gutiérrez, María Alicia, 124
gynecomastia, 154, 283n20, 285n31

hair removal procedures, 15, 55, 285n31
Hall, Stuart, 13, 109
harassment: clinic waiting-room, 252; at *consultorios inclusivos,* 238; police, 26
harm reduction, 194, 315n9
HBIGDA (Harry Benjamin International Gender Dysphoria Association), 69, 191, 297n19
health, population, 114–15, 130–36, 141, 143
health bureaucracies, state, 42–43
"Healthcare for All" (video series), 150, 176
Health Care for All! coalition, 147, 154, 167–68, 171–72, 174, 178, 179, 180, 311n19
"Healthcare Professional Calls for Care for All" (video), 150
health-care reform in Argentina, 297n17
Health Care Rights Law, 294n4
Health Communism (Adler-Bolton and Vierkant), 290n67
Health Disparities Working Group, 165, 166
Health Information Technology Certification Criteria, 302n31
Health Liberation Now!, 265
health outcomes, population-level, 114–15, 134, 151–52, 154, 165–66, 177, 304n6
health records, electronic, 302n31
health risks. *See* risk
healthscapes, 293n85
health system in Argentina, three-tier, 23
health-system management, 164
hedge funds, 246–47
heterogeneity of care, 11, 105
heterosexuality, 195
HIV: and AIDS activism, 243; infection, 163; status, 104, 115, 124–25; treatment and prevention paradigms, 313n5
homelessness, 163
homeless shelters, 172, 235, 310n16
homophobia, 173, 310n16, 311n18
homosexuality, 45, 57, 296n10
horizontalism, 43, 231, 241–42, 244, 246, 251, 252, 255
hormone treatments: to affirm gender identity, 58; choice to receive, 213, 214; consent-driven care and, 190–91, 193, 202, 220, 313n5; gatekeeping and, 67, 69; Gender Identity Law and, 187; incarcerated people and, 74, 298n26; informally procured, 203, 220; informed-consent and, 193–94; Medicaid and, 102–3, 146, 294n3, 308n1; medical necessity of, 55; requirements to receive, 192; scarcity of affordable, 322n45; work-arounds for, 51–52, 100
hospital systems in Argentina, safety-net public, 4, 7, 23
hospital systems with integrated transgender care, 3, 281n7
Hotel Bauen, 2, 36, 290n66
hotels in Buenos Aires, reclaimed, 36

housing: access, 288n48; affordable, 310n16; deprivation, 168, 173
human rights, 225, 226
Human Rights Campaign (HRC), 247–48, 281n8, 324n14
human rights campaigns, transnational, 118
human-rights law, 188, 214
human rights networks, transnational, 199, 316n14

Ibarra, Vilma, 129
ICD (International Classification of Diseases): about, 87–88; adding trans-sexualism to, 78; classificatory changes to, 257–58; depathologization shaped changes in, 9; *DSM* and, 289n55; Endocrine Disorder-NOS in, 52, 100–102; evolution of trans- diagnoses in, 90–91; removing transsexualism from, 45; revisions, 33–34, 83, 94–97, 99, 108, 299n6; version 9, 88, 90, 102; version 10, 46, 59–60, 90, 95, 102, 266; version 11, 46, 52, 83, 88, 90, 94, 95
identification cards, New York City's municipal, 73
identification documents, 24, 41, 267, 289n57, 292n79
identification documents, legal, 2–3, 30
identity, legal right to, 195, 315n11
illness–care conundrum, 34, 46, 48, 53–54, 57, 80, 266
immigration detention centers, 93, 261, 323n9
immigration policies, racist, 310n16
immiseration: in bioethical frameworks, 227; depathologization activism and racialized, 106; endangering trans- life, 38; pathologization and, 108; racialized, 106, 141, 153, 227; structural, 143; systemic, 210; of trans- and travestis, 116, 153, 211; travestis subject to systemic, 140, 141
imperialism, 269
imperialist nationalism, 291n71
imperilment, conditions of, 113, 130, 142, 147, 180
imprisonment, 106, 270
incarceration, 163, 238
income equity, 270
Indigenous populations: erasure of Indigeneity, 23, 304n3; exclusion of trans- therapeutic coverage for, 314n6; gender expression subordination of, 86; genocide against, 291n71; health-care access for trans-, 6; "human" status and, 320n34; irreducibility of Indigeneity, 306n24; racialized medical care for childbearing, 60; self-determination and, 215, 320n35; sovereignty and Green Tide movement, 63; as study participants, 22; travestis racialized as, 14; violence against activists, 62
individualism, 218
infographics in Medicaid campaign, 167–71, 174, 175, 179, 311n21
informed consent: approach to care, 190, 192; bioethics and, 189–90, 227, 317n21; boundary object of, 219–20, 226; contracts, 222–23; driven care, 70; ensures personal choice, 205; forms, 193, 198, 221; Gender Identity Law and, 187–88, 196; guidelines, 204–5; in Ministry of Health guide, 197; models, 194, 263, 316n15; protocols, 39–40, 194–95, 219, 220–21, 223, 225, 226, 318n24; providers and, 318n23; for therapeutic coverage, 51; transnational advocacy for, 199, 316n14
Informed Consent for Access to Trans Health Care (ICATH), 28, 47, 49, 50–51, 72, 199–201, 321n43

infrastructures: binary, 292n79; biomedical and regulatory, 221; of care, 98–99, 104–5; durability of, 266–67; health-care, 81–82, 262; public-health, 29; of regulation, 224
Institute of Medicine, 164
insurance: coverage for trans- therapeutics, 2, 51, 156, 177, 283n20; diagnostic codes and, 267; disparities between trans- and nontrans-, 11; limited flexibility of biomedical practices due to, 193; psychotherapy not covered by, 191; reimbursements for trans- therapeutics, 201; risk and, 152–53; Z-codes and, 60. *See also* coverage, health-care
Inter-American Commission on Human Rights, 128
International Classification of Diseases (ICD). See *ICD (International Classification of Diseases)*
International Lesbian, Gay, Bisexual, Trans and Intersex Association, 95
International Monetary Fund (IMF), 297n17, 323n10
International Women's Strikes, 62
intersectionality, 81, 299n5
intersex people, 85, 188, 207, 239, 283n20, 295n6, 313n3, 318n24
intersex rights advocacy, 203, 316n14
Ireland, 187
Irving, Dan, 37, 40, 239, 291n69
It's War in Here (study), 308n2

Jacob (nurse practitioner), 73
Jarrín, Carmen Alvaro, 295n5, 295n7
Joaquín (trans- advocate), 74, 196, 198, 222, 261
Johnson, Marsha P., 211, 212, 232, 318n28
Joly, Eduardo, 64, 65
justice, as a term, 324n17

kidney transplantation, 282n5
Kirchner, Néstor, 248, 297n17
Krafft-Ebing, Richard von, 30

labor exclusions, 24, 36, 129, 140, 253, 261. *See also* employment
labor movements, 230
Labor Quota Law for Travestis and Trans People in the Public Sector, 211, 319n30
labor quota laws, 243, 270
Lacanian psychodynamics, 29, 30
Lamarckian frameworks of heritability, 28–29, 288n52
language: change in clinical, 78–79; of depathologization, 98–99; gendered, 295n6; gender-neutral, 63. *See also* terminology used
Latin America, 115, 126, 205, 284n21, 297n17, 323n8
Latinx populations, 60, 323n9
law, administrative, civil and criminal, 31
law, human-rights, 188, 214
laws, provincial, 129
lawsuits, class-action, 42, 294n3
lawsuits, state-level, 138
lawyers, poverty, 163, 310n14
legal action, Medicaid and, 158–63
Legal Aid, 158
legal control, 28, 30, 42
legal systems, international, 213, 319n32
legitimacy and self-determination, 224
León, Mónica, 126, *127*
letters of authorization, 68, 70, 192, 193, 201
letters to providers, ICATH sample, 199–201
Leveille, Lee, 265
Levine, Rachel, 1, 7
Lewis, Vek, 37, 238–39, 291n69
LGBQ people, 172, 234–35
LGBT health disparities, 164, 179
LGBT politics, 247–48

life chances, 33, 137, 236, 249, 307n32
life expectancy of trans- and travestis, 38, 113, 116, 117, 126–28, 129–30, 141
life span of trans- people, 177, 311n22
LILACS (database), 115
Lisette (trans- activist), 244
Logroño, Sol, 131
Loyd, Jenna, 69, 71, 249
Lugones, María, 59, 206–8, 213, 284n21, 318n26

Macri, Mauricio, 7–8, 54, 237, 297n17, 307n29, 323n12
Madres de la Plaza de Mayo, 131, 139, 307n34, 315n11
Madrigal v. Quilligan, 318n24
Make the Road New York (group), 163
"Making New York the Healthiest State" population-health summit, 145–47, 171
Malatino, Hil, 32, 207, 318n27
malpractice: claims, 194, 199, 220, 315n8; suits, 69, 267
Malta, 187–88, 292n78
Mamo, Laura, 294n2
managed health care, 68
manifesto, Traps, 1–2, 6
Marcus (social worker), 52
Marea Verde (Green Tide). *See* Green Tide (Marea Verde) feminist movement
marginalization, 14, 26, 65, 138, 236, 239, 240, 252, 253, 294n2
Mark (advocate and attorney), 73, 109–10, 217, 232–33, 235, 238, 239, 261, 321n43
Martínez, Juliana, 133, 307n28
Marx, Karl, 183
Marxists, 237, 238
masculinity, 138, 298n21
Massad, Joseph, 319n33
Mastercard, 183–84, 312n27
material conditions, 172
material relief, 113, 117, 137, 139, 140
McReynolds-Pérez, Julia, 296n11
McRuer, Robert, 245, 291n68
media campaign by Health Care for All!, 167–71
Medicaid: about, 25, 287n44; access campaign, 154–55, 184; ban lifted but with exclusions, 147, 158–59, 178, 179, 287n45, 294n3, 302n26, 309n9; exclusion of coverage for trans- therapeutics, 308n1; future of, 183; infographics to end exclusion ban by, 169–70; legal action against, 158–63; in New York, 249; population-level health outcomes and, 151; reimbursement requirements of, 193; savings, 168–70, 174; section 1557 of ACA and, 310n15; section 1983 of, 310n14; trans- therapeutic coverage and, 3, 26, 41–42, 51–53, 71, 102–3, 147, 165, 235, 294n3, 309n6, 311n19
Medicaid exclusion: access campaign and, 154–55; activists and advocates challenge, 4, 150, 153; broad-based community mobilization against, 160, 161–62; explanation of, 146; fact sheet and, 162, 164–65, 167, 174–75, 179, 311n21; focus on economic risk to challenge, 180–82; Health Care for All! coalition and, 172; infographics and, 167–71, 179; legal action to overturn, 158–63; lifting of, 147–50, 178, 258; Medicaid Redesign Team and, 165–66; providers use work-arounds due to, 101; as state racism, 39; videos produced to challenge, 176–77
Medicaid for All, 138
Medicaid Redesign Team (MRT), 145, 157–58, 165, 166, 167
Medi-Cal, 191
medical charting, 77–78, 80–81, 104, 299n2, 302n31
medical diagnoses. *See* diagnoses

medical-industrial complex, 63, 65, 297n15
medicalization: distinguishing pathologization from, 28, 57–58; expansion of, 58; preserving, 50
medical necessity for trans- therapeutics: activists' views, 50; government agencies' views on, 181; infographics and, 168–71; insurance coverage and, 53, 55, 156, 224; legal standpoint of, 163; Medicaid and, 160, 165, 174–75, 193, 309n13
medical paternalism, 60, 103, 190, 201, 204, 222, 226
medical power, 27
medical regret, 263–66
medical tourism, 35
Medicare, 3, 25–26, 42, 53, 151, 287nn44–45
medicolegal power, 307n32
Mendelian frameworks of heritability, 288n52
Menem, Carlos, 131, 297n17
menopause hormone treatments, 176–77
mental health: crises of trans- people, 153; diagnoses of trans- people and, 93, 190; infographics and, 171, 311n21; negative outcomes of, 175; trans- therapeutics for improved, 147
mental illness: stigmatization of, 93, 99; transsexualism as, 45–46, 49
methods and methodology, 16–19, 149–50, 286n34
Meyer-Bahlburg, Heino, 92, 301n17
"militant mixed methods," 140, 173, 307n35
Mingus, Mia, 64–66
Ministry of Health (Argentina), 54, 124, 197, 201, 316n13
minors: gender-affirming care for, 281n9; Gender Identity Law and, 41; Medicaid and trans- care coverage for, 42. *See also* youth
Miranda (nurse practitioner), 92–93
misogyny, 264
misogyny, racialized, 138
Money, John, 85
Mount Sinai hospital system, 3, 26, 178
Moyano, Laura, 111–12
Moynihan Report, 157
Mukerjee, Ronica, 176, 177–78
Muñoz, José Esteban, 241
"murderous inclusions," 136, 140, 142
Murphy, Michelle, 39, 135, 142, 148, 181, 222–23, 237, 256, 321n39

Nadia Echazú Textile Cooperative, 246
National Commission on Correctional Health Care, 298n24
National Front for the Gender Identity Law (Frente), 322n2
National Institutes of Health, 164
National Ministry of Labor (Argentina), 304n10
National Transgender Discrimination Survey, 177, 311n22
Nelson, Alondra, 50, 217, 320n35
neoconservatives, 157, 309n8
neoliberalism: activists and, 39, 292n74; class struggle and, 238; in India, 182–83; macroeconomy and, 312n25; public-health infrastructures and, 151; racial, 37, 291n70; trans- health and, 245, 252, 269; welfare reform and, 309n8
neoliberal reforms, 69, 124, 234, 246, 248, 297n17, 323n10
neoliberal regimes, 181, 182
New York City: austerity politics in, 157–58; hospital transgender health programs in, 3; identification card in, 73; Medicaid battle in, 4, 155, 157; municipal budget

of, 249; social movements in, 26–27; as study site, 16–17, 24–26
New York Department of Health, 42, 171
New York Human Resources Administration, 164, 172
New York Post, 166–67
New York State: health-care providers, 52, 178; jail-based care in, 74, 308n2; Medicaid and, 4, 25, 41, 51, 193; Medicaid exclusions in, 51, 150, 155–57, 258, 309n6
New York State Department of Health, 145–46, 150, 158–59, 161, 175–76
New York Times, 7
NGOs, 243–44, 247
Ni Una Menos (Not One Less), 62, 112, 303n1, 303n2
NML Capital Ltd., 246
nonnormativity, sex/gender, 72, 84, 121
nontrans-, as a term, 283n16
nontrans- people, 11, 283n20, 313n3
normalization therapies, 188
normativity, 294n2, 295n6
"Nuestros Cuerpos, Nuestra Salud" (Our bodies, our health) (study chapter), 125

Obama administration, 25–26, 138, 310n15
objects, boundary, 189, 219–20, 223, 226, 321n40
O'Brien, Michelle, 203
oncology, 264
Onganía, Juan Carlos, 315n10
Orgulla Disca (organization), 64
out-of-pocket care, 53, 55, 103, 106

Página 12, 211
Pandemonium, Eire, 64, 65
"Parent Calls for Healthcare for All, A" (video), 150
Patel, Geeta, 148, 181–82
paternalism: medical, 60, 103, 190, 201, 204, 222, 226; Orgulla Disca and, 64
pathologization: ableist, 61, 65; activists and, 217, 256; biomedicine and, 31, 86; damage of, 232, 236; of disability, 59; eugenic, 59, 63; histories of harm led to, 43; medicalization and, 28, 57–58; persistence of travesti, 325n2; of pregnancy, 61; of queerness, 56–57; racialized, 63, 208; regimes of, 28–30; self-determination and, 210. *See also* depathologization
patients, trans-, 206, 322n45
patients, travesti, 197, 322n45
Patients' Rights Act, 205
people of color, 22, 26, 60, 102, 208, 320n34
people of color, trans-, 6, 71, 103, 146, 154, 157, 176, 191, 259, 302n29, 310n16, 314n6
Perón, Eva, 23
Perón, Juan, 23, 323n10, 324n15
Peronismo (Peronism), 23, 248, 324n15
Personal Responsibility and Work Opportunity Reconciliation Act, 156
personhood, 206, 317n22
petitions, 45, 59, 168
Pfäfflin, Friedemann, 92, 301n17
Philadelphia (Penn.), 286n33
physical aggression of police, 122, 126, 128
piquetero movement, 131, 230, 259
plasticity of sex, 85, 260, 325n4
plastic surgery industry, 55
Plemons, Eric, 55, 94
police abuse: data from *Cumbia,* 128t; in epidemiological studies, 121–22, 126, 127; of travestis by region, 128
police harassment, 310n16

police profiling, 71
police violence: activists use examples of, 140; data from *La gesta,* 125–26; epidemiological biographies and, 117, 120; "A Fabulous Attitude" study and, 173; health and, 132–33; in New York City, 26; and sexual abuse, 122, 126, 128; against trans- and travestis, 24, 131, 235, 307n29; Trans March centers, 288n48
political action, collective, 113, 131, 132
political economy: and activist claims, 108, 142, 211, 231, 238; racialized, 142, 211, 238; as structuring condition, 269, 294n2; as trans-specific, 37, 238–39, 291n69. *See also* trans political economy
politicization of psychiatry, 289n56
poner el cuerpo (putting one's body on the line), 230, 244, 245, 323n9
poor populations: in clinic waiting rooms, 237; consultorios inclusivos for, 232; gatekeeping and, 191–92; health-care coverage for, 71, 102–3, 314n6; Medicaid and, 310n14; medicalization of childbearing, 61; state bureaucracies and, 302n29; welfare reform and, 157; work-arounds for trans-, 103. *See also* poverty
popular health (*salud popular*), 131
popular media views on trans- therapeutics, 39, 144, 148
population health: events related to, 145–47, 171; health-system management and, 151–52, 164; knowledge, 130–34; outcomes, 177; prevention policy, 154; shift from trans- health to, 143; state violence and, 38, 114–15, 141; statistical collectivization and, 134–36, 147
poverty: affecting health, 114; in Argentina, 246, 323n10; class struggle and, 238; as danger to the U.S., 291n71; eugenic politics of, 211; knowledge, 173, 174, 179, 184; racialized, 40, 61, 106; transgender people living in, 169; trans- people living in, 172
poverty law organizations, 311n17
poverty lawyers, 163, 310n14
power dynamics: in clinical interactions, 197–98, 199, 203, 316n16; hierarchical, 189; horizontal, 119, 231, 242
pregnancy, 59–60, 61, 303n1
prevention: -based care, 52; population-level health, 145–46, 154, 177
prison abolition, 183, 240–41, 312n26, 323n9
prison- and jail-based health care, 3, 73–74, 93, 261, 298n24, 298n26, 308n2
prisons and jails, 216, 235, 310n16
problem list on medical charts, 77–78, 299n2
Professionals Concerned with Gender Diagnoses in the DSM, 92
providers, health-care: activist, 75, 298n27; autonomy and, 203, 219; boundary objects and, 219; and care without pathology in practice, 189; classificatory revision and, 79, 81; consent-driven care and, 190–93, 199, 203, 220, 223, 226; contain HIV infection rates, 313n5; gatekeeping and, 56, 216; general demographics of, 22; hierarchical dynamics and, 222; informed consent and, 205–6, 219, 318n23; interviewed by author, 20–21, 287n39; medical paternalism and, 226; obstructing access to care, 103; orientation to care of, 195; primary-care, 68; sample guidelines for and letters to, 199–201; scarcity of affordable hormones and, 322n45; self-

determination and, 223–24; supportive of trans- health, 296n8; sympathetic to trans- health activists, 321n41; view of trans- health by, 10–11, 283n17; work-arounds and, 52
providers, mental health, 288n54
providers, trans- health, 31
provincializing, as a term, 284n21
psychiatric diagnoses. *See* diagnoses
psychiatric imperialism, 39
psychiatric institutions, 93
psychiatry, 28–30, 69–70, 197, 289n56, 289n59, 296n10
psychoanalysis, 29–30
Psychopathia Sexualis (Krafft-Ebing, von), 30
psychotherapists as gatekeepers, 55, 56, 66
psychotherapy, 191, 192, 201–2
Puar, Jasbir, 235, 325n2
public-health infrastructures, 29, 151–52

queer, as a term, 15, 281n1, 323n8
queer and trans-justice movements, 323n9
queerness, 56–57
queer people, 26, 173–74, 234, 318n28
queer politics, 235, 241, 323n9
Queers for Economic Justice, 150, 172

race: administrative definition, 23; Argentine national politics and, 23, 288n53, 291n71, 304n3; and coconstitutiveness with other forms of difference, 206, 241, 317n22; disability and, 206; eugenic "unfitness" and, 29, 85; health stratification and, 60–61; medical pathologization and, 61; sexual differentiation and, 85, 87; as statistical classification, 135–36, 173, 179
racialization, 43, 128–29, 139, 291n71
racism: ACA reform and, 69; and conditions of life, 38; gendered/sexualized, 61; guardianship and, 296n13; prison-based health care and, 93; state, 38, 113–14, 135, 293n84; structural, 114, 240, 282n10
Radi, Blas, 63, 296n12
Ravenwood v. Daines, 160, 310n14
Raymond, Janice, 155–56, 308n5
Reagan administration, 292n74
Reagon, Bernice Johnson, 242–43, 245
Redacción La Tinta (media collective), 238
referrals as gatekeeping, 68, 70
regret, medical, 263–66
regulators, New York, 180–81
regulatory changes, 160–61, 310n15
regulatory control, 28, 42
reimbursements for trans- therapeutics, 33, 48, 53–56, 60, 82, 98, 102, 193
reparations for trans- people and travestis, 24, 37, 39, 72, 129–30, 142, 211, 270
repression, state, 84, 320n35
reproductive-health activism, 255
reproductive justice (RJ) movements, 28, 48, 59, 61–63, 66, 239, 241, 256, 288n49, 296n12
reproductive technologies, 294n2
Republic of Argentina v. NML Capital Ltd., 323n11
researchers, community-based: affected by criminalization and violence, 130; in Buenos Aires, 121; epidemiological biographies used by, 132; statistical collectivization and, 135
researchers, travesti and trans-, 113–14, 117–18, 120–21, 142
research publications, trans- health, 115
revision: constancy of, 34, 78; diagnostic or classificatory, 33, 42,

46, 54, 60, 75, 79, 83, 88–89, 105, 108, 110; as a process, 34, 87; as related to practice, 33, 58, 75; of trans- health, 33, 257, 267–68
Ridge, Maureen, 176–77
Right to Protect Mental Health Law (Arg.), 292n77
right-wing ideologies, 9, 10
risk: activists and advocates developed new narratives about, 153–54, 168; defining, 152–53; economic, 147, 174, 177, 180; "A Fabulous Attitude" study and, 172; factors, 114, 124–25, 304n6; new narratives about, 268; population-health, 147; social, 154–55
risk-pooling, 148, 180, 181–82
Rivera, Sylvia, 211, 212, 318n28
Rizki, Cole, 131, 292n73, 323n8
Roberto (nurse practitioner), 100, 103
Robinson, Cedric, 291n70
Ross, Loretta, 61

Sacayán, Diana, 124, 319n30
same-sex marriage, 247
San Francisco, 191, 313n5, 322n4
San Francisco Department of Public Health, 191, 313n5
Schevers, Ky, 264–65
Schneider, Eric, 50
scholars, trans- studies, 136
science and technology studies (STS), 17–18, 87, 286n35, 302n27
Section 1557 of Affordable Care Act, 54, 137–38, 270, 287n46, 294n4, 310n15
securitization, state, 38, 139–40, 142–43, 304n5
self-determination: activists and, 189, 208, 321n41; boundary objects of, 226; coalitional depathologization and, 240; collective, 217, 227, 271; collective claim of, 213, 319n31; constraints of, 221; depathologization and, 66; formal principles of, 319n33; freedom from racially stratified constraints, 219, 321n42; gender, 73, 209–12, 213, 215–16; Green Tide movement and, 63; ICATH and, 201; individualist/collectivist tensions of gender, 215–16, 320n36; informed consent and, 187, 226; legitimacy and, 224; leveling relationship between provider and patient and, 58; power relations in, 40; referrals undermine trans- people's, 67; RJ movement and, 61–63; sovereignty and, 215, 320n35; synonymous with bodily autonomy, 218; tensions surrounding, 256; transforming care relations and, 217; *Yogyakarta Principles and,* 188
self-medication, 169, 171, 175, 311n21
self-perceived need, 3, 54, 96, 216, 224–25, 321n38
settler colonialism, 291n71, 319n33
sex binary, 8, 10, 29, 84–86, 285n27, 292n79, 310n15, 320n36
sex differentiation, 85, 87
sex discrimination, 294n4
sex/gender nonnormativity, 71, 72, 84, 301n20
sex/gender reclassification, 102, 195–96, 207, 292n79
sexological paradigms, U.S. and European, 84
sexological research, 57
sexology: and the concept of sexual inversion, 30, 57, 85; as a field, 28–29, 84–86, 260, 288n50; pathologization and, 84–87; research, 57; U.S. and European paradigms, 28, 84
sex reassignment, 66, 155, 295n5, 297n16
sexuality: and coconstitutiveness with other forms of difference, 317n22; criminalization of, 30

sexualized profiling by police, 71
sexual orientation, 188
sex work: abolishing, 323n7; in Argentina, 86, 121, 303n1, 319n30; and criminal law, 30, 289n57; economies, 313n5; racialized criminalization of, 73, 137; travestis and association with, 14, 24
sex workers: consultorios inclusivos for, 232, 252; state violence inflicted on, 139
Shah, Nayan, 323n9
Shah, Nirav, 145–46, 147, 158, 162, 166, 168
shelters, 216
Shim, Janet, 294n2
"Should Medicaid Cover Transgender Healthcare" (infographic), 150, 170, 171
shuster, stef, 206, 261, 283n17, 287n39, 318n23
side effects of hormone treatments, 193–94
Singer, Paul, 246–48
Singer, T. Benjamin, 8
SisterSong (organization), 61
Sitrin, Marina, 242
situational analysis, 18–19, 287n40
Snorton, C. Riley, 241, 293n84, 320n34, 321n42
social epidemiology, 114–16
social health, 50, 141–42, 217
social-media campaign, 154
social movements: in Argentina, 249, 292n73; differences in approach in, 37; in New York City, 26–27; population-health knowledge and, 130–34; queer and working-class, 26
social travesticide, 112, 116, 136–38
social welfare systems, 152
Soledad Cutuli, María, 245, 287n42, 304n10, 325n2
Somos Dueñxs/os de Nuestros Cuerpos (drawing), 213, 214
Sonya (nurse practitioner), 103, 106
Spade, Dean, 137, 235, 244
"Spider Model," 98
standards of care in trans- medicine, 315n8
Star, Susan Leigh, 17, 32, 40, 50, 219, 267, 286n34, 321n40
"Starfish Model," 46, 59, 97–99
Starr, Paul, 325n3
state securitization, 38, 304n5
state violence: acknowledgement of, 304n7; activists use statistics to show, 112–13; Black women and, 208; in contemporary Argentine social movements, 292n73; endangering trans- life, 38; epidemiological biographies and, 116–17, 132–33; gender policing as tool of, 212; gender self-determination and, 209–10; neglected variable of concern, 135; population health and, 113–14, 141–42, 143; as primary health risk, 129–30, 142, 153, 168; reparations for, 37; social travesticide and, 138; statistical collectivization and, 134
statistical collectivization, 38, 113, 134–41, 143–44, 147, 149, 153, 182, 253, 307n31
statistics: of health of trans- people, 177–78, 311n22; state power and, 135; of travesti violence in Buenos Aires, 112–14
Steptoe, George Liam, 145
sterilization: coerced, 30, 318n24; forced, 203–4; forced or coerced, 59, 60; freedom from forced, 239; Gender Identity Law and, 296n12; gender reclassification previously required, 24; refusal of, 188
stigma: activists focus on, 82, 109; conceptual limitations, 82, 106; of a psychiatric diagnosis, 94, 99, 100, 101, 106; singularity of transness and, 107

Stoller, Robert, 85
Stone, Sandy, 49, 81
Stonewall Rebellion, 26
Stop Trans Pathologization (STP), 49, 50, 72, 95, 99, 294n1
Strangio, Chase, 93, 106
Strauss, Anselm L., 19
Street Transvestite Action Revolutionaries (STAR), 212, 245, 318n28
structural violence, 38, 114–15, 116, 135, 168, 267
"studying across" approach, 17–18
study methods of author, 20
study sites, 23–27
subordination, racialized, 30, 86–87, 293n81, 317n17
Suess, Amets, 49
suicide, nontrans- people, 311n22
suicide, trans- people: attempts, 177; conditions for, 182; rates, 147, 169; risk, 153, 171, 175, 311n21; statistics used to pathologize, 177–78
surgeries: aesthetic, 55; choice to receive, 213, 214; Endocrine Disorder work-around not applicable to, 103; facial, 55; facial feminization, 292n80; gender-reassignment, 193; genital, 2, 55, 79, 326n5; on intersex children, 283n20, 295n6; proof of, 315n10; reassignment, 187; reconstructive, 55; requirement of, 2–3; sterilizing, 24, 30, 195; trans- health, 58; transsexual, 155; trans- therapeutics requiring letters of referral, 66–67
surveillance: in gatekeeping model of care, 190; nontrans- people and, 313n3; trans- people and government, 217
surveillance, political, 131
suspicions, health-care provider, 69–70, 73
Sutton, Barbara, 230
Sylvia (social worker), 218, 233–35, 238, 249–50, 261
Sylvia Rivera Law Project (SRLP), 145–46, 150, 158, 162, 164, 169–71, 176, 308nn1–2, 311n17

Talackova, Jenna, 45
Talia (nurse practitioner), 51–52, 94, 194–95, 217, 220–21, 315n9, 321n43
taxpayers and funding for trans- therapeutics, 37, 145, 149, 153, 166, 168, 174
templates for patient self-advocacy, 199–201
TERFs (trans-exclusionary radical feminists), 9–10, 263, 264, 265. *See also* feminists, gender-critical
terminology used, 12–16
theory-method packages, 17–20, 286n34
Theumer, Emmanuel, 251–52
"third gender," 86, 300n9
Tierra Violeta Cultural Center, 266
Tina (nurse practitioner), 100–101
Title IX antidiscrimination rules, 138, 287n46
Title VII federal employment discrimination prohibition, 294n4
Tom Waddell Health Center, 191, 221, 313n5, 322n4
torture by police, 122, 128
Tourmaline (organizer and advocate), 176, 318n28
trans*, as a term, 14–15, 98–99, 285n27
trans- activists. *See* activism and activists
trans and gender-nonconforming (TGNC) people of color, 310n16
trans-, as a term, 13–15
Trans Day of Action for Social and Economic Justice, 310n16
trans- depathologization. *See* depathologization
trans- diagnoses: activists working

to revise, 105; evolution of the classification of, 88, 89–90, 300n15; Gender Identity Disorder, 87
trans-exclusionary radical feminists (TERFs), 9–10, 177–78, 263, 264, 265
transfeminine activists, 1
transfeminine people, 1, 14, 117, 120, 282n11
transfemininity, 128, 141
transfeminism, 43, 215–16
transfeminist biopolitics. *See* biopolitics
transfeminist care, 210, 211, 221, 222–23, 228
transgender, as a term, 7, 12–13, 14–15, 98, 284n21
Transgender Europe, 95
Transgender Tuesdays, 191
Transgender Tuesdays (documentary), 313n5, 322n4
trans- health: available in health-care delivery systems, 236; care standards for, 1; as commodity, 259–60; confidentiality within study of, 22; consent-driven care in, 226; contributions of care without pathology to, 267; coverage through lens of economic rationality, 175, 311n21; depathologization one part of, 240; described by Mark, 233; described by Sylvia, 234; emergence of, 269–70; financial costs of, 35–36, 200–201; fraudulence and, 299n3; Gender Identity Law and, 190; growing institutionalization of, 27; infographics, 169–70; informed consent and, 188; infrastructures, 70; within large health-care systems, 35; legitimacy of, 79; New York advocates and activists campaign for, 146–47; not only gender affirming care, 217; no treatable illness in, 239; pathologizing providers in, 290n61; prioritized by health and poverty law organizations, 311n17; public coverage for, 4–5, 35–36; as public good, 159; public systems of care and, 4–5; questioning the emergence of, 12; revisions of, 257; revisions to transsexual medicine by, 266; self-determination in, 58, 66; shift from individual to population, 113; situational analysis to study, 19; as social good, 6, 36, 259; state violence and, 134; steps to address well-being of trans- people and, 270; as a term, 16; transsexual medicine shifts to, 256–57, 260; wellness instead of curative treatment for illness, 47, 51
trans- health research publications, 115
TransJustice (group), 162–63, 171, 176, 288n48, 310n16
"trans maladjustment," 32
Trans March, 288n48
transmasculine activism, 305n14
transmasculine people: epidemiological biographies and, 120; erroneous intent of, 9; images not included in "Expectativa" campaign, 118; owners of their own bodies, 213–14; subtle bureaucratic or state violence experienced by, 140
transnational depathologization activists, 94, 105
transnational feminisms, 43
transnational transfeminism, 44, 105
trans necropolitics, 136, 293n84
transness: as condition of the psyche, 94, 301n21; defined through frameworks of psychiatric pathology, 8;

depathologization of, 46; developing new classification for, 46; evidence of, 10, 283n17; feelings associated with, 32; psychiatric pathologization of, 31; singularity of, 107; as a term, 284n23, 284n25
trans- of color, 260, 283n19, 293n84
trans- patients, 52, 58, 77–78, 206, 222, 322n45
trans- people: access to health care, 179; autonomy of, 40, 210; consultorios inclusivos for, 197, 232; coverage for gender-affirming care, 283n20; in epidemiological biographies, 141; in "A Fabulous Attitude" study, 172; hired in public sector, 211, 243; labor quota laws and, 211, 319n30; legislative bombardment of, 7; legitimacy of, 196; marginalization of, 240; mental health diagnoses and, 190; minors, 41, 42, 281n9; a new welfare state for, 234; post–Gender Identity Law and, 42; self-perceived need and, 225; state violence and, 122–23, 140, 304n5; youth, 9, 26, 281n9, 318n28
trans- people, poor: barriers to accessing trans- therapeutics, 191; Department of Health abandoning, 176; dismissal of legal cases affecting, 160–61; embodiment of gender nonnormativity, 259; Health Care for All! coalition and, 154; redefining issues of concern for, 173–74; stakes of health-care access for, 6; trans- therapeutic coverage exclusion and, 157
trans- people, women, 1, 281n1
trans- people of color, 154, 157, 176
transphobia: ableism and, 69; in bioethical frameworks, 227; biomedicine and, 50, 217; detransition and, 264–65; earlier state, 159–60; elimination a social good, 175; health care and, 155, 256, 294n1; Medicaid and, 182; pathologization beyond, 245; pervasiveness of, 310n16; power relations and, 240; public benefits and, 164; state security and, 138; talking about, 270; transfeminism and, 216; welfare and, 173
trans political economy, 37, 238–39, 291n69
trans- politics, 7, 9, 13, 218, 244, 246–48, 284n22, 304n3
trans- population health. *See* population health
Transsexual Empire, The (Raymond), 155, 308n5
Transsexualism: classification protested in *ICD*, 45–46; as *DSM* diagnosis, 78, 88–89; as gender nonnormativity, 34; as *ICD* diagnosis, 90; revised to Gender Identity Disorder, 87
Trans-sexualism, as *ICD* diagnosis, 78, 88, 90, 300n11
transsexual medicine: in 20th century vs. present-day, 69, 297n18; beginnings of, 8–9, 282n13; classification and, 33; the need to make fundamental changes to, 70; shifts to trans- health, 256–57, 260, 266–68
transsexuals: in Brazil, 295n7; demographic information of, 120; no subgroup distinction in epidemiological biographies, 141; violated by the state, 122–23
trans- studies, 135, 136, 206
trans- therapeutics: activists and advocates for, 147–48, 163, 165, 227, 239; and broader conditions of life, 257, 258–59; called gender-confirming procedures, 308n4; considered a public right

in Brazil, 295n7; coverage of, 4–6, 38–39, 41, 46–47, 51, 54, 68, 146–47, 176, 181, 261, 295n6; criminal action against providers of, 7, 9; debts of democracy and, 249–50; evidence required for gender reclassification, 71; exclusion clauses for, 155–56, 161; fact sheet and, 164–65; freedom of access to, 217; gatekeeping and, 66–67, 206, 314n6; Gender Identity Law and, 2, 190; Health Care for All! coalition and, 179–80; for incarcerated trans- people, 74; less accessible, 3; Medicaid and, 25–26, 146, 158, 309n6; medical necessity and, 55; Medicare and, 25–26; as monetizable, 35; opponents of, 263–64; population-level health outcomes and, 177; proclamation of heterosexuality for, 195; as "the regular health care," 176–77; self-determination and, 54, 210; sex reassignment and, 297n16; as a social good, 153–54, 180; as a term, 15–16, 285n32; in the U.S., 144; video and infographics to support, 168–70; visit codes for, 59–60; wellness-based rather than curative, 27

transtopia, 15, 285n29

transvestism, 85, 90, 306n24

trans- women, 140, 308n5, 313n5

Trans Women of Color Coalition, 163

traps, 1, 281n1

Traps (collective), 1–2, 6

"travar el saber," 133, 307n28

travesti activists. *See* activists, trans- and travesti; activists, travesti

travesticide, 111–12, 116, 136–38, 253, 303n1

travestis: about, 282n11; anticapitalist struggles related to, 251–52; autonomy of, 40; avoidance of health care sites, 124; in Brazil, 285n26; care denied to, 295n5, 295n7; consultorios inclusivos for, 232; criminalization of, 24, 72, 119; demographic information of, 120; embodiment of gender nonnormativity, 259; employment exclusion of, 304n10; epidemiological biographies and, 132, 141; in "Expectativas" campaign, 117–19, 128; expulsion from public spaces, 30; Gender Identity Law and, 292n79; hierarchical dynamics with providers, 222; hired in public sector, 211, 243; HIV-positive, 124–25; labor quota laws and, 211, 319n30; legitimacy of, 196; marginalization of, 240; mental health diagnoses and, 190; post–Gender Identity Law and, 42; public surveillance of, 118, 131; reclaimed Gondolín hotel, 36, 290n65; restrictions on, 30, 301n20; self-perceived need and, 225; sex work and, 121; stakes of health-care access for, 6; subject to systemic immiseration, 140; as a term, 14; terms for, 307n28; under transgender umbrella, 13; trans- people and, 129; travesti femininity, 135; violated by the state, 122–23; violence against, 111–12, 117–23, 139, 140, 304n5; work and housing for, 246

"Travestismo and Police Violence" (study chapter), 120–21

travesti textile cooperative, 118, 304n10

Triple Aim approach: of New York Department of Health, 145–46, 151, 165, 175; of trans- health activists, 147, 154, 171, 177

Trouillot, Michel-Rolph, 320n35

Trump administration, 7, 25–26, 138, 270, 294n4, 310n15

TSQ, 209

"undone science," 132, 140, 141, 149, 164
United States: paradigms of racialization in, 37–38, 291n71; psychoanalysis in, 29–30; RJ movements in, 61; surgical requirements for gender reclassification in, 79
United States Federal Bureau of Prisons, 74, 298n26
United States Tea Party, 69
universal health care, 270
University of Buenos Aires, 36
unruliness of trans- diagnoses, 105, 109, 302n32
upstream factors affecting health, 114–16, 134, 152, 164
urban focus of book, 19
U.S. Department of Health and Human Services, 1, 25, 54
U.S. Professional Association for Transgender Health (USPATH), 290n61

Valerie (attorney), 158–161, 166, 178, 181
Velocci, Beans, 69, 228, 263
vertical relations of care, 199, 242
Vidal-Ortiz, Salvador, 133, 307n28
Videla, Jorge Rafael, 323n10
Videla dictatorship, 130–31, 315n11
videos, Health Care for All! coalition, 176, 179
Vierkant, Artie, 290n67
violence: administrative, 164, 290n63, 302n29, 307n32; gendered, 250; institutional, 117, 123; as key term in journal articles, 115; racialized, 66, 113, 136, 140; sexual, 140; structural, 116; against trans- and travestis, 304n5; against women and trans- people, 62, 111, 303n1, 303n2
violence, police, 113, 117, 120, 132–33, 140, 307n29
violence, state, 38, 112–16, 117, 123, 133, 134, 138, 141, 143, 304n7
violence, structural, 38, 114–15, 116, 135, 168, 267
"Violencia" (study chapter), 122–23
visit codes, 53, 59–60
voice coaching, 15, 55
vulture funds, 39, 246–48

waiting rooms, clinic, 236–37
"walking while trans," 30, 289n57
"walking while travesti," 72, 289n57
Washington Consensus, 297n17
Washington State Medicaid, 309n6
Wayar, Marlene, 124
wealth: insulates subjects from criminalization, 298n21; out-of-pocket care and, 106, 227; redistribution, 259, 269, 271
"We are Trans* Not Sick" petition, 45–46
Weber, Max, 307n32
"Welfare Justice" campaign, 171–72, 174, 179
welfare reform, 156–57, 309n8
Welfare Reform Act of 1997, 156
welfare warriors, 259
Welfare Warriors Research Collaborative, 150, 172, 179, 210, 311n20
whiteness, 23, 137, 259, 290n64, 291n71, 298n21, 302n32, 325n4
whitening regimes, 23, 288n53, 291n71, 304n3, 306n24
white supremacy, 31, 85, 106, 320n35
Willkie Farr & Gallagher, 158
Winter, Sam, 78
Winters, Kelley, 92
women: Black, 60–61, 86–87, 157, 173, 208, 304n3, 311n20; of color, 61, 103, 208; poor trans-, 313n5; trans-, 1, 140, 281n1, 308n5; violence against, 62, 111, 303nn1–2
work-arounds, diagnostic, 52, 80, 100–104, 192–93, 294n3, 302n27, 302n29

Work Group on Sexual and Gender Identity Disorders, 92
working-class movements, 26, 64, 245, 249
Working Group on the Classification of Sexual Disorders and Sexual Health (WHO), 94–96, 99
World Health Organization (WHO), 9, 45–46, 59, 78, 88, 94–95, 97, 108, 289n55
World Professional Association for Transgender Health (WPATH), 55, 67, 191, 194, 197, 201, 297n19, 301n17, 316n15
WPATH *Standards of Care*, 55, 67, 69, 70, 201

xenophobia, 23, 86, 289n60, 310n16

Yogyakarta Principles, 188, 199
youth, 9, 26, 281n9, 318n28. *See also* minors

Zachs, Maxwell, 45, 59
Z-codes (visit codes), 59–60, 98
Zevin, Barry, 191
Zucker, Howard, 158
Zucker, Kenneth, 92, 290n61

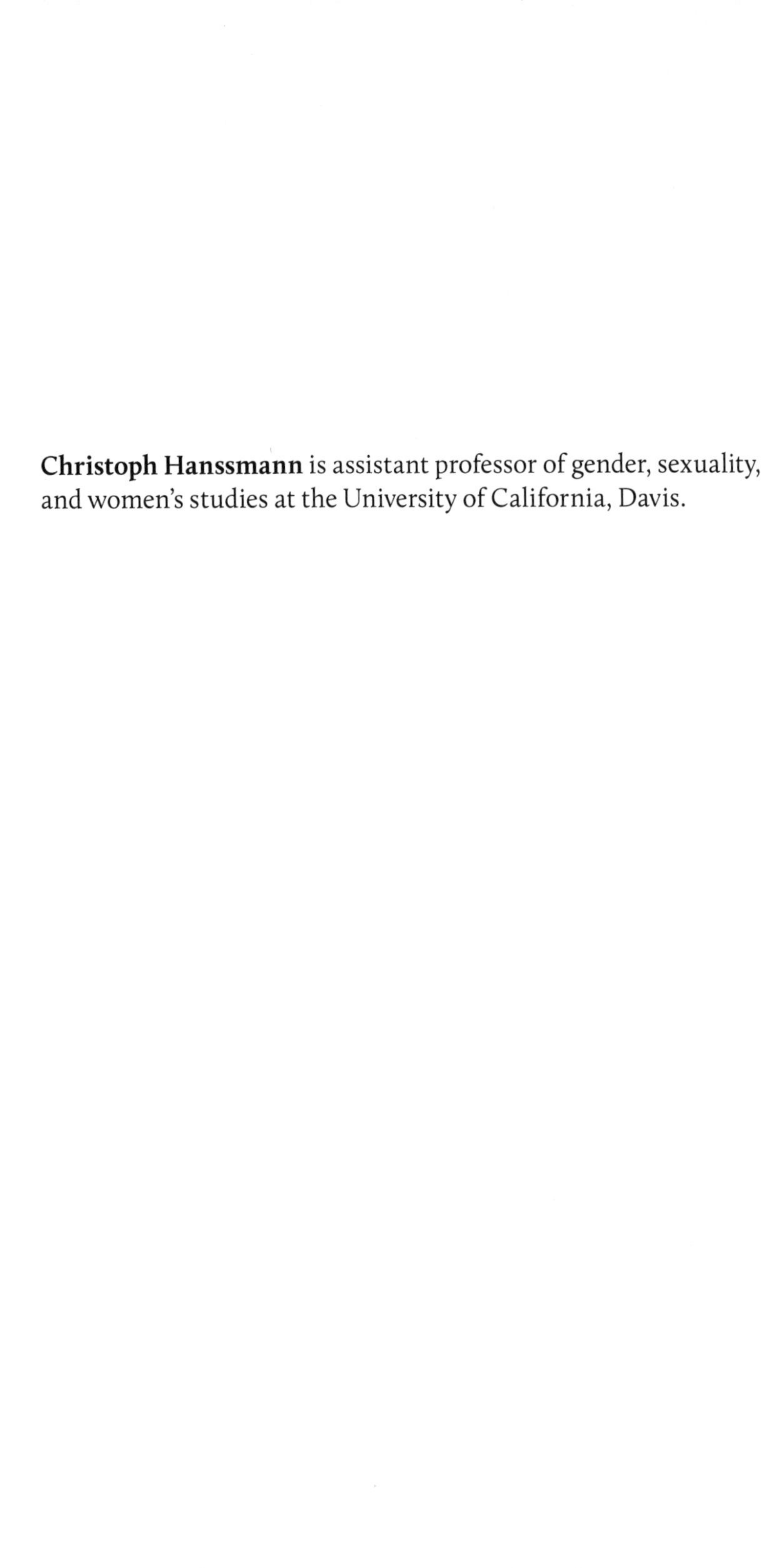

Christoph Hanssmann is assistant professor of gender, sexuality, and women's studies at the University of California, Davis.